Dr Patrick Treacy is one of the first pioneers of the field of Aesthetic Medicine. He was awarded 'Top Aesthetic Practitioner in the World' (2019, Las Vegas) as well as 'Top Medical Aesthetic Practitioner UK & Ireland' (2019), earning himself a lifetime achievement place in the MyFaceMyBody Aesthetic Medicine Hall of Fame. He has contributed to many new techniques and protocols and has been given specialist research awards by the British College of Aesthetic Medicine (London), Irish Healthcare Awards (Dublin), IMCAS Scientific Committee (Paris), AMWC Scientific Committee (Monaco), Azerbaijani College of Aesthetic Medicine (Baku), and the CMME Medal of 'Medical Excellence' (Mexico). He has been cited amongst the 'Ultimate 100 Global Aesthetic Leaders' for the past four years.

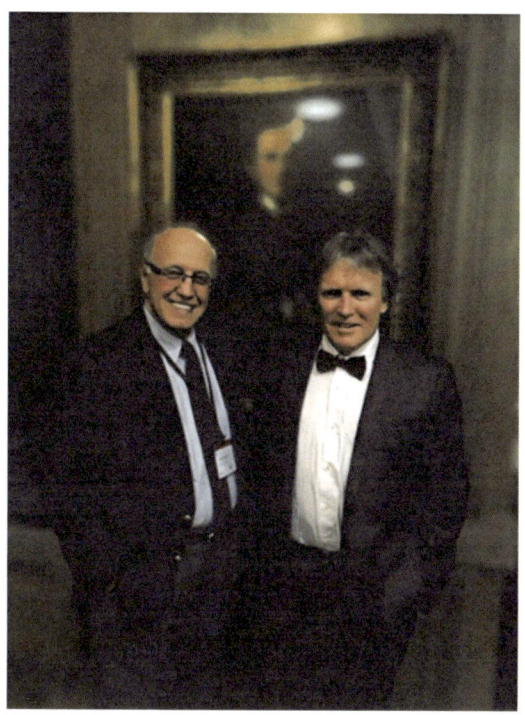

The author and Dr Ercin Ozunturk

This book is dedicated to my deceased good friends and colleagues, Dr Ercin Ozunturk (Istanbul) and Dr Moses Herzenhorn (UK), who both succumbed to COVID-19 during the pandemic. May they rest in peace!

Dr Patrick Treacy

THE EVOLUTION OF AESTHETIC MEDICINE

The Evolution of a New Field of Medicine by a Pioneer Voted the Top Aesthetic Doctor in the World

AUSTIN MACAULEY PUBLISHERS™

LONDON * CAMBRIDGE * NEW YORK * SHARJAH

A CIP catalogue record for this title is available from the British Library.

ISBN 9781398417489 (Paperback)
ISBN 9781398417496 (Hardback)
ISBN 9781398417502 (ePub e-book)

www.austinmacauley.com

First Published 2022
Austin Macauley Publishers Ltd®
1 Canada Square
Canary Wharf
London
E14 5AA

To my mentors and friends, Dr Pierre Fournier, Dr Yves-Gerard Illouz, dec; Dr Hugues Cartier, Dr Benjamin Ascher (France), Dr Bruce Katz, Dr Rod Rohrich, Dr Neil Sadick, Dr Rox Anderson, Dr Arnold Klein, dec; Dr Frederick Brandt, dec; Dr Richard Fitzpatrick, dec; Dr Randy Waldman, Dr John Cole, Prof Seb. Cotofana (United States), Dr Ronald Feiner (Australia), Prof. Peter Velthuis (Nederland), Drs Marlen and Giorgio Sulamanidze (Georgia), Dr Shimon Eckhouse (Israel), Prof. Christopher Roland Payne (United Kingdom) and to Patrick Druggan, University of Brighton who helped with proofing.

"The greatest good you can do for another is not just to share your riches but to reveal to him his own." – Benjamin Disraeli, Former Prime Minister of the United Kingdom.

Table of Contents

Foreword

During the nineties, minimally invasive surgery became popular and accessible to many aesthetic patients. This evolution from aesthetic surgery allowed many people to access rejuvenation techniques not previously available to them. Among the numerous methods of minimally invasive aesthetic surgery, articles on thread lifts methods began to be published in reputable periodicals, and lectures were given at congresses, symposia, and scientific conferences. The first mention of using threads for lifting the soft tissues of the face and neck in the scientific literature, probably started with Buttkewitz. Then Guillemain, Mario Gonzales Ulloa, Sergio Capurro, Sassaki and other colleagues developed thread methods in aesthetic and plastic surgery. An invaluable contribution to the popularization of thread lifting methods was made by the famous Frenchman Pierre Fournier, whose publications and presentations at various congresses and scientific conferences facilitated the spread of these methods. However, these threads were smooth and lacked a proper method of tightening the facial structures. I proposed the use of barbed threads for the purpose of facial rejuvenation in 1996. Of interest, was the simultaneous discovery that some mummies in Egypt were found to have golden threads in their face, presumably used for cosmetic reasons.

Dr Patrick Treacy, in his book on the evolution of Aesthetic Medicine shines a worthwhile light on this period. He describes how the Egyptian School of Alexandria influenced the future development of cosmetology as well as philosophy and medicine. It is suggested that high ranking females of this period may have had threads inserted in their face by latter-day aesthetic surgeons. The assumption was based on the well-known axiom that the noble metal gold has a beneficial effect on human tissues: it resists the occurrence of infection, does not decompose under the influence of body juices, and contributes to the strengthening and rejuvenating of body cells. Based on this, some of my colleagues began to implant the finest gold threads under the skin of their patients, but they proved ineffective at lifting ptotic skin being smooth and subjected to migration during facial expression. Because of this, I initially decided to use barbed threads, and now we use over thirty different types of thread products used on the face, body, female breast, intimate sphere, and in general surgery as well.

Dr Patrick Treacy provides a wonderful historical narrative of how botulinum toxin, dermal fillers, and laser technologies made their way into the emergent field of aesthetic medicine, and this book is very timely as he monitors its evolution into a separate faculty. The fact, he has been awarded by his international colleagues for scientific research in this area, and his contribution to new protocols and techniques, means this impressive book will be of historical interest to all who practice in the field of aesthetic medicine.

Dr Marlen Sulamanidze MD, Ph.D.,
Plastic Surgeon and Inventor of APTOS Threads

International medical awards 2016-2020

- Winner - MyFaceMyBody 'Top Global Medical Practitioner' 2019 (Las Vegas) November 2019
- Winner - MyFaceMyBody 'Top UK & Ire Medical Practitioner' 2019 (Las Vegas) November 2019
- Winner - AMEC Anti-aging & Beauty Trophy 'Best Global Clinical Case' (Monaco), October 2019
- Winner - Irish Healthcare Award 'Best Medical Aesthetic Clinic (Dublin), Sept 2019
- Winner - MyFaceMyBody Specialist Award 'Scientific Contributions to the Aesthetic Industry' (London), March 2018
- Winner - Irish Healthcare Award 'Best Medical Research Award' (Dublin), March 2017
- Winner - MyFaceMyBody Award 'Ultimate 100 Global Aesthetic Leaders' (Los Angeles), August 2017
- Winner - British College of Aesthetic Medicine 'Quality & Research Award'(London) September 2017
- Winner - AIDA Trophy 'Best Clinical Case in Aesthetic Medicine in Dermatology & Aesthetics' (Abu Dhabi) Oct 2017

- Winner - AAAMC Trophy 'Contribution to Development of Aesthetic Medicine' Azerbaijan Nat. Organizing Committee (Baku) Oct 2017
- Winner - John Bannon Award for the "Best Clinic in Ireland" at the Aesthetic Awards (London), December 2017
- Winner - Irish Health & Beauty Award 'Best Cosmetic Surgery Clinic in Ireland 2016' (Dublin), June 2016
- Winner - Safety in Beauty Award Aesthetic Doctor of 2016' (Highly Commended) (London), June 2016
- Winner - AMEC Anti-aging & Beauty Trophy 'Best Clinical Research Case in Aesthetic Medicine' (Paris), September 2016
- Winner - CCME Mexican Congress Medal for' Excellence in Medical Aesthetics' (Mexico), November 2016
- Winner - MyFaceMyBody Award 'Best medical research for wound healing' (London), November 2016

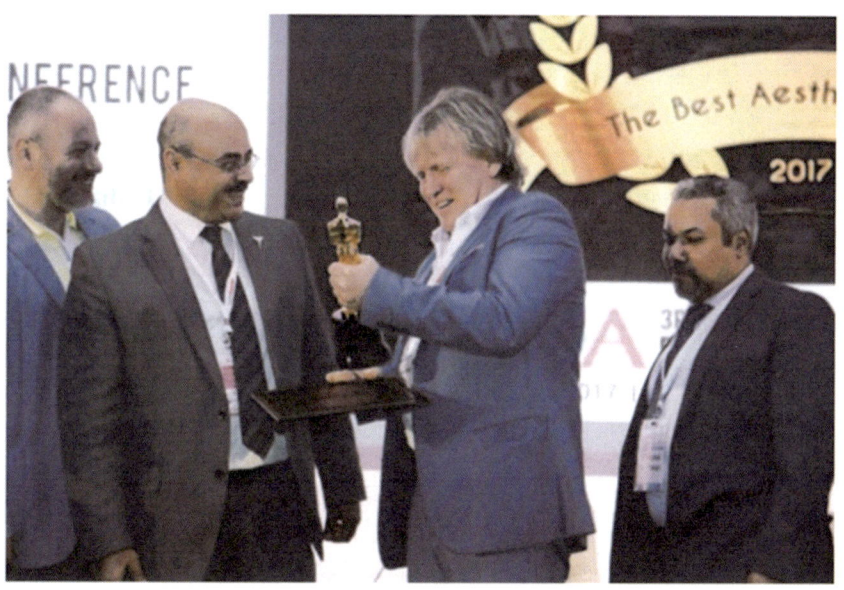

Winner – AIDA Trophy (Abu Dhabi) Oct 2017

Prologue

The history of aesthetic medicine is a recent one, largely forged through the advent of twentieth century technology. It was the emergence of three new technologies: hyaluronic acid dermal fillers, botulinum toxin and the IPL laser at the turn of the last century, which gave us the possibility of creating a whole new field of medicine. In that period, I was working in a dermatology clinic in Queensland, Australia but appreciated that a whole new era of medicine could now be created and returned to Ireland to do so. The twenty first century brought novel energy-based technologies, which pushed new boundaries, and scientists and engineers experimented with every wavelength to try and help us achieve eternal youth. These new sciences effortlessly moved across the energy-based spectrum from fractionalised laser skin resurfacing (FLSR) to radiofrequency (RF), and onwards to high intensity ultrasound (HIFU). Gone were the days of medicine where an old theory was abandoned to favour something new as evidenced in theGalen, Harvey, and Osler tradition.

In these early years, I met and learned techniques from pioneering doctors, many who are mentioned in this book. They include a few famous French plastic surgeons, such as the late Yves-Gerard Illouz and Pierre Fournier, innovators like Russian plastic surgeon, Marlen Sulamanidze as well as his son Giorgio. It includes Canadian ophthalmic surgeon Jean Carruthers, who iscredited with noting the cosmetic effect of botulinum as well as hair transplant specialists, Dr John Cole, Dr William Rassman, and Greek entrepreneur KostasGiotis. It is within recent memory that I have enjoyed their wonderful hospitality in each of their respective countries, and more often, also in their homes. Manywould say that I have contributed to this pioneering development myself over the years, being acknowledged of being amongst the first to treat HIV lipodystrophy patients with facial endoprosthesis, to develop new botulinum techniques for migraine and trigeminal neuralgia, for establishing hyaluronidaseprotocols for reversing vascular occlusion and experimenting with using PRP (platelet rich plasma) in androgenetic alopecia and facial rejuvenation. I am forever grateful to my medical colleagues who have given me numerous international awards over the years in respect of these developments. Last year was an important one for me, as I won 'Top Aesthetic Practitioner in the World'(Las Vegas) as well as the UK and Ireland'(London). I was honoured with laureates in aesthetic medicine from Russia and Azerbaijan, winning the AIDA Trophy (Abu Dhabi), the Anti-Aging and Beauty Trophy (Baku) and a medal for excellence in medicine by CCME (Mexico). I am grateful also to MyFaceMyBody (London) for giving me a specialist award for my scientific contributions to the development of aesthetic medicine.

The term Aesthetic Medicine now encompasses a more generalised term covering procedures that tend to focus on altering cosmetic appearance. These include conditions such as skin laxity, wrinkles, excess fat, cellulite, unwanted hair, skin pigmentation and broken vessels. Traditionally, for thousands of years there has always been conflict as to which specialism owns this territory. It is only in the early part of the 20th century some of these cosmetic procedures gradually were included in the medical discipline and differences of opinion date back five hundred years before the birth of Christ to the School of Alexandria.

Although medicine, was included in the school of Alexandria, along with astronomy and philosophy, the practice of cosmetology was not as it was considered by these physicians to be minor, without healing purpose, and left to lay practitioners. In 1745, George II created a legal separation between physicians and barber-surgeons. Initially this new field of Aesthetic Medicine included aesthetic physicians, dermatologists, reconstructive and plastic surgeons but now includes dentists, nurses and more recently beauticians, each specialism pushing the boundaries of what the regulators allow them to do. Surgical procedures (liposuction, facelifts, breast implants) have largely remained within the realm of doctors, but non-surgical procedures (radio frequency skin tightening, non-surgical liposuction, high-intensity focused ultrasound, radio frequency fat removal and chemical peels) are now being done by many aestheticians, especially in countries with weaker regulation. In fact, I find the subject so interesting that I have dedicated a chapter of this book to this.

Aesthetic Medicine procedures are usually elective and are increasing year by year. There were 50 million aesthetic type procedures performed globally in the period 2019-2020, and these numbers increased during the Covid pandemic. The way patients access these services has also changed. This has created its own challenges for the industry. I am writing this prologue during lockdown isolation in my Dublin home as the Covid-19 pandemic sweeps across the world. At the beginning of last year, we looked forward to the start of a new decade, and nobody knew that SARS-CoV-2 even existed. Now the virus variants, from Alpha to Omnicron have spread to almost every country, infecting over two hundred and fifty million people, devastated economies, and disturbed modern society on a scale that most of us have never witnessed. The recent authorisation of mRNA vaccines has been a landmark achievement for modern medicine. More especially, as this technology had only been involved in cancer treatment up until the pandemic began. Isolation is the ideal time for introspection. History shows us that pandemics often change the world for the better. They shine a light on what is broken in our society and possibly also how to fix it. I have decided to illustrate some of the chapters with actual case histories taken from the Ailesbury Clinic in Dublin and I am thankful to the patients for allowing this privilege.

I write this prologue on the night that Ireland lifts its Covid restrictions and announces, 'Freedom Day'. The Covid journey is hopefully now over. Gustav Flaubert once said to 'focus on the journey, not the destination. Joy is found not in finishing an activity but in doing it'. In this instance, I must politely disagree and focus on the destination and not on the journey. The joy here is found finishing the activity.

Dr Patrick Treacy, Dublin Jan 2022

Chapter 1: Botulinum Toxin

Botulinum toxin (Botox®) consists of 7 types of neurotoxins; however, only toxins A and B are used clinically. Botox A is used for several disorders in the field of medicine, particularly in dermatology, for cosmetic purposes. It is produced by the bacterium Clostridium botulinum *and can be used as a treatment to reduce the appearance of wrinkles in the upper areas of the face, elevate the eyebrows and treat problems such as migraine, hyperhidrosis, lichen simplex, pompholyx (dyshidrotic eczema) and acne vulgaris.*

The Long History of Botulinum

1793 was an eventful year by any standards. It started with the French King Louis XVI being guillotined in front of a cheering crowd in Paris and ended later that year with the execution of his wife, Marie Antoinette. The fact that Louis had tried to escape and was captured while trying to make a purchase at a store, where the clerk recognised his face on the coinage, only added to the drama. It was around the time that the British Admiralty began to supply citrus juice to its navy ships to prevent scurvy and the Holy Roman Empire decided to declarewar on France after it banned Roman Catholicism. Across the Rhine, in Southern Germany, a food poisoning epidemic caused by eating uncooked blood sausages was claiming the death of over the half of those patients who fell ill. The symptoms of the disease included malaise, nausea, vomiting, diarrhoea, double vision, dilated pupils, fatigue, unsteady gait, difficulty swallowing, thirst and, when fatal, unconsciousness, rigor and ultimately death. The disease and the remnants of the century passed, and the Acts of Union of 1800 united the Kingdom of Great Britain with the Kingdom of Ireland. The nineteenth-century started off with the armies of Great Britain, Prussia, Austria, and Russia finally ending the Napoleonic wars and subsequently dismissing the French armies to their homes after twenty two years of war.

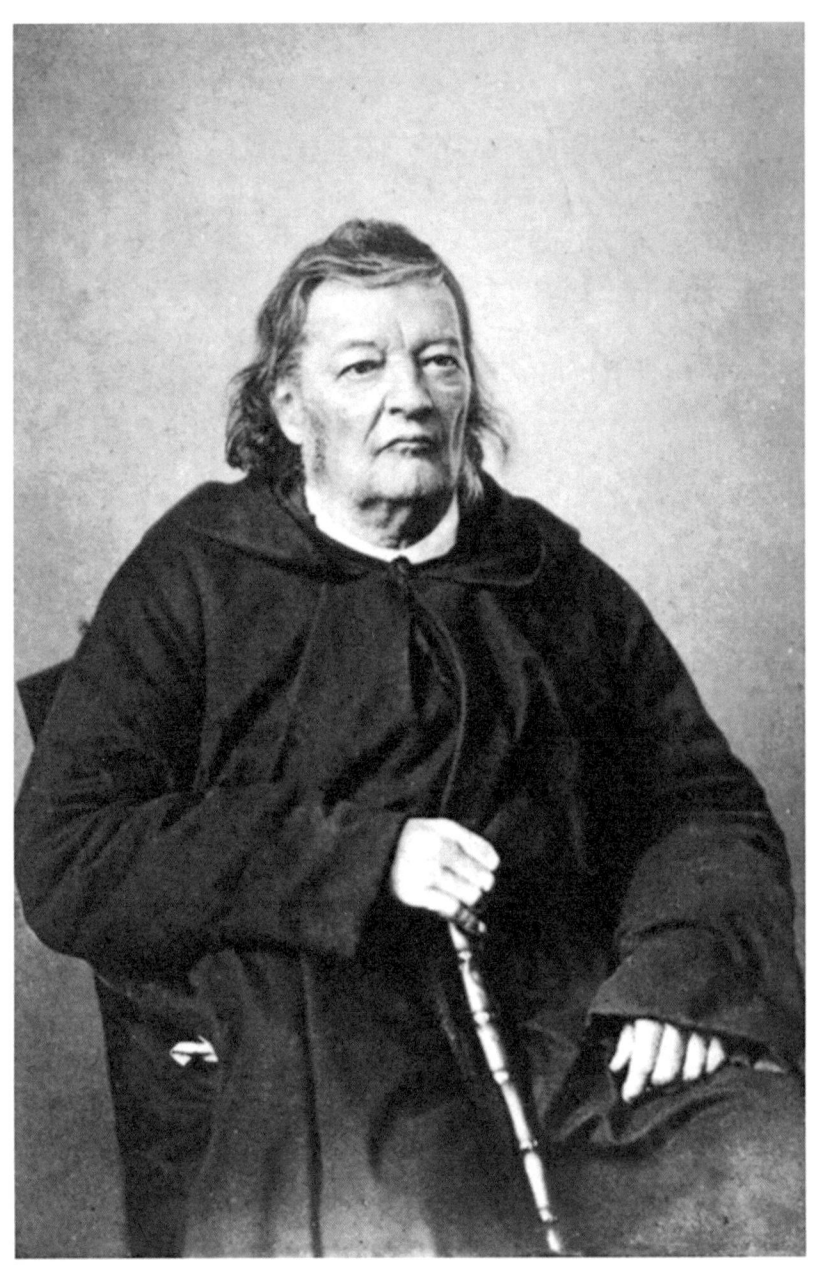

Justinus Kerner (1786-1862) German physician

However, in this poverty-stricken landscape, disease and pestilence was never far away and in 1817, the dreaded uncooked sausage food poisoning returned to the town of Baden-Wurttemberg. All this mention of disease and food poisoning in the days before antibiotics would have passed idly into history except for the actions of a meticulous medical doctor called Justinus Kerner. Justinus, who later became one of Germany's greatest romantic poets, was born in the small town of Ludwigsburg in 1786, the same year that the first British convict ships set sail to Botany Bay in Australia. During his teenage years, he was apprenticed in a cloth factory but in 1804, he entered the University of Tübingen to study medicine. In 1808, he graduated and settled as a practicing physician in Wildbad. In 1815, he obtained the official appointment of district medical officer in Gaildorf, and three years later, he was transferred to Weisberg, where he was to spend the rest of his life. The local townspeople gave him a house at the foot of the historical Schloss Weibertreu and within these walls, he dedicated all his spare time to discover the cause of the dreaded food poisoning, which was killing half of his patients.

Between 1815 and 1820, Kerner investigated 155 cases, treated 12 patients, performing autopsies on some of them. He also gave extracts from sausages that had been confiscated by the police to different animals and observed their reaction before dissecting the remains. In 1822, he published the first systemic description of the clinical picture of botulism, a lethal type of food poisoning known since the era of the Roman Empire. At the end of his publication, he concluded that there was no cure for sausage poisoning and recommended that 'all blood sausage and liverwurst still on the fireplace by February should be thrown out by the chimneysweep with the other rubbish'. With great foresight, in the dying throes of his seminal paper, the poetic doctor also noted that small amounts of the sausage poison might be useful for neurological conditions such as St Vitus' dance. St Vitus' dance or Sydenham's chorea is a disorder characterized by rapid, uncoordinated jerking movements primarily affecting the face, hands and feet. It is an autoimmune disease that results from childhood infection with Group A beta-haemolytic Streptococcus.

Without knowing it, Justinus Kerner laid the opening shots in the greatest contribution of biology to the world of cosmetic medicine… he was describing the neurological action of Botulinum toxin, later to be known to in another century as Botox®! Kerner could isolate the toxin and use it to kill other animals, but he was lacking the biggest piece of the jigsaw – what was it and how was it formed.

The next part of the botulinum toxin journey takes us back across the Rhine to meet one of the greatest scientists that the world has ever known, …. Louis Pasteur.

The Influence of Louis Pasteur

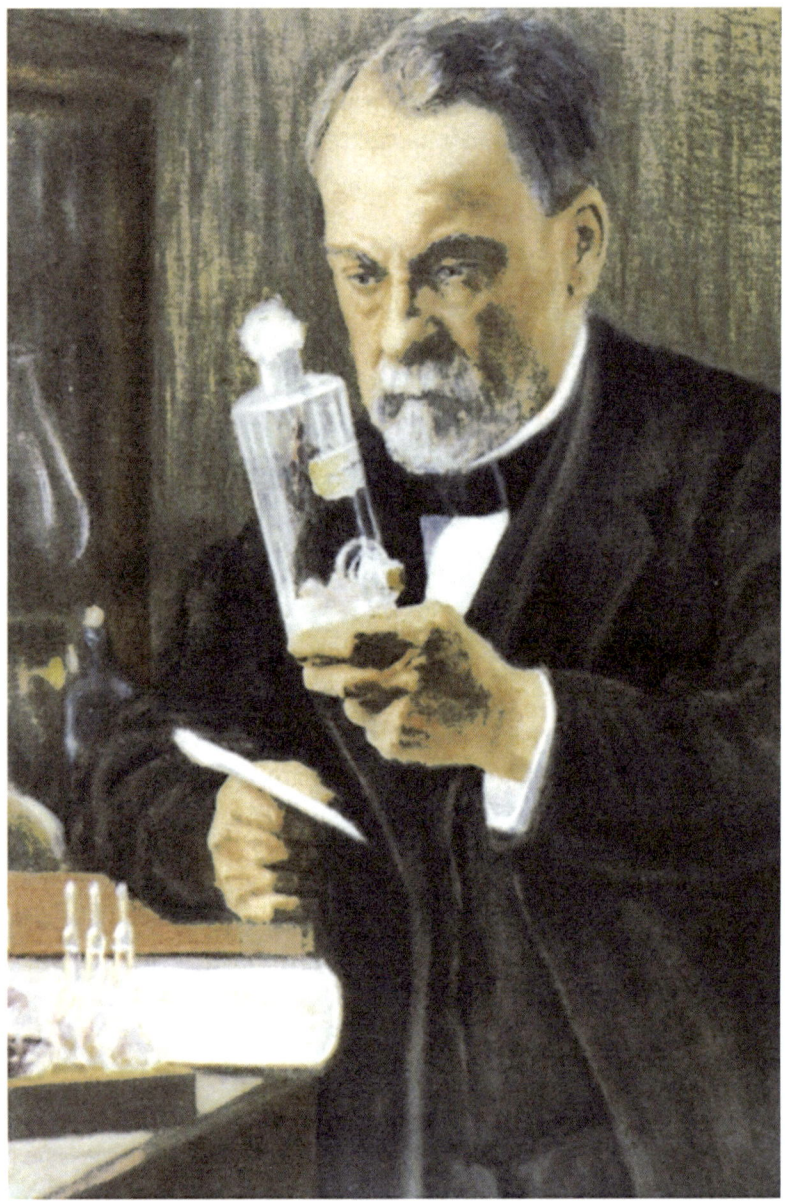

Louis Pasteur

Louis Pasteur's seminal work from the late 1850s proved that milk became sour because of yet unknown living organisms; by verifying the 'germ theory', This work would change the whole outdated post-Aristotelian pathology and surgery forever. Of course, this great thesis led to the discovery that the bacteria van Leeuwenhoek found in his microscope slides in 1668 couldcause disease and illness. Pasteur died in 1895, and in that year, the dreaded disease struck again, and this time in the exalted company of the salted pork dishat the annual gathering of the Music Society in the town of Ellezelles in Belgium.

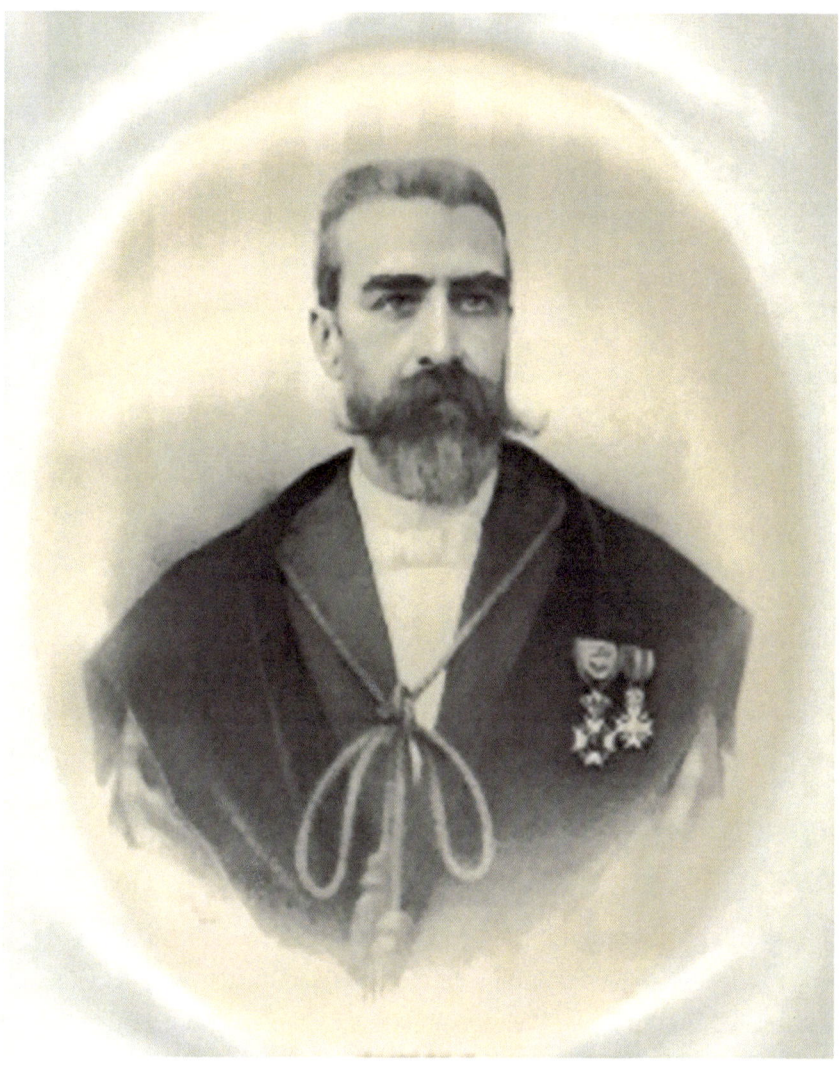

Émile van Ermengem (1851-1932), Belgian bacteriologist

Three people eventually died from the resultant food poisoning, amongst them a close friend of one of society's eminent members – the microbiologist, Professor Emile P. Van Ermengem.

The professor took the death of his friend personally and armed with the twin technologies of van Leeuwenhoek's microscope and Pasteur's closed flasks, and in 1896 became the first person to isolate the microbe Clostridium botulinum from both the food and the post-mortem tissue of victims who had died. He also knew that the disease process was caused by a toxin produced by this bacterium.

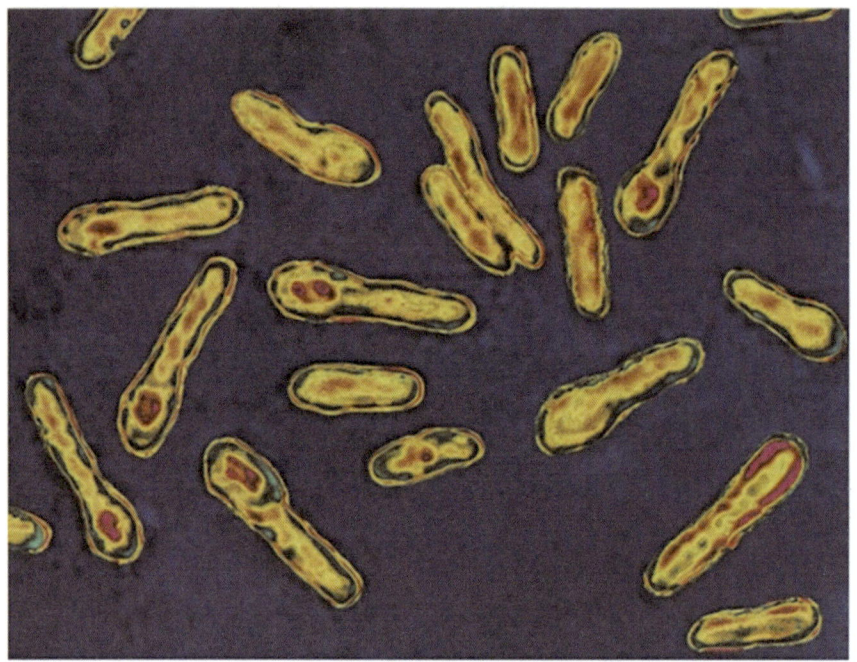

Clostridium botulinum

It is worth mentioning Behring (an assistant of Robert Koch), Behring, who in the early 1890s, together with his university friend Erich Wernicke, managed to develop the first effective therapeutic serum against diphtheria. At the same time, together with Shibasaburo Kitasato he developed an effective therapeutic serum against tetanus. But this knowledge remained unheralded within the dusty pages of science books, because at the end of the nineteenth century, the sexy end of microbiology was tropical disease, increasingly important with the ever-expanding colonial empires, thrusting young soldiers into evermore unfamiliar climates. evermore unfamiliar climates. In 1898, Robert Ross proved mosquitoes were the cause of malaria, and in the same year, the Spanish American War prompted new research into yellow fever. The new century came and, with it, more effective ways for the soldiers to kill their enemies. The first chemical agent to be used was chlorine gas, on 22 April 1915, near the Belgian village of Ypres. Over 5,000 Allied troops died in that first attack and a similar number in a second attack at Ypres two days later. Overall, about 113,000 tons of chemical weapons were used in World War I, killing around 92,000 soldiers and creating a total of 1.3 million casualties. But the biggest problem with chemical attacks during this time was that their effective ability could change rapidly if the winds shifted, and they often did. The use of biological agents in warfare has been known since time immemorial.

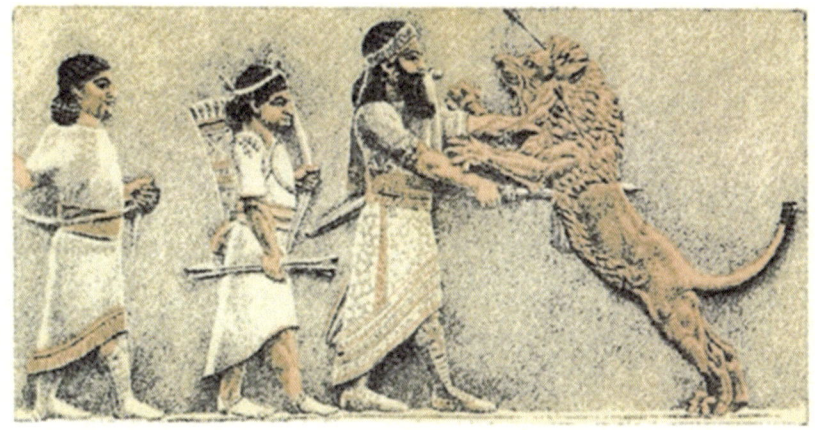

A LION HUNT

Ancient Assyrians hunting a lion

The use of biological agents in warfare

During the sixth century, the Assyrians poisoned their enemies' wells with ergot and in 1346, the Tartars threw the bodies of their bubonic plagued soldiers over the cities' walls to force surrender during its siege of Kaffa. Russian soldiers used the same tactic against the Swedish in 1710. And it did not end there. Pizarro is known to have given biologically contaminated blankets to South American natives in an earlier period and the British used the same tactic against the native Indians loyal to the French in the Indian War of 1754 to 1767.

The smallpox eventually caused widespread disease amongst the natives defending Fort Carillon, allowing Sir Jeffery Amherst's plan to work with great effect. There is little reason to see why the powerful toxin from Clostridium botulinum would remain in the dusty pages of a Belgian book whenever the armies of the Anglo-Saxons were on the march. And so, it came to pass that these scientists and others began to try and harness the power of the Botulinum bacterium in the use of warfare. In 1916, the British set up a chemical warfare complex in 7,000 acres of scrubland at Porton Down in Wiltshire and research into the ability of Botulinum toxin as an agent went underground.

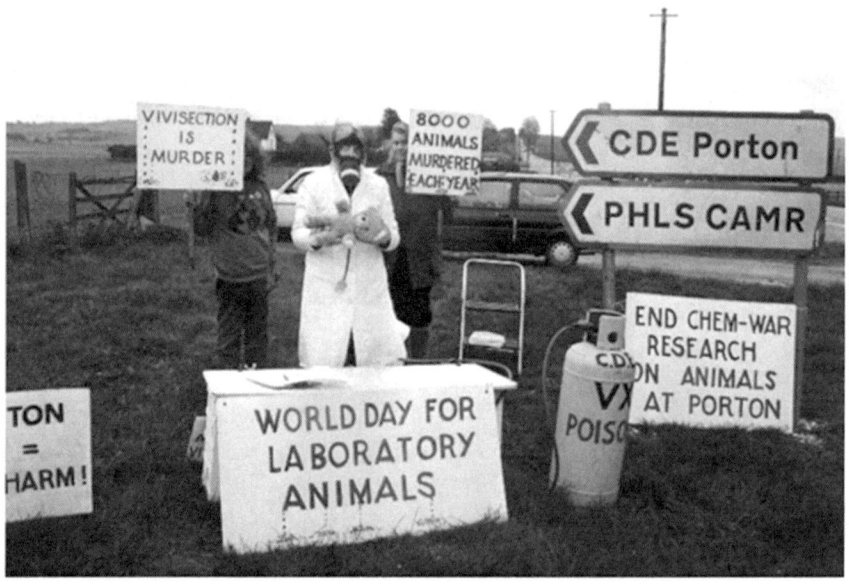

Porton Down in Wiltshire

In many ways, Botulinum toxin would appear to be an ideal agent for this type of warfare as it is an anaerobic organism. This means that its use is rather short-lived, and the bombed area can clean itself within a short period, allowing friendly troops to enter the area. But this apparent benefit also made it impractical as an easy agent for British and American armies to use as aerosol disposal. It was also known that vast quantities of Botulinum bacteria would have to be produced for it to become effective.

In 1937, as the German airship Hindenburg crashed at Lakehurst, New Jersey, the Japanese formed a biological warfare group called Unit 731, who poisoned prisoners in occupied Manchuria with Clostridium botulinum. In 1942, a high-ranking German SS and police official, Reinhard Heydrich, was assassinated by a bomb explosion in Prague by Czech patriots who were trained and equipped by the British. At first, Heydrich appeared to recover but later succumbed to an interesting disease. It was widely speculated at the time that he was killed by a bomb containing a biological agent after British scientist, Dr Paul Fides, confided to one of his colleagues that Heydrich's death was "the first notch on my pistol". Many state he died of a pulmonary embolism, and the association with botulinum toxin is mythical.

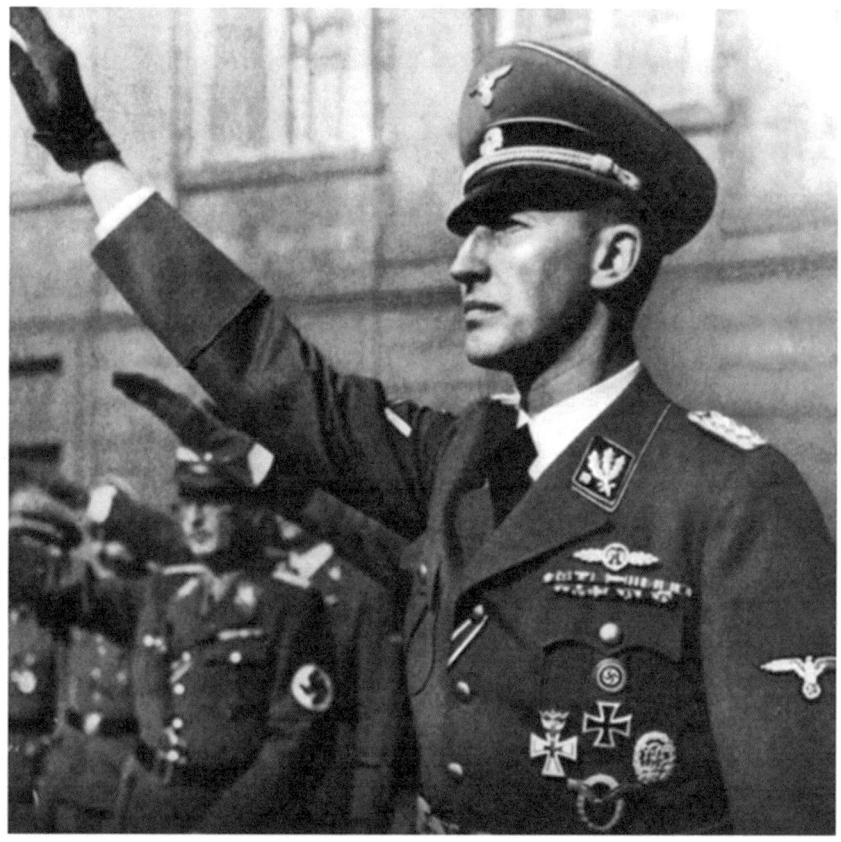

Reinhard Heydrich

Botulinum toxin during World War II

In 1944, more than 1 million doses of Botulinum vaccine were made for Allied troops in preparation for D-Day as intelligence sources indicated that Germany was interested in developing Botulinum toxin as a type of cross-channel weapon. In the same period, it is known that a group of British scientists led by the same Dr Paul Fides concentrated on using Botulinum toxin as a bioweapon. Their research at Porton Down eventually gave rise to the increasingly popular strain of Botulinum toxin known to the world today as Dysport®. In 1946, the RAF placed a request code-named 'Red Admiral' with the renamed Microbiological Research Department for a biological warfare bomb. The project aimed for a production capacity of 200 cluster bombs a week, providing a reserve of 10,000 bombs by 1955.

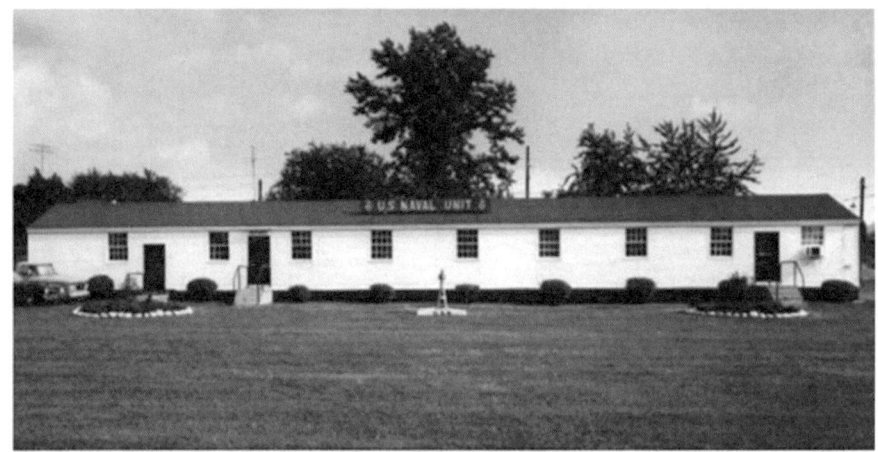

Naval Unit, Fort Detrick, MD

In the United States, research into Botulinum toxin began in earnest during the same period in a place called Fort Detrick in a militaristic bid to address the threat to the American nation from biological warfare. It is now known that members of the Special Operations Division conducted more than 200 biological warfare tests, some on ordinary subjects, from 1943 until the mid-1960s.

In 1969, President Richard Nixon banned the offensive research program and instead set up a defensive biological research program under the US Army Medical Research Institute of Infectious Diseases. When the experiments with Botulinum bacterium became public knowledge in 1977, American citizens became outraged that their government had exposed them to live organisms without their consent or knowledge. It was the same year that the rock 'n' roll entertainer, Elvis Presley, died at his home in Memphis, Tennessee. US military authorities during World War II were interested in the use of Botulinum as a weapon, and they recruited scientists to help produce it and evaluate its potential. One of the biochemists who gained employment at Fort Detrick during this period was a scientist called Dr Edward J. Schantz who had developed an interest in a highly lethal toxin called saxitoxin, which was found in clams and other shellfish. Schantz was born in Hartford, Wis., and grew up on his family's dairy farm. He received his primary and postgraduate biochemistry degrees from the University of Wisconsin and Iowa State University.

In 1946, he became chief of chemistry at Fort Detrick with the specific task of producing the different types of Botulinum toxin in their pure crystalline forms.

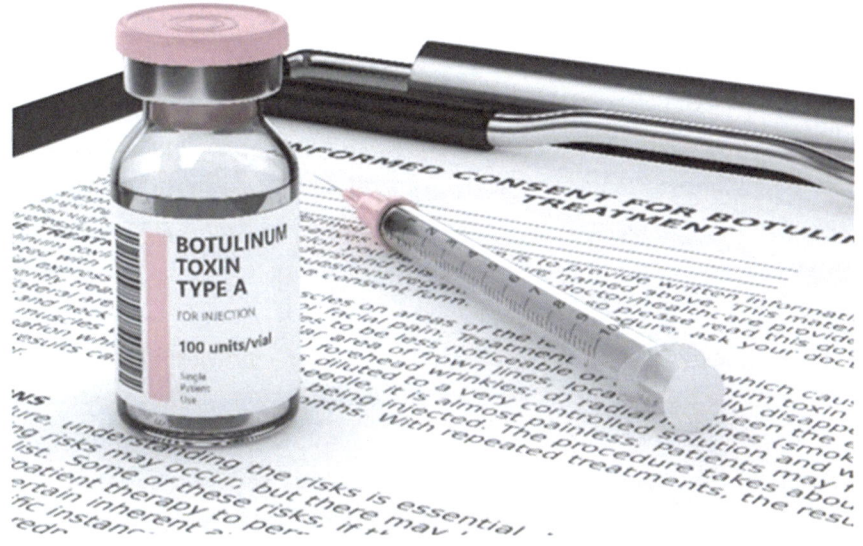

Botulinum Toxin Type A

It was the same year that Sir Winston Churchill warned the world about the threat of the Soviet's ideology in Europe and said, "An iron curtain has descended across the continent."

Botulinum toxin and medicine

In his first year at Fort Detrick, Dr Edward J. Schantz isolated the first crystalline form of the neurotoxin serotype BTX-A. Three years later, Arnold Burgen discovered that Botulinum toxin blocked neuromuscular transmission through decreased acetylcholine release. It was 1949, the same year that Mao Tse-Tung proclaimed China a Communist Republic. Indeed, the batch (79-11) originally prepared by Schantz was still used by Allergan Inc, Irvine, Calif., until December 1997 and marketed as the miracle anti-ageing drug, Botox.

During the 1960s, Schantz continued his research into BTX-A while the rest of America decried Bob Dylan for playing an electric guitar. It is known that the CIA used some of his pure batch to saturate some of Fidel Castro's favourite cigar type and when they were tested many years later, the neurotoxin was still found to be effective. It was during these years, as the Vietnam War waxed and waned, that Schantz became more and more convinced that Botulinum toxin would probably never become an effective biological warfare weapon and instead, he convinced his military leaders to market his discovery for the purpose of scientific research within the wider community.

One of the first people to attempt to use Botulinum toxin in the treatment of human disease was a scientist called Dr Alan B. Scott, who worked at the Smith-Kettlewell Eye Research Institute in San Francisco. Scott was looking for an agent like BTX-A for some time as he was convinced that he could use it to provide a new non-surgical treatment for the disease of strabismus, commonly known as cross-eyes. During the seventies, he injected a sample of the drug into the rectus muscles of cross-eyed monkeys to find a cure for the condition. The procedure was successful and within a short period, he had progressed to trying the neurotoxin on humans with similar eye conditions, including blepharospasm or eyelid spasm. The experiments were again successful, and his work led to the FDA to approve the use of Botulinum toxin to treat two eye muscle disorders – uncontrollable blinking (blepharospasm) and misaligned eyes (strabismus). The cosmetic effect of BTX-A on wrinkles was originally documented by a plastic surgeon from Sacramento, California – Richard Clark – and published in the journal, *Plastic and Reconstructive Surgery*, in 1989. It was the same year that I stood on the Berlin Wall, witnessing the fall of communism.

Botulinum toxin and aesthetic medicine

During the late eighties and early nineties, the Soviet Union and Iraq produced Botulinum toxin for weapons use, despite signing the 1972 Biological and Toxin Weapons Convention, prohibiting offensive research and manufacturing of biological weapons. In 1990, Iraq invaded Kuwait and deployed 13 specially designed missiles with a 370-mile range and 100 bombs, filled with the toxin. It admitted, after the Gulf War, that it produced 19,000 litres of concentrated Botulinum toxin, with about 10,000 litres loaded into weapons. I became a prisoner of Saddam Hussein's regime in that same year, being held for five days in prison. In 1992, Canadian husband and wife ophthalmologist and dermatologist physicians, JD and JA Carruthers, published the first study on BTX-A for the treatment of glabellar frown lines. Similar effects were apparently being observed by several other independent groups.

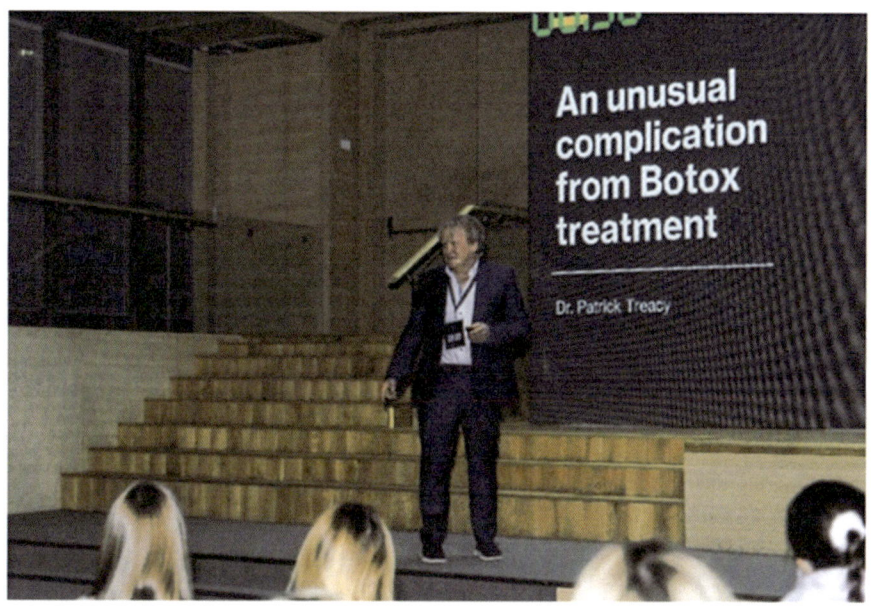

The author teaching Botox techniques at S Congress Kiev, Ukraine 2021

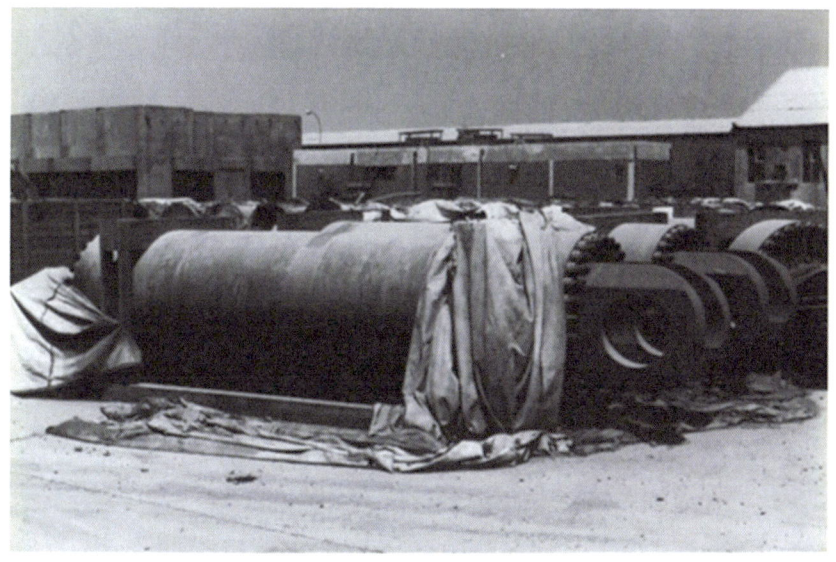

Iraq's Chemical, Biological and Nuclear Weapons

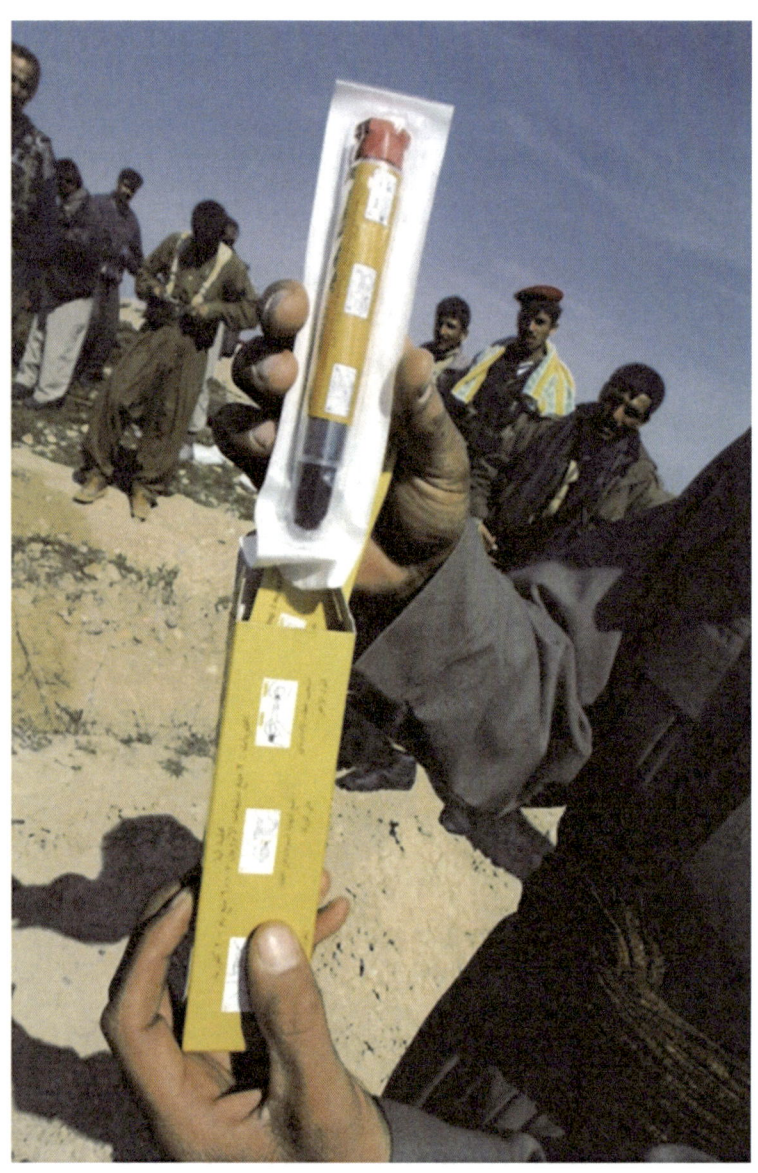

An Iraqi Kurd peshmerga holds an atropine injector, a drug used in combatting the effects of chemical or biological agents.

From here, I would like to look at this publication a little closer. It was, after all, the decisive observation in 1987 of Jean Carruthers that frown lines disappeared following treatment of blepharospasm that ignited the explosive cosmetic application of this product today and without her, I probably would

never have penned this article. Jean once told me that she had been using Botox®
for five years on eye patients, when she was struck with the idea that her patients
noticed that it smoothed out their facial lines.

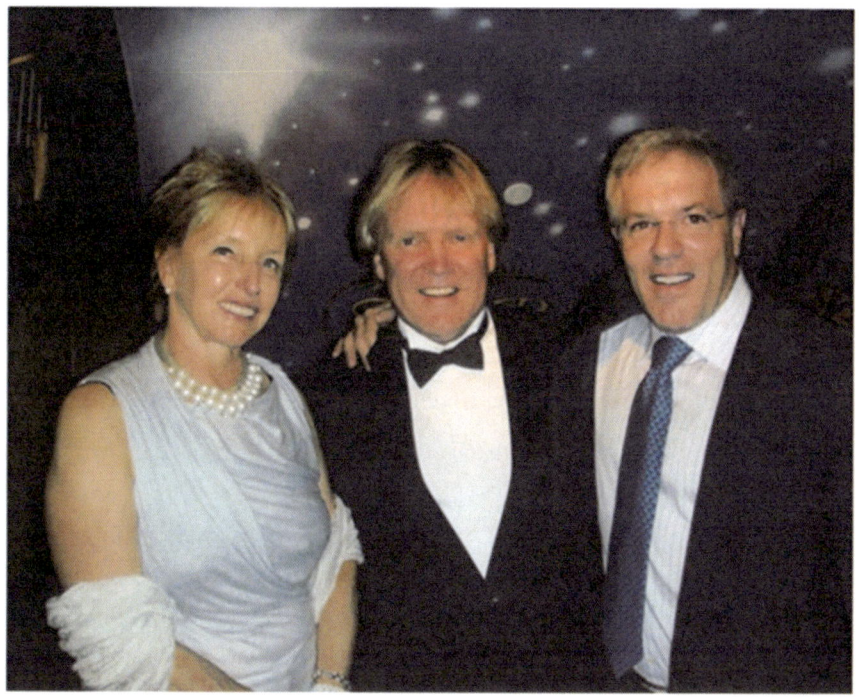

With Dr Jean Carruthers and Dr Tim Flynn Face Conference London 2007

She shared this seminal observation with her husband, Alistair, who was a
dermatologist, by saying, "My poison will get rid of your patients' wrinkles."
Jean Carruthers was familiar with Alan Scott's laboratory and was aware of the
potential cosmetic applications for the product. When she mentioned her findings
to Alan Scott, she discovered that he had apparently used the preparation for such
purposes in 1985. The first person that Alistair injected was their joint
receptionist, Cathy Bickerton Swann, who was only thirty at the time but had
always had deep frown lines. All were pleased with the result. And the rest, as
they say, is history.

The treatment was so successful that other researchers started looking at
using Botulinum toxin A in larger muscle groups and it quickly became
recognised that the drug was effective in the treatment of dystonia and spasm in
cerebral palsy. In 1995, as Michael Jackson was slipping down the charts with

You Are not Alone, the Japanese terrorist group Aum Shinrikyo was busy planning their gas attack on Tokyo's subway system. A follow-up operation discovered they had built a plant for producing Botulinum toxin. In 2000, the toxin was FDA-approved to treat a neurological movement disorder that causes severe neck and shoulder contractions, known as cervical dystonia.

As the century changed, President George Bush tried to convince his nation and a sceptical world that Iraq was involved in industrial-scale fermentation to produce large quantities of the neurotoxin for use as a biological agent. After formal trials, on 12 April 2002, the FDA announced regulatory approval of Botulinum toxin type A (Botox® Cosmetic) to temporarily improve the appearance of moderate-to-severe frown lines between the eyebrows (glabellar lines). Subsequently, cosmetic use of Botulinum toxin type A has become widespread. Botox® is the most popular non-surgical cosmetic procedure performed. Onabotulinum toxin A (trade name Botox) received FDA approval for treatment of chronic migraines on 15 October 2010.

****

Dr Edward J. Schantz became despondent with American civilian opposition to his biological warfare program, and he left Fort Detrick to become Professor Emeritus at the University of Wisconsin. He died at the ripe old age of 96 from congestive cardiac failure. He had lived long enough to see the toxin he isolated become known to the world as the wonder medicine that could erase lines and wrinkles on the faces of ageing patients. What he thought of how this potential military warfare product had become remains unknown.

Can botulinum work for depression?

Depression affects over 120 million people globally, making it one of the leading causes of disability in the world. A recent search of MEDLINE, EMBASE, Cochrane, and Scopus through May 5, 2014, for studies evaluating the efficacy of botulinum toxin A in depression showed it can produce significant improvement in depressive symptoms and is a safe adjunctive treatment for patients receiving pharmacotherapy for depression. Only randomized controlled trials were included in the meta-analysis. A pooled mean difference in primary depression score, and pooled odds ratio for response and remission rate with 95% confidence interval (CI) were estimated using the random-effects model.

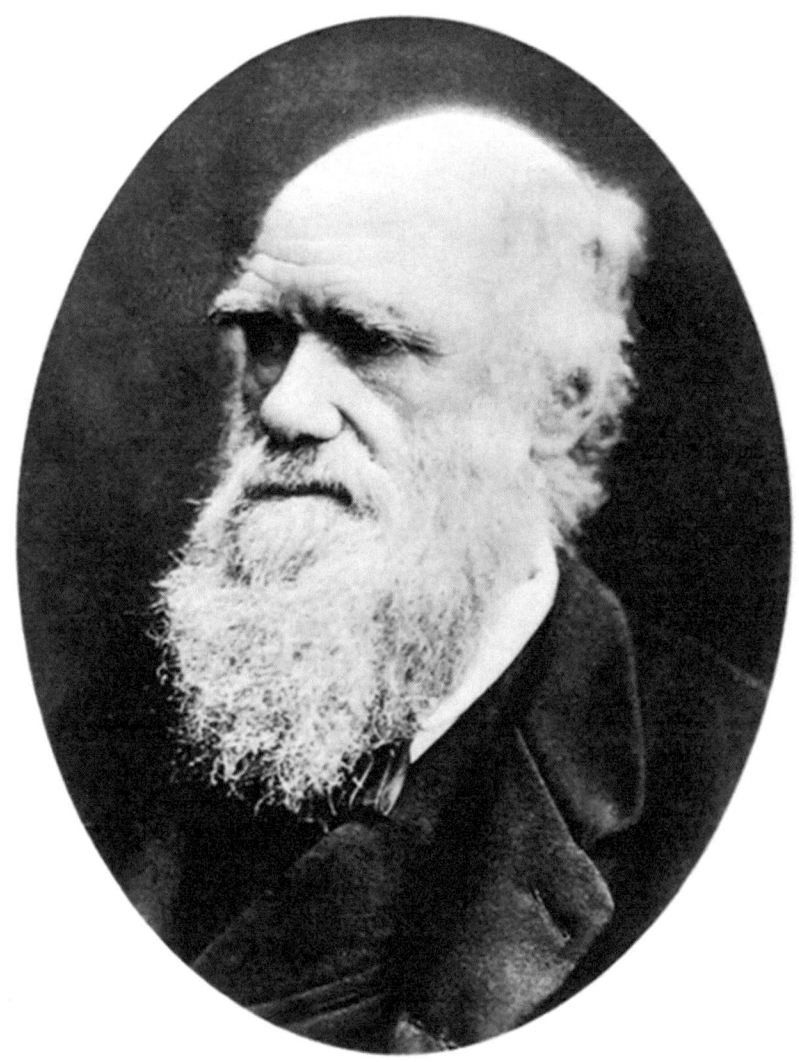

Charles Darwin (1809-82), English Naturalist, circa 1878

In 1872, Charles Darwin recognised these features as a specific expression of sadness and attributed them to the activity of so-called 'grief muscles' in the frown area. Negative emotions, such as anger, fear, and sadness are prevalent in depression and are associated with hyperactivity of the corrugator and procerus muscles in the glabellar region of the face. Darwin formulated a new theory called the 'facial feedback hypothesis', which implied a mutual interaction between emotions and facial muscle activity. Although there are various effective treatments, therapeutic response remains unsatisfactory, and depression can develop as a chronic condition in a considerable proportion of patients.

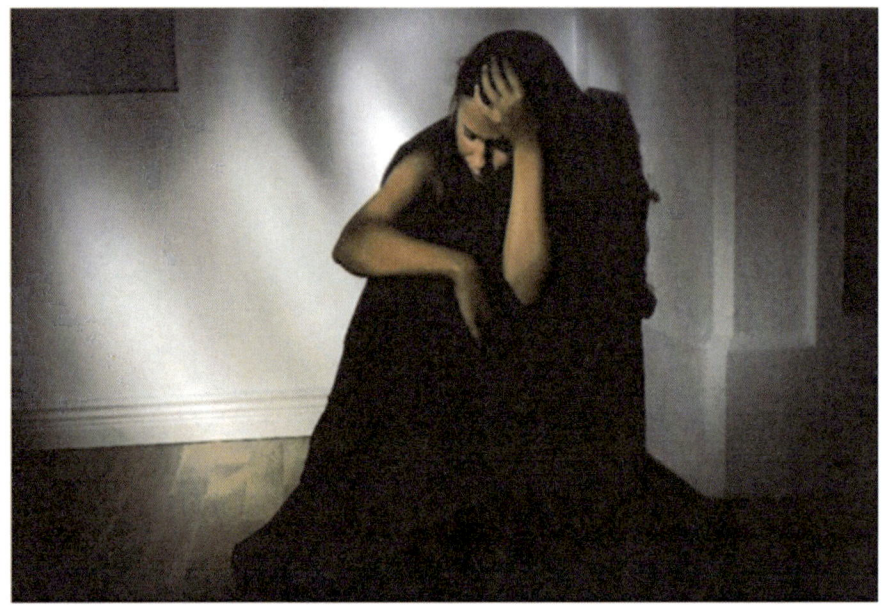

120 million suffer from depression

More recently, Larsen showed experimental evidence that voluntary contraction of facial muscles can channel emotions, which are conversely expressed by activation of these muscles. Heckmann published data suggesting that treatment of the glabellar (frown) region with botulinum toxin produces a change in facial expression from angry, sad, and fearful to happy and this can impact on emotional experience.

Many therapists, including Sommer (2003) have shown that patients who have been treated in the frown area reported an increase in emotional wellbeing and reduced levels of fear and sadness beyond what would be expected from the cosmetic benefit alone. Hennenlotter (2009) went one stage further and showed that botulinum toxin treatment to the frown area stopped the activation of limbic brain regions normally seen during voluntary contraction of the corrugator and procerus muscles.

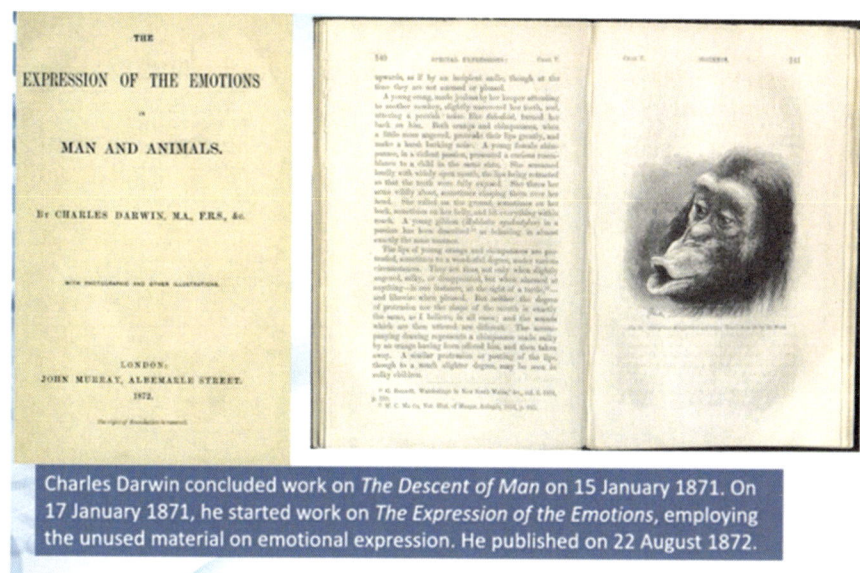

Darwin's book The Expression of Animals

This indicated that feedback from the facial musculature in this region in some way modulated the processing of emotions. Many other researchers have continued down this road with Havas (2010) noting that the processing time for sentences with negative affective connotation was prolonged in women after botulinum toxin treatment of the frown area Neal and Chartrand (2011) speculated that the treatment interfered with the ability to decode the facial expression of other people. This is where things were until recently with many authors suggesting that this capacity to counteract negative emotions could be put to some clinical use during the treatment of depression. There were some papers, including one with ten female patients in the Journal of Derm. Surgery by Finzi and Wasserman (2006) that postulated that botulinum toxin in the frown area demonstrated a reduction in the symptoms of depression.

However, a footnote by editor Alastair Carruthers stated that the report must be considered anecdotal as there were no appropriate methods of control utilized.

I noted by letter at the time that patients' self-report of depressive symptoms by administration of the Beck Depression Inventory (BDI-II) introduced a significant self-report bias. This is of more concern because of the potential for secondary cosmetic gain. While the BDI-II is an accepted method of evaluating an individual's level of symptoms over time, self- report in isolation was not considered an acceptable method of diagnosing depression. It was concluded that to ensure that patients' psychiatric symptoms are accurately classified, a thorough psychiatric interview must be conducted. More recently, two centres, the Psychiatric University Hospital of the University of Basel, Switzerland and the Medical School Hannover, Germany conducted a randomised, placebo-controlled, double-blind trial.

THE 'BOTOX PARADOX': IS IT EFFECTIVE FOR DEPRESSION?

Patrick Treacy considers the conflicting evidence of botulinum toxin use as a therapy for depression, and proposes that it all comes down to *where* the toxin is injected

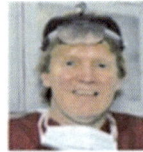

The 'grief' muscles

Article about botulinum toxin from PRIME Magazine

40

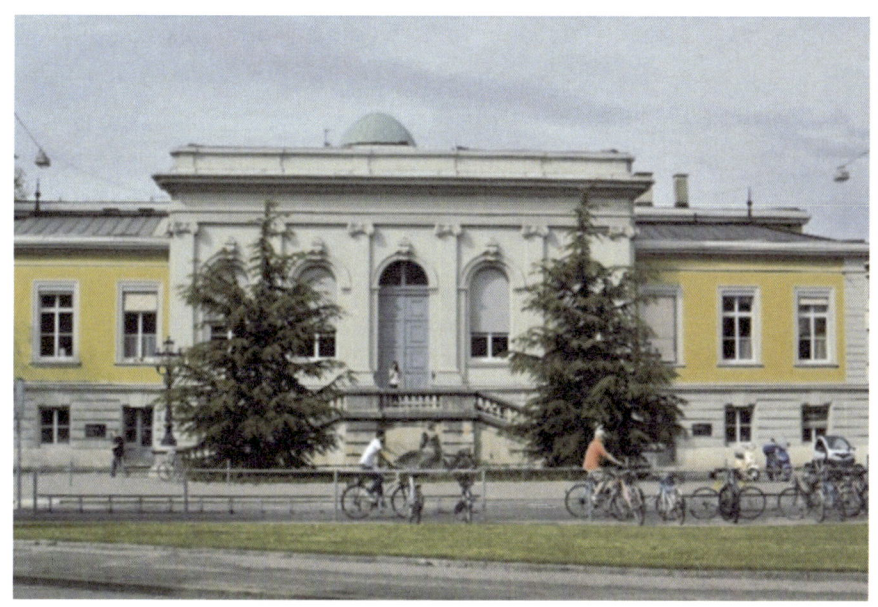

University of Basel, Switzerland

The authors hypothesised that facial psychomotor features associated with depression are not just epiphenomena but integral components of the disorder and may be targeted in its therapy. To explore, they conducted a randomised controlled trial of botulinum toxin injection to the frown region as an adjunctive treatment of major depression. The study was carried out independently of any commercial entity. Participants in the study were recruited from local psychiatric outpatient units and psychiatrists in private practice. To avoid attracting candidates who were primarily motivated by receiving this treatment for cosmetic reasons, botulinum toxin treatment, was not explicitly mentioned. At each study visit participants were assessed using the Hamilton Depression Rating Scale with Atypical Depression Supplement (SIGH-ADS), the Beck Depression Inventory (BDI) self-rating questionnaire and the Clinical Global Impressions Scale (CGI).

The study concluded for the first time that a single botulinum treatment of the glabellar region with could reduce the symptoms of major depression. This effect developed within few weeks and persisted until the end of the sixteen-week follow-up period. The effect sizes in the study were large and the response and remission rates were high. There is now enough evidence to suggest evidence that botulinum toxin injection to the glabellar region may be an effective, safe, and sustainable intervention in the treatment of depression. The reason for this has not yet been fully evaluated but we must consider the concept that the facial musculature not only expresses, but also regulates, mood states. Because of the long treatment intervals, it may also be an economic treatment option and the safety and tolerability record of botulinum toxin injections to the glabellar region is excellent.

****

There also have been recent studies investigating the possibility of botulinum toxin for bipolar disorder and post-traumatic stress disorder (PTSD). There is a certain irony to the fact that soldiers returning from combat zones at risk of chemical warfare been treated for PTSD may be now treated with botulinum toxin. Even to the uninitiated, it would appear to have turned the full circle.

****

Treating Axillary Hyperhidrosis with Botulinum Toxin

1n 1960, US Presidential debates were televised for the first time. Nixon battled an infection, and the studio lights caused the sweat to run down his brow. He repeatedly mopping his forehead with a handkerchief. Kennedy was tanned, healthy and looked like he had just stepped off the cover of a magazine. At that time, iontophoresis was the only treatment for the condition. However, things changed during the nineties, when local injections of botulinum toxin were found to result in a safe and effective solution for primary axillary hyperhidrosis. Although its pathophysiology was not clear and somewhat controversial, the beneficial effect of Botox® in inhibiting localised sweating temporarily is now well established. Before the procedure, one must correctly identify the affected area to avoid drug wastage and to enhance efficacy, as the area of sweating may not always match the hairy axillary region.

The maximum effect for Botulinum toxin type A (BTX-A) is seen quickly, often the next day. In many cases, the recommended dose will provideadequate suppression of sweat secretion for between three to nine months.The time point for further applications should be determined on an individual basis according to clinical need.

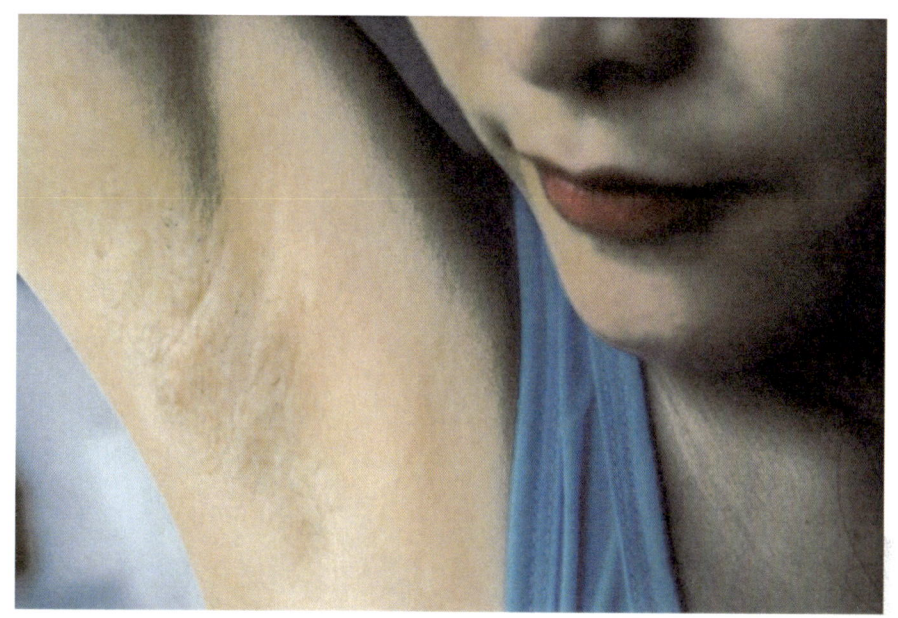

Dysport® for axillary hyperhidrosis

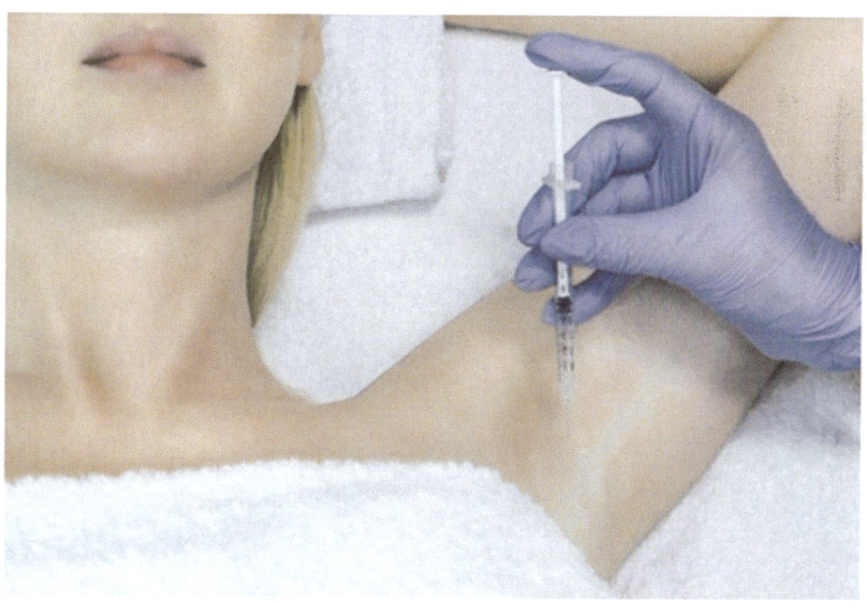

Injecting Botox® for sweating

Injections should not be repeated more frequently than every 12 weeks.

There is some evidence for a cumulative effect of repeated doses so the time of each treatment for a given patient should be assessed individually.

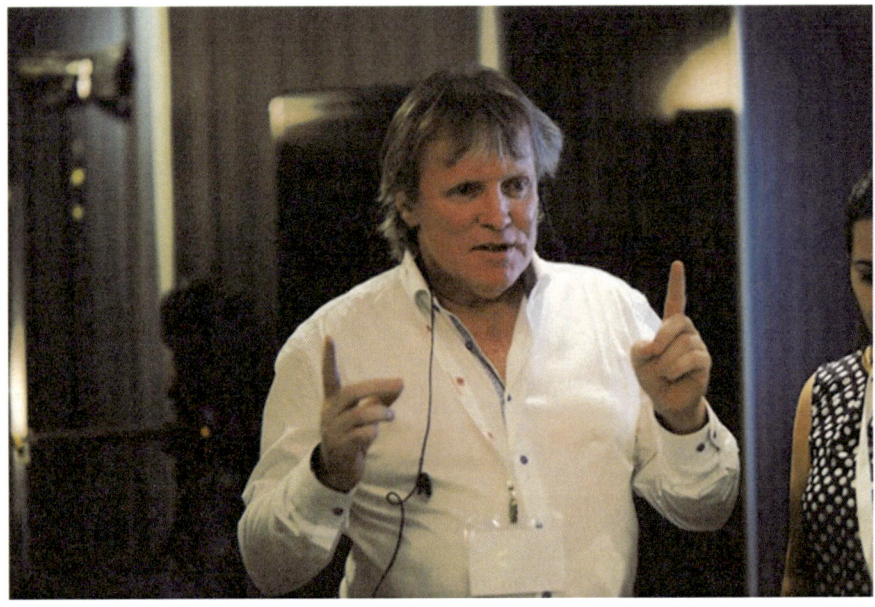

The author teaching how to use botulinum toxin for chronic migraine in Budapest 2018

****

Can we use botulinum in children?

I have treated a few patients ranging between nine and eleven years presenting with both migraine and axillary hyperhidrosis very successfully with botulinum toxin over the past years. As a migraine prophylaxis, botulinum is only approved by the US Food and Drug Administration (FDA) for adult patients.

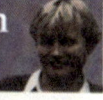

The Cutting Edge

BTX Type A and its application in the treatment of chronic pain

Dr Patrick Treacy says that while this series on BTX-A has been well received, there is some scepticism – but this is both a healthy and welcome sign.

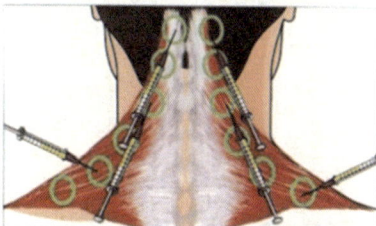

Diagram 2: Trapezius muscle group – injection points included by some practitioners

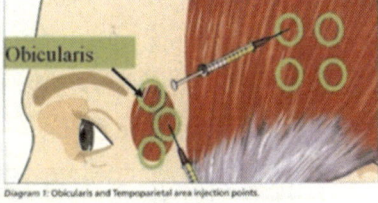

Obicularis

Diagram 1: Obicularis and Tempoparietal area injection points.

Article about botulinum toxin in the treatment of chronic pain by the author from the Irish Medical Times 2001

Chapter 2: Dermal Fillers

Many different hyaluronic acid-injectable fillers are available on the market and differ in terms of hyaluronic acid concentration, particle size, cross-linking density, requisite needle size, duration, stiffness, hydration, presence of lidocaine, type of cross-linking technology and cost. Hyaluronic acid soft-tissue fillers include a range of products (Juvederm Ultra, Juvederm Ultra Plus, Voluma, Restylane Defyne, Restylane Refyne, Restylane Lyft and Belotero Balance) that are used commonly for facial rejuvenation and enhancement of facial features. Although these products are similar in many ways, they are not interchangeable and have unique characteristics that need to be considered. Hyaluronic acid is a natural component of many soft tissues and is identical across species minimising immunogenicity.

The Discovery of Hyaluronic Acid

In 1934, while Nazi Germany and Poland were signing a 10-year non-aggression treaty, Germans Karl Meyer and John Palmer wrote in *Journal of Biological Chemistry* about an unusual polysaccharide with an extremely high molecular weight isolated from the vitreous of bovine eyes. Karl Meyer was born in the village of Karpen, Germany, near Cologne. In 1917, he was drafted into the German army and served in the last year of World War I. After the war, he entered medical school at the University of Cologne and received the MD degree in 1924. He then went to Berlin for a year of study in medical chemistry and met several promising young biochemists, including Fritz Lippman, Hans Krebs and Ernst Chain.

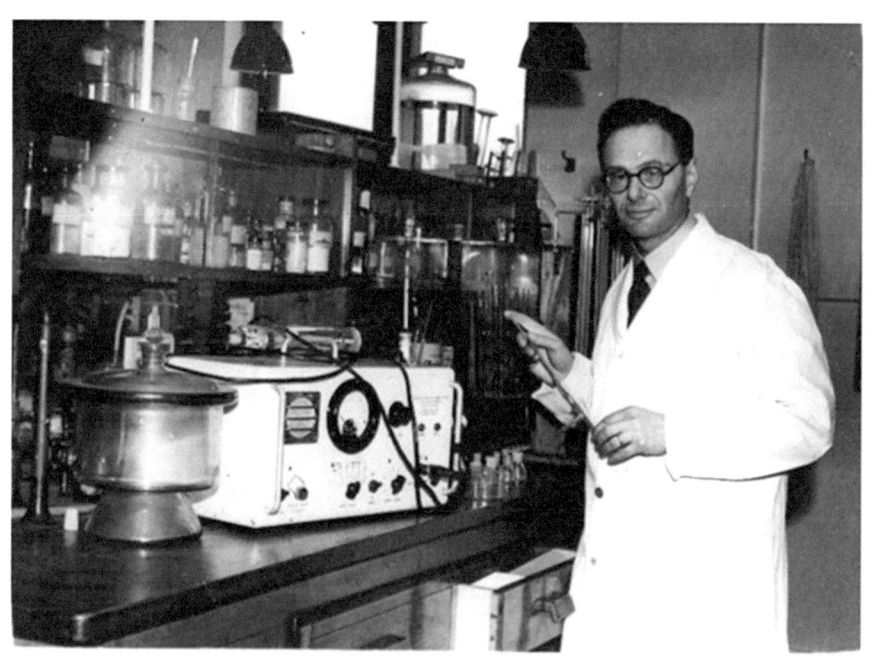

Sir Hans Adolf Krebs

Sir Hans Adolf Krebs was born at Hildesheim, Germany. In June 1933, the National Socialist Government terminated his appointment, and he went to the School of Biochemistry, Cambridge, where he researched the complex chemical processes that provide living organisms with high-energy phosphate by way of what is known as the Krebs or citric acid cycle. The Nobel prize in physiology or medicine in 1953 was divided equally between Hans Adolf Krebs 'for his discovery of the citric acid cycle' and Fritz Albert Lipmann 'for his discovery of co-enzyme A and its importance for intermediary metabolism'. Ernest Chain was another German-born British biochemist, who became a 1945 co-recipient of the Nobel prize for physiology or medicine for his work on penicillin.

Meanwhile, Karl Meyer decided, no doubt in part because of the rising anti-Semitism in Europe and the increasing probability of war, to go back to the US. He received a position as assistant professor in the department of ophthalmology at the College of Physicians and Surgeons. In part because of the mission of his department, Meyer began to study the lysozyme present in tears and undertook to identify a physiological substrate for the enzyme.

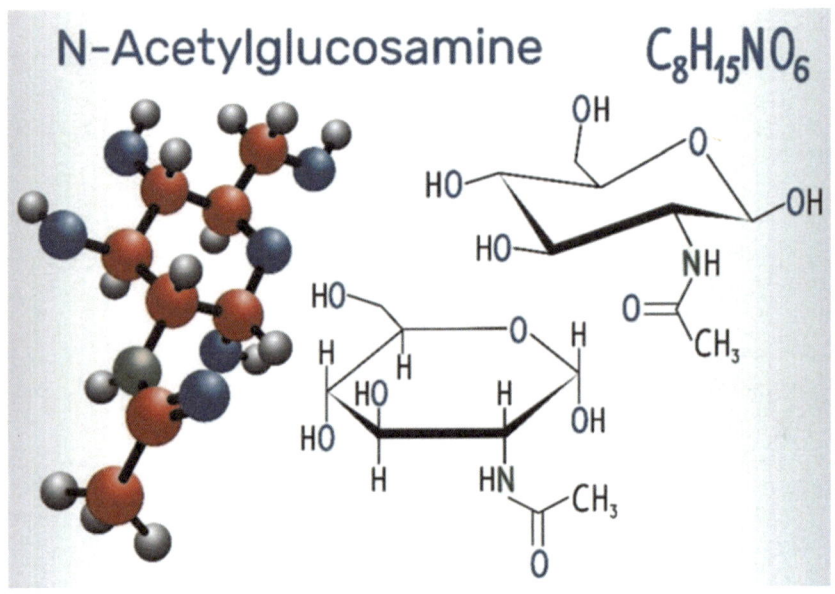

N-Acetylglucosamine $C_8H_{15}NO_6$

N-Acetylglucosamine (NAG) molecule, is the monomeric unit of the chitin and polymerized with glucuronic acid, it forms hyaluronic acid

Examination of the viscous vitreous humor of the eye as a plausible source of substrate quickly led to the discovery of hyaluronan, which is reported in this Journal of Biological Chemistry (JBC) classic. While there, Meyer and his assistant, John Palmer, isolated a novel, high molecular weight polysaccharide and reported that it was composed of 'a uronic acid and an amino sugar'.

Being the first to mention it, they gave the new substance the name *hyaluronic acid* (HA, the modern name 'hyaluronan') derived from 'hyaloid' (glass-like in appearance) and 'uronic acid'. Nearly 25 years of work were required to establish the structure of the repeating disaccharide that is the basic unit of the hyaluronan polymer, namely, glucuronate-β-1,3-N-acetylglucosamine-β1,4-

In 1958, while the US launched its first satellite, Explorer I, and NASA was established, Meyer chaired the annual meeting of the American Society of Biological Chemists and stated in his opening remark:

It is my opinion that the mucopolysaccharides will never be a highly popular field in biochemistry, but they will probably not be relegated again to the insignificance and disregard in which they were held not so long ago.

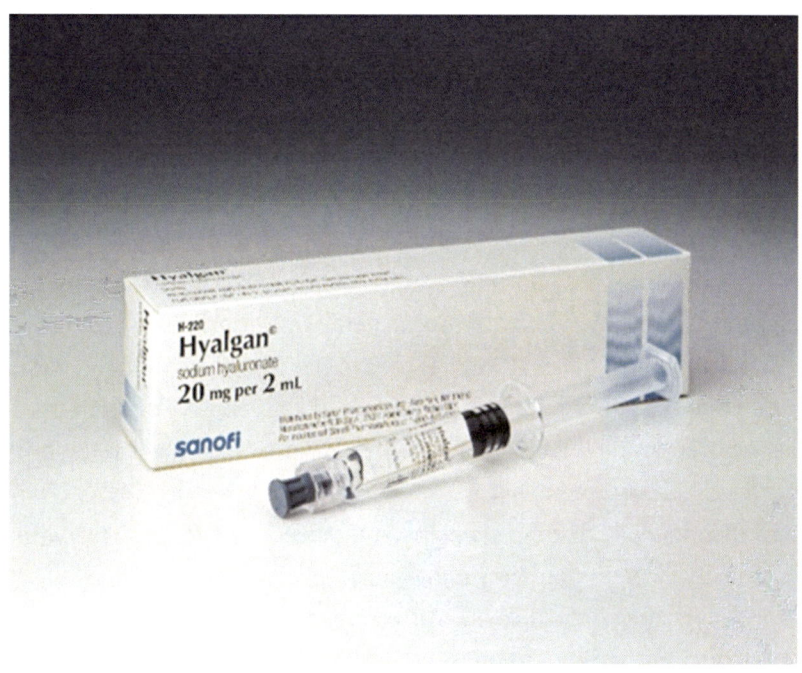

The drug Hyalgan a strong arthritis drug

How wrong he was; like the Beatles and computers being originally turned down, hyaluronic acid was to become one of the most important chemicals in the world.

While Meyer and Palmer are generally considered to have discovered hyaluronic acid, it is fair to mention that as far back as 1918, just as World War I ended, Levene and Lopez-Suarez had isolated a new polysaccharide from the vitreous body and cord blood that they called 'mucoitin-sulfuric acid'. It consisted of glucosamine, glucuronic acid, and a small amount of sulphate ions. It is now clear that this substance was hyaluronic acid extracted together with a mixture of sulphated glycosaminoglycans.

At the time of the discovery of hyaluronan, the polysaccharides, which represent a major part of the organic material on our planet, were already quite well known. Several so-called mucopolysaccharides, currently known as glycosaminoglycans, had already been discovered. Hyaluronic acid is known to belong to this class as well. Mucopolysaccharides were isolated from mucus, to which they give viscous lubricating properties. These properties, in turn, are related to glycosaminoglycan's ability to bind to a significant amount of water.

Over the next decade, Meyer, and others, isolated hyaluronic acid from various animal organs. It was found to exist in joint fluid, the umbilical cord and, recently, it has become possible to extract HA from almost all vertebrate tissues. In 1937, as the Golden Gate Bridge opened to pedestrian traffic, F. Kendall was busy isolating hyaluronic acid from the capsules of Streptococci groups A and C. I feel this was the biggest breakthrough for hyaluronic acid fillers, as even today in 2020, Streptococci groups are the most economical and reliable source for the industrial production of hyaluronic acid. Finding a use for hyaluronic acid in medicinal practice did not actually occur until 1943, during the Second World War. The start of World War II (WWII) led to the deployment of combat troops in several continents and fatalities and casualties among both the military and civilians became an inevitable consequence. A large amount of injured people needed life-saving treatment and a speedy return to duty. The Soviet Union, its allies and its opponents had no specialised medical units for patients with burn injuries in military or civilian hospitals when the WWII began. Intensive studies of the specific issues of diagnosis and treatment of thermal and frostbite injury were conducted in the Soviet Union before the war. The first special units for patients with burn injuries were created, and the first specialists received their first clinical experience.

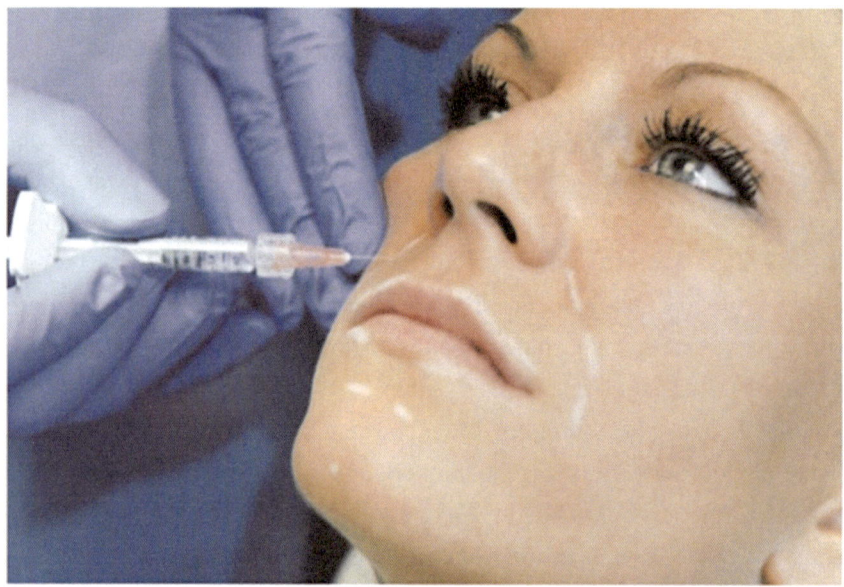

Beauty treatment on woman with hyaluronic acid

The contributions of famous Soviet scientists in the development of the treatment of burns and frostbite in WWII is well documented. N.F. Gamaleya (Н.Ф. Гамалея) created a new type of bandage to treat the frostbitten soldiers in the military field hospital No 1321. The main component of the bandage was an extract from the umbilical cord, which he called a 'factor of regeneration'. The method was later approved by the USSR Ministry of Health and the drug received the name 'Regenerator'. It is apparent that HA was a major contributor towards the positive effect of the treatment, given that the human umbilical cord contains a significant amount of Ha. Several practical ventures that explored HA's medical applications followed. Research into finding practical applications to match the physico-chemical properties of hyaluronic acid is considered to have begun in 1951 with the publication of a series of five volumes under the title, Hyaluronan: From Basic Science to Clinical Application, by Balazs et al. It was the same year that the North Korean offensive pushed beyond the 38th parallel as truce negotiations failed.

In the 1950s, E.A. Balazs initiated experiments with HA to investigate its potential as a prosthesis for the treatment of retinal detachment. In 1953, Roseman and co-workers published an article in which they describe the precipitation of HA from the cultural liquid (CL) of Group A streptococcus. They reported the yield 200-300 mg from 4 l of CL. Later, Warren and Gray found the semi-synthetic media for the cultivation of the HA producers was preferable. In 1970, hyaluronan was first injected into the joints of racehorses that suffered from arthritis with a clear and positive outcome observed. It was the same year that the Beatles broke up and US President Richard Nixon ordered an invasion of Cambodia, widening the war in Vietnam.

In 1982, R. Miller started to use hyaluronic acid in implanted intraocular lenses. It was the same year that the first CD player was sold in Japan. Since these ground-breaking cases, hyaluronan has become one of the most important components in ophthalmology and has found extremely wide application in aesthetic medicine.

****

In 1996, while Mad Cow Disease hit Britain, causing the mass slaughter of herds of cattle and new laws to stop beef being sold on the bone, a Swedish company called Q-Med released to the world NASHA technology (Non-Animal Stabilised Hyaluronic Acid). For the first time, hyaluronic gel particles within a viscoelastic medium, subjected to a physiological salt solution, could be used as a soft-tissue augmentation facial implant. The process was invented by Bengt Ågerup, who was born in Uppsala (1943) and studied renal physiology at a university there. He had previously worked for many years as a researcher at Pharmacia. In March 2011, he sold his shares in Q-Med to Galderma SA, a French-Swiss pharmaceutical company. In 2018, a new breakthrough skin treatment called Profhilo® was developed by IBSA, which introduced a new category in the injectables market – bio remodelling. It is an injectable, stabilized Hyaluronic Acid based product, produced without the use of chemical cross-linking agents (BDDE) according to a patented technology (NAHYCO), designed to remodel multi-layer skin tissue.

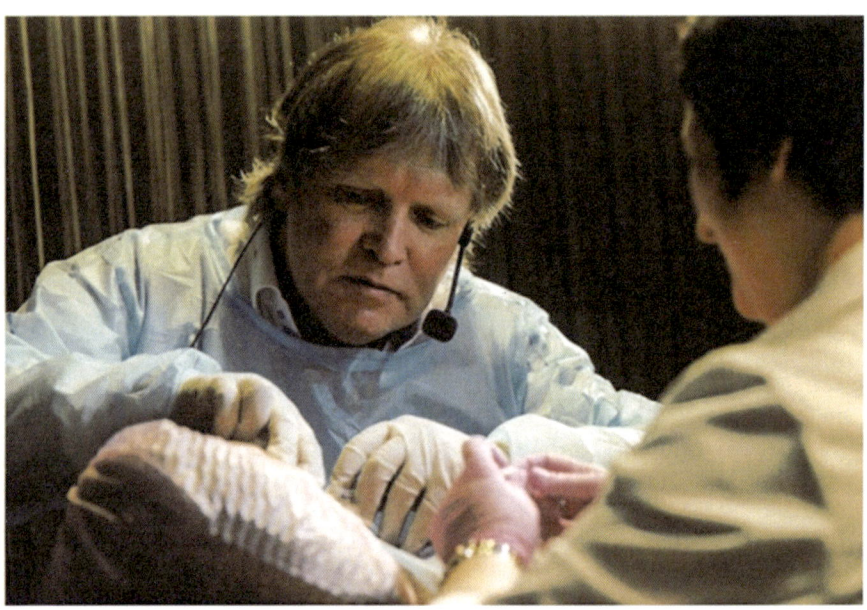

The author demonstrating his dermal filler cannulation injection techniques to Russian doctors on board the 'Sovereign of the Seas' in Italy

'Lip Augmentation with hyaluronic acid fillers'

The techniques for injection of HA for lip augmentation are dependent on the filler, area to inject, and the physician and patient preference. These include serial puncture and linear threading, which may be antegrade or retrograde.

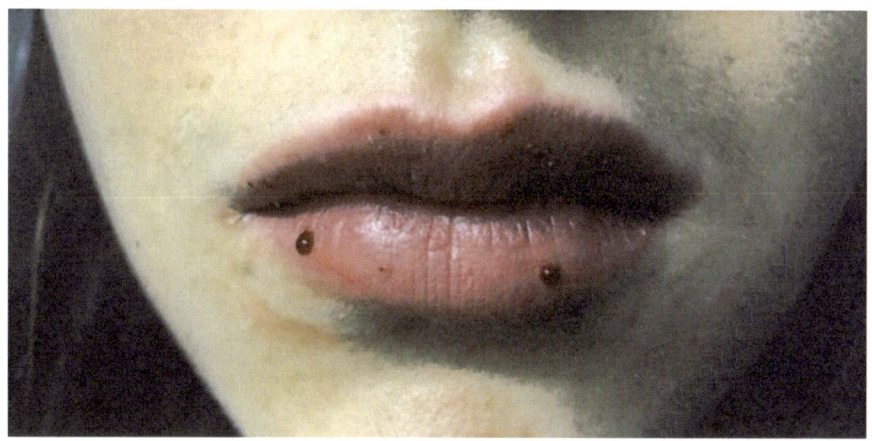

The author's 'PT' lip augmentation technique

The operator can perform the technique either with a needle or the use of a cannulae. The use of cannulae is recommended but it takes time to learn the technique and the use of a 27G needle has been involved in some vascular occlusions. A needle is probably faster, but a skilled operator can soon reduce the procedure time involved. To reduce injection and filling related pain, topical anaesthetics or nerve blocks may be used. Some fillers contain lidocaine to reduce injection pain. The author recently demonstrated his 'PT' lip augmentation technique to an audience of 350 doctors in the Fairmont Hotel in Kiev in October 2021.

The History of Treating HIV Lipoatrophy Patients (HLS)

During the turn of the twenty-first century, (HIV)-lipodystrophy syndrome was a major problem for many HIV patients undergoing long-term use of highly active antiretroviral therapy (HAART). The psychological effects of the condition (both abnormal fat loss and abnormal fat accumulation) were distressing, as it created low self-esteem, depression, anxiety, reduced confidence as well as social withdrawal and isolation secondary to perceived social stigma. A study of the period showed that 53% of patients with HLS had abnormal scores for depression and 45% for anxiety. Patients presenting with facial lipodystrophy were twice as likely to feel recognizable as HIV-positive by their physical appearance. The condition was characterized a loss of subcutaneous fat, especially in the cheeks, temples and around the eyes.

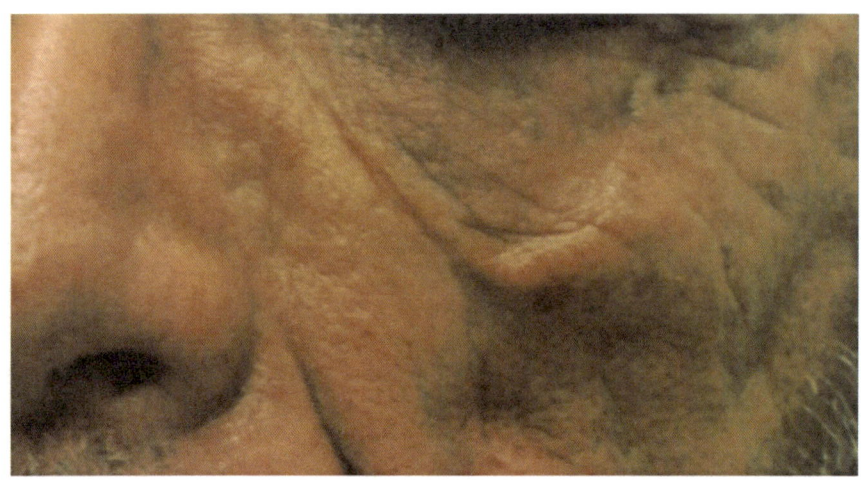

HIV lipoatrophy before treatment

The cause of the condition was not fully understood. While some researchers focused on a multifactorial phenomenon, others said that the HIV infection was the most likely cause of the pathology. Others, like myself believed that HLS was caused by the pharmaceutical drugs, d4T and to a lesser extent AZT. What made me convinced was the fact that I never saw the condition amongst any of the HIV patients whom I had treated in Africa.

Either way, there was no available pharmacological therapy to manage this complex condition and medications such as rosiglitazone, pioglitazone, metformin, and growth hormone proved to produce no significant benefit. Most currently used strategies of the period tended to compensate for facial fat loss. These included a range of dermal fillers including bovine collagen; but the effects declined after 3 months. The use of Hyaluronic Acid was limited due its expense and the fact it had continually replenished on a periodic basis. In that period the most widely used product for facial HLS was a slowly degradable polylactic acid (PLA) called Sculptra®.

By 2000, Sculptra® had some found favour in HIV lipodystrophic patients as it had certain advantages over other more permanent dermal fillers in respect to its safety record and efficacy. However, it was difficult to inject, required hundreds of injections and took many months to see the eventual effect. It also required up to five sessions to administer and the resultant contouring effect lasted only last two years. In addition, it did not actually restore lost fat mass where it was injected, but rather it expanded the thickness of the skin by forming

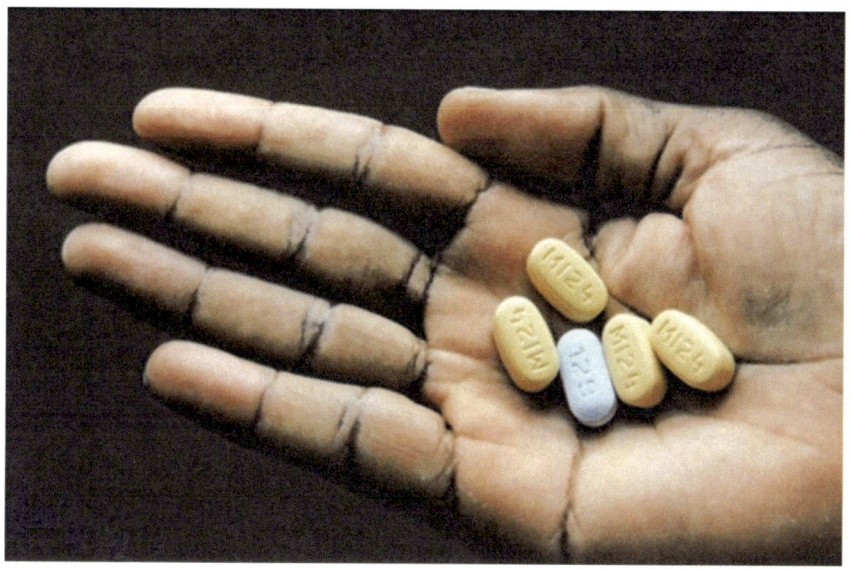

Daily ration of Antiretroviral Medicine to fight AIDS

new collagen. In 2001, the only other means of restoring facial contour was by autologous fat transfer. This method was limited by the availability of patient donor sites and the fact that the transferred fat also disappeared as it was further metabolized by the on-going lipodystrophic process. In this period, I did a study evaluate the efficacy, immediate aesthetic effect, and eventual safety of a new permanent, injectable gel polyalkylimide (Bio-Alcamid™) in HIV-infected patients with facial lipodystrophy. The injected material comprised of a network of alkyl-imide groups (approximately 4%) and water. It did not tend to migrate post-injection as it became coated by a 'thin collagen capsule', which transformed into what was called an endogenous prosthesis.

The introduction of Bio- Alcamid™

The compound has been used since 2000 in over twenty countries and did not require any sensitization test as no allergic reaction has ever been reported. Bio-Alcamid™ claimed to have been the subject of numerous specific scientific documents as well as multi-centre clinical evaluations in major hospitals and universities, including a 2000 patient study demonstrating the safety, efficacy, and biocompatibility of the product. The compound had already some popularity in Europe in the treatment of road collision or cancer patients requiring facial reconstruction.

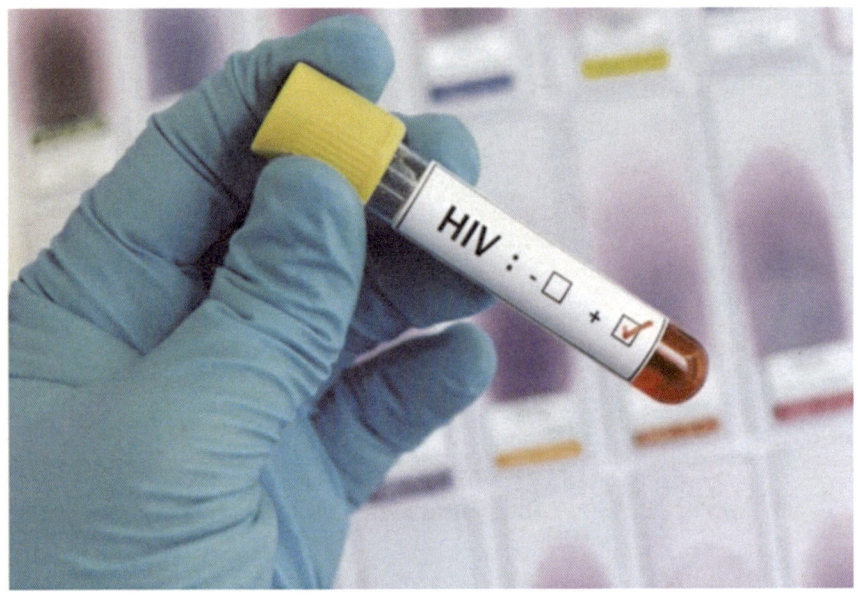

HIV prevalence at the turn of the century

One of the advantages of this endoprosthetic material was the fact that large quantities of up to 200mls could be injected at one session. Its polymeric structure meant it didn't contain free monomers, and it appeared to be devoid of the risk of undesirable effects such as toxicity, lumps and pigment changes that are associated with similar materials. The manufacturers, Polymekon, (a researcher of medical polymers headquartered in the Science and Technology Park, National Centre for Research and Development of Materials, in Brindisi, Italy) claimed that this process means it can be extracted from surrounding tissue and a copy of the removal procedure can be obtained directly from them. In 2001, reactions to polyalkylimide gels appeared to be rare.

The manufacturing company claimed that many years of rigorous clinical and laboratory analyses show that the compound was non-toxic, non-sensitizing, non-mutagenic, biocompatible, permanent, removable, and physically and chemically stable. In addition to this, the compound was also radio-transparent and hypoechoic, thus allowing X-Rays and ultrasound to be used. These properties tend to suggest to me that it could become an effective long-term alternative to adipose tissue auto transplantation for HIV-infected patients.

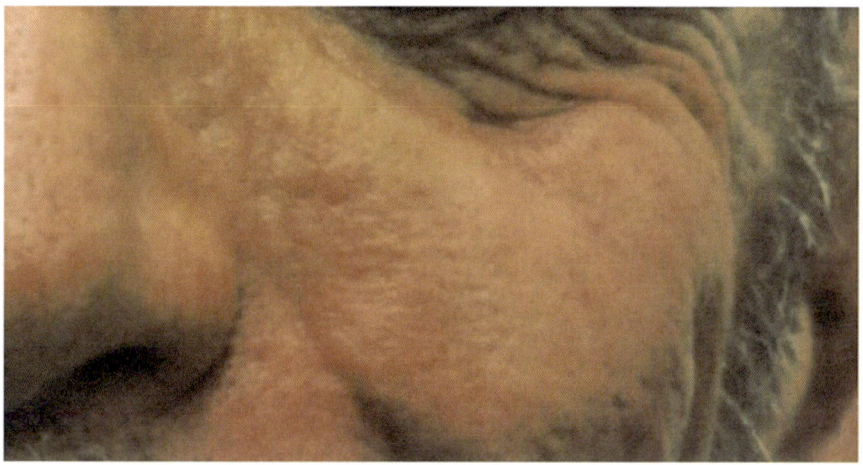

HIV lipoatrophy after treatment

Patient with severe facial lipodystrophy after treatment. The patient was injected bilaterally into the buccal, malar, and temporal areas of his face with 23mls of the polyalkylimide gel (BioAlcamid®)

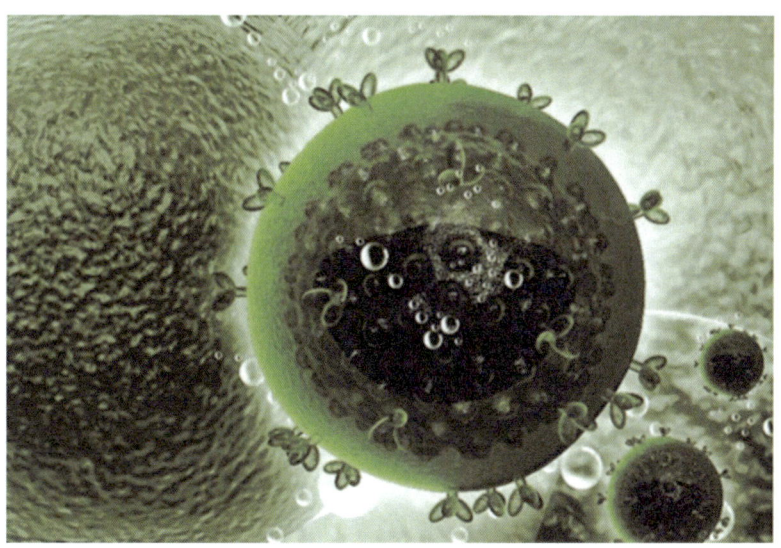

HIV Virus

I treated over forty HIV patients and my results showed that polyalkylimide gel injections could lead to significant clinical improvement in, (HIV)-lipodystrophy syndrome (HLS) patients as well as improving their anxiety, and depression. In a 2006 publication of my results in the *Journal of Dermatological Surgery*, I stated that larger studies were required to determine long-term safety of this gel. In that year, I switched to Radiesse to treat these HLS patients. In the next few years, between 2008-2010 reports emerged of higher-than-expected rates of complications were found with Bio Alcamid. Members of the Dutch Society of Cosmetic Medicine conducted a survey of plastic surgeons to find out some of the issues associated with Bio Alcamid. They found that 3,196 patients received 4,738 treatments with this product. Of the 3,196 patients, nearly 5% developed complications broadly grouped in the categories noted below.

The later complications of using Bio- Alcamid™

(1) Inflammation – This was the most common problem occurring years after implantation and "mainly after surgical procedures in the face, such as dental procedures," noted the Dutch doctors. Inflammation associated with the implant also occurred after patients experienced infections in their head and neck.

(2) Accumulation – In some cases, Bio-Alcamid™ seemed to build up in one area, typically many years after implantation.

(3) Hardening of the capsule – Another complication was hardening of the capsule of collagen surrounding the implant. The doctors stated that this was "generally a visible and disturbing disfigurement for patients."

(4) Migration – In some cases, the implant would move to another area. This was a problem, particularly in the cheeks.

In January 2004, I went to Miami to learn about thread-lifting and while there, met the famous French plastic surgeon, Dr Pierre Fournier, considered by many to be the father of cosmetic surgery. During that Miami visit, I also met Dr Abdala Khalil and his wife, Carol, and spent one evening with them drinking some wine and watching the sunset in the environs of their beautiful Miami beachside home. Little did I know, as we sipped wine on their boat deck that evening, that fifteen years later, I would be inviting Carol over to speak to my medical colleagues in London. There, in my capacity as chairman of the

Aesthetics Conference of the Royal Society of Medicine, she would tell us her story of how she developed a major aesthetic complication resulting in her having to get a forehead transplant after damage done to her by somebody injecting a silicone filler into her face. It was during this period that I developed an interest in treating complications, and her husband sent me over some cases for management and treatment. Ms. Donna Corden followed her persuasive speech and Lindsey McEnroe, clinical director of True You Skin Clinics, both gave a similar lecture on 'How a flesh-eating bug caused me to require an autologous partial face transplant.'

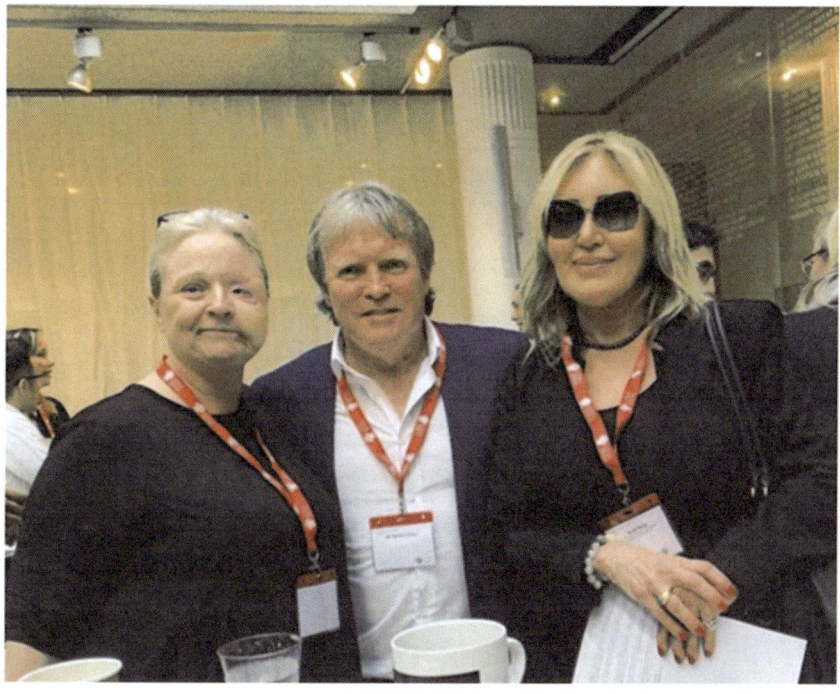

With partial autologous face transplant patients, Ms Donna Corden, Ms Carol Bryant
Royal Society of Medicine Aesthetic Conference London 2019.

Chapter 3: Aesthetic Lasers

The word 'LASER' is an acronym for 'Light Amplification by Stimulated Emission of Radiation'. Lasers generate light energy in the form of a beam of photons emitted from the laser medium, which usually gives the laser its name and determines the precise wavelength produced by the laser. For example, a ruby crystal gives the ruby laser its name, and emits at red: the CO_2 laserhas carbon dioxide gas as its medium and emits energy at far infrared. Current medical lasers emit wavelengths from the ultraviolet to the mid-infrared portions of the spectrum. Intense pulsed light (IPL) is a technology used by cosmetic and medical practitioners to perform various skin treatments for aesthetic and therapeutic purposes, including hair removal, the treatment of skin pigmentation, sun damage and thread veins.

It is ironic now to think that in 1951, when American scientist, Charles Townes, showed that a MASER could theoretically be made to operate in the microwave region of the spectrum, his colleagues told him that 'his work would have little relevance to the real world'. The year was 1951, and Kellogg's introduced Sugar Corn Pops Cereal and the first Ford Consul was manufactured by Ford in Britain. I am sure the world had changed a lot when Charles Townes received the Nobel prize in physics thirteen years later. In that year, three civil rights workers were murdered in Mississippi the president signed the Civil Rights Act of 1964. Today, lasers are used in every aspect of life including an ever-increasing number of cosmetic treatments, such as skin resurfacing for wrinkle reduction and acne scars, removal of tattoos, removal ofhair, removal of pigmented blemishes (age spots and moles) and the treatment of vascular lesions (port-wine stains and spider veins).

In fact, the real story of lasers started many years before. In the year 1917, the great physicist, Albert Einstein, postulated that atoms could be persuaded to emit tiny packets of energy called 'photons' in his treatise, *On the Quantum Theory of Radiation.*

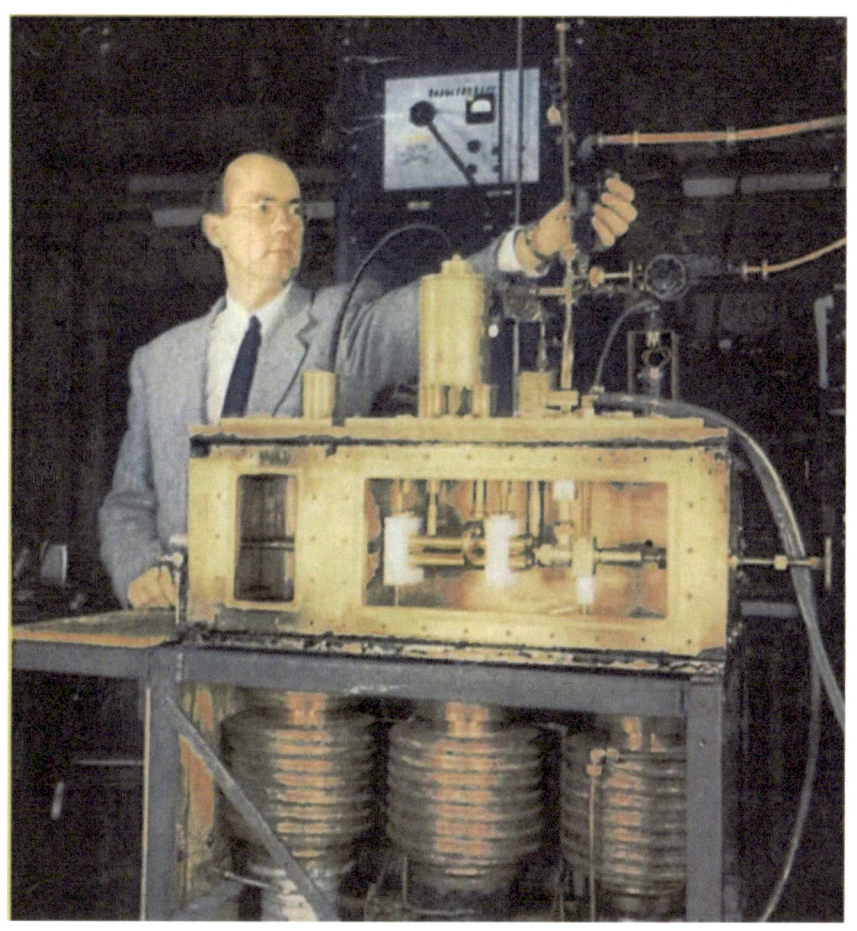

Charles Townes and first MASER

This seminal piece of physics laid the groundwork for the theory of stimulated emission of radiation, which was later used by American physicist, Gordon Gould, to coin the acronym LASER.

The word is an abbreviation of the phrase: light amplification by stimulated emission of radiation. The year was 1957 and the Russians had just launched Sputnik 1 into the skies above a horrified US nation. Senator Lyndon Johnson spoke for the nation when he said, "Soon, they will be dropping bombs on us from space like kids dropping rocks onto cars from freeway overpasses!"

The newspaper headlines of the day reflected his fear when one stated, *Soviet satellite circles globe every 90 minutes.*

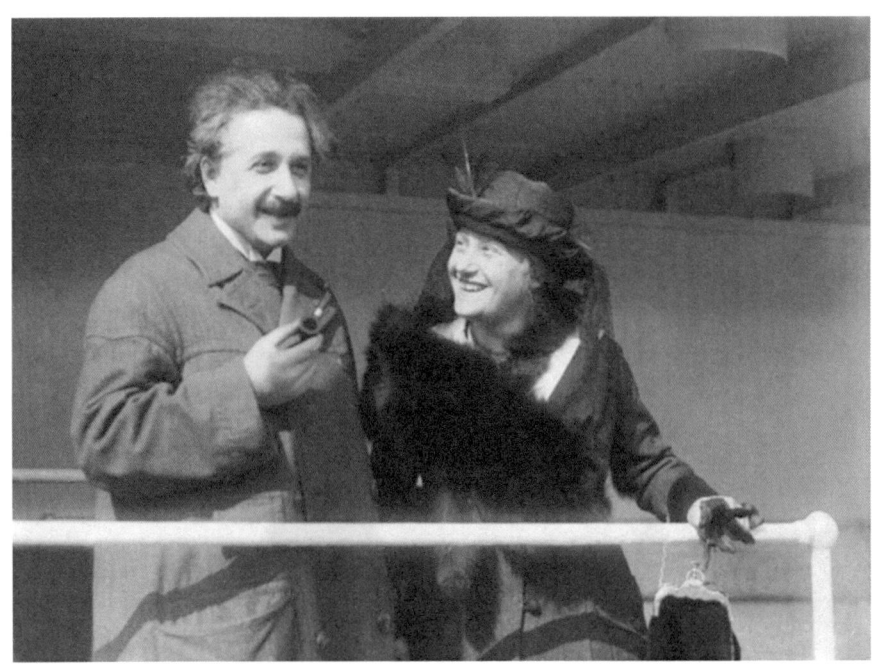

Albert Einstein and his wife, Elsa

In that year, plans were made to start the space race and America ushered in a new age of political, military, technological and scientific developments. The government formed the Pentagon's Defence Advanced Research Projects Agency and huge grants were poured into private and public laboratories across the US to fund the creation of a new spacecraft and the first working laser.

In 1960, their efforts paid off when a physicist called Theodore Maiman, working with the Hughes Electric Corporation in California, created the world's first working Ruby laser. The acronym LASER, although appearing theoretical, is of more than passing interest, because it means that a laser device must be able to make a new form of light. This light must be composed of one wavelength (colour), it must pass in one direction (coherent) and its waves must be parallel. These unique characteristics can be used by doctors to achieve different results. We know the different wavelengths can penetrate various depths of skin and they can also cause dissimilar effects by targeting differing-coloured lesions. This means the laser could act independently on different chromophores deep in the skin. Hence, laser A could be used to target haemoglobin (red) in broken blood

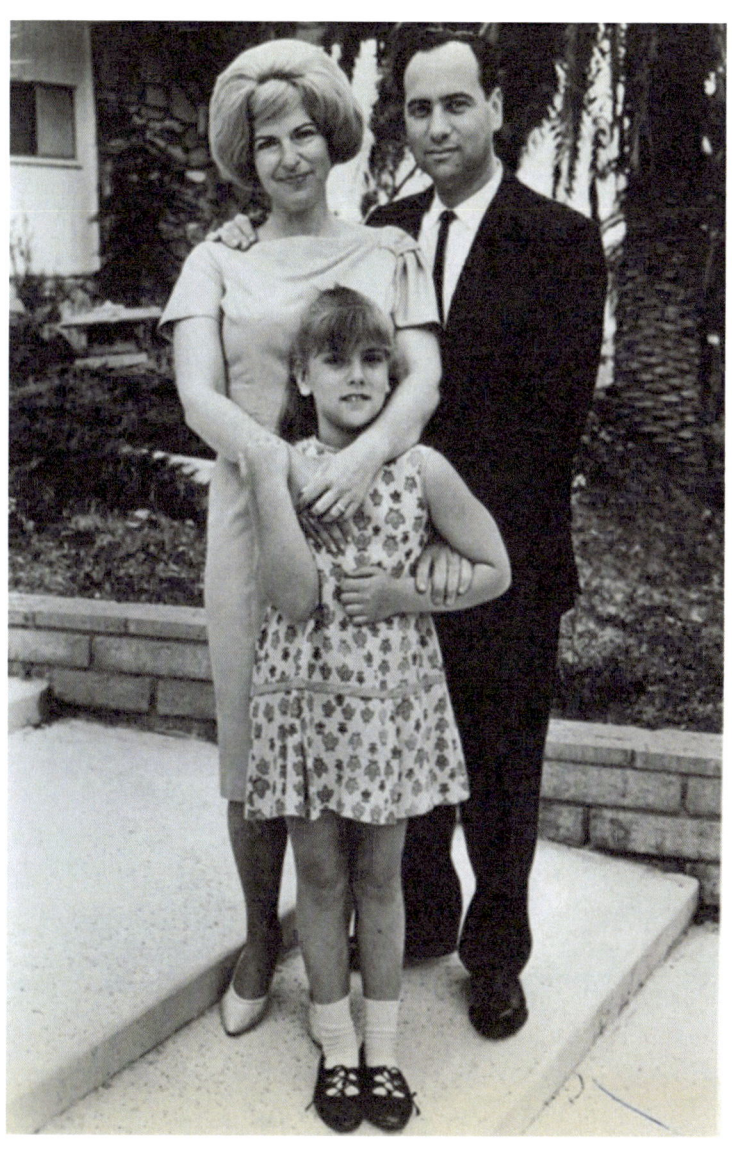

Theodore Maiman and family

vessels (telangiectasia) of rosacea, while laser B may be used to target melanin (brown) in the hair on an upper lip of a female with hirsutism. It also meant that lasers could be used to vapourise water in tissues, thereby causing resurfacing and later collagen stimulation with significant improvementsto wrinkles in the skin.

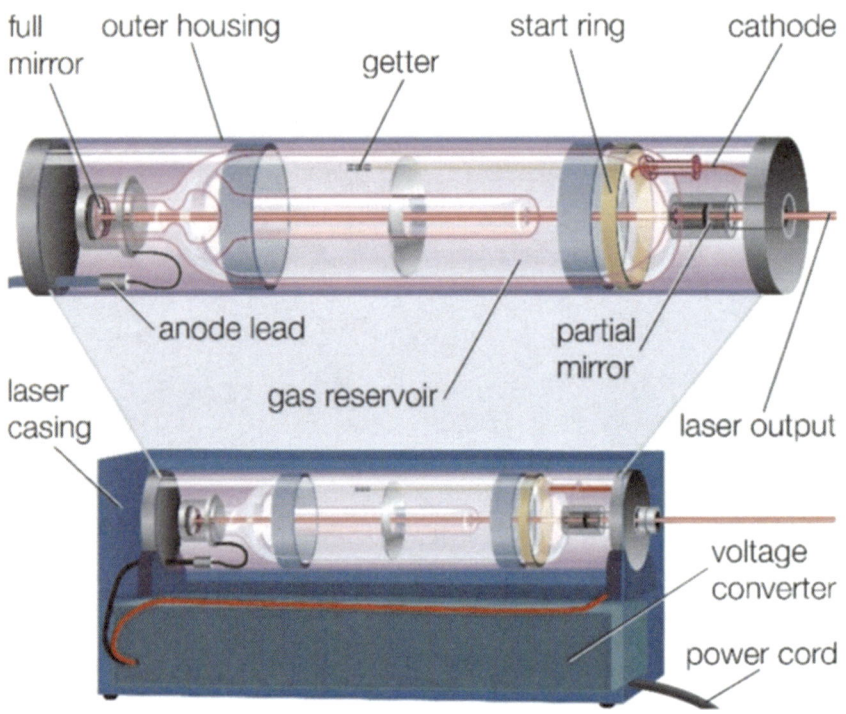

The basic components of a laser

In 1961, research was focused on this new technology continued with the production of a new laser made from crystals of yttrium-aluminium-garnet treated with 1-3% neodymium. The world's first NdYAG laser was developed. This laser emitted energy in the near infrared (IR) spectrum at a wavelength of 1,060 nm. Although many Americans felt safer to have more powerful lasers being developed, doctors tried to harness its power as they found its high- penetration emission to be useful for vapourising tissues and thermally coagulating large blood vessels. The laser is still widely used in cosmetic medicine today. It has even found a new role targeting hair follicles in darker coloured skin. The following year, the first experiments into depilation by laser took place when Dr Leon Goldman used the principle of selective target destruction with ruby lasers to destroy the melanin in hair follicles.

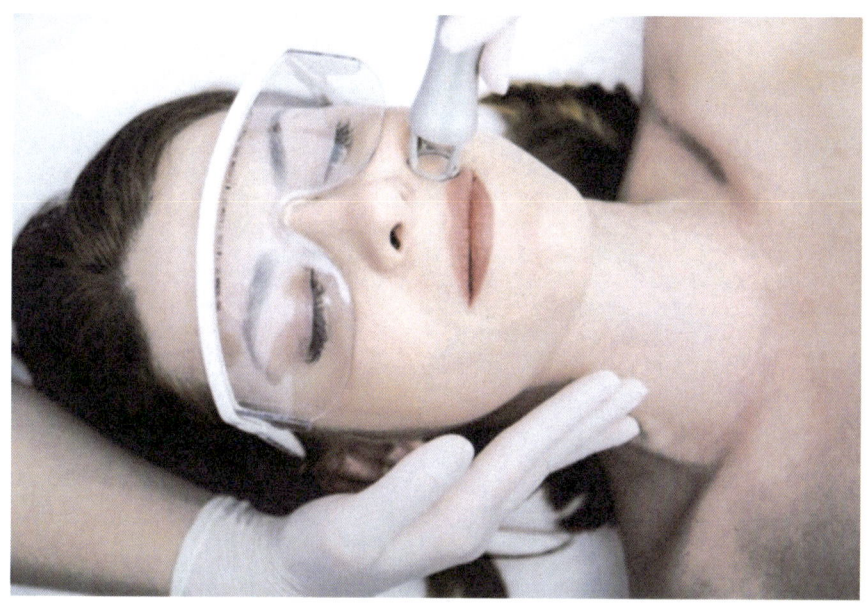

Using an ablative laser for skin rejuvenation

Unfortunately for him, although the idea was good, he did not consider that the laser emitted a continuous wave more adept at shooting down Sputnik and it also targeted melanin in the skin and burnt his patients.

The other patients in the experiment suffered from post inflammatory hyperpigmentation and the experiment was abandoned. In that year, the argon laser was also developed. This laser emitted energy in the blue-green portion of the visible spectrum, making it more readily absorbed by melanin and haemoglobin than by the surrounding tissue. It was 1962 and the American public waited with bated breath as President Kennedy and Soviet Premier Nakita Khrushchev waged a battle of nerves over the Cuban missile crisis.

In 1963, the ruby laser became the first medical laser when Francis L'Esperance from the Columbia-Presbyterian Medical Centre used it to coagulate retinal lesions. In 1965, he began working with Bell researchers Eugene Gordon and Edward Labuda to design a better laser for eye surgery as the blue-green light of the argon laser is more readily absorbed by blood vessels than the red light of the ruby laser. After further refinements and experiments, they developed a laser that is still used to this day to treat patients with diabetic retinopathy.

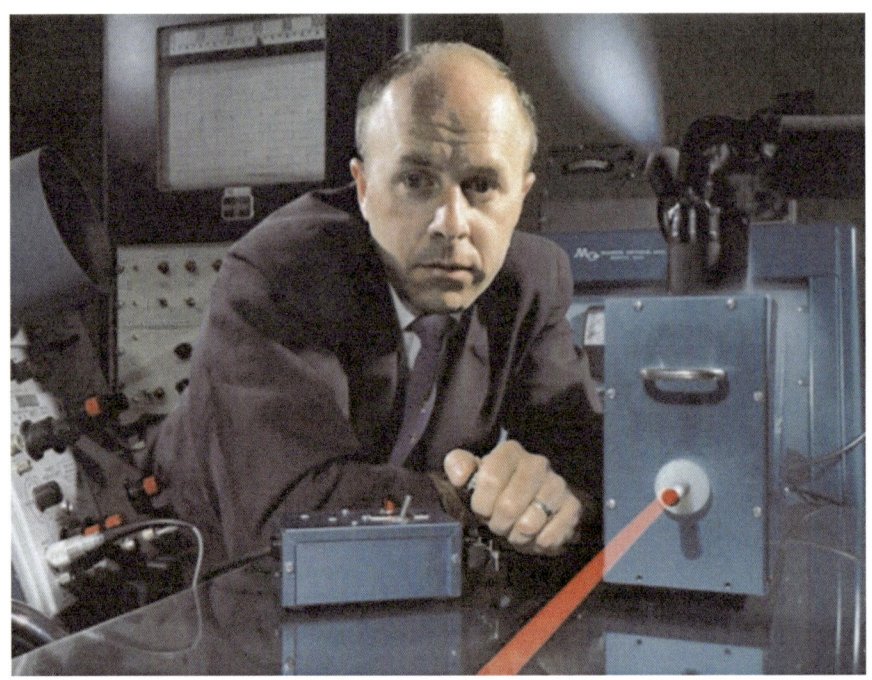

Ruby laser beam

It also has a use in the treatment of port-wine stains. As the cold war developed, the US government funded projects that covered research into more powerful lasers, ones that had the power to cut through steel. In 1964, Patel at Bell Laboratories developed the CO_2 laser.

This laser operated at 10,600 nm and it was like the NdYAG in that it could be used for cutting materials like stainless steel. The advantage was that it could also be focused onto a smaller spot; a function that one day could be useful in space. Thankfully, for cosmetic medicine at this wavelength, energy is also heavily absorbed by water, which everyone knows is the primary constituent of cells in living tissue.

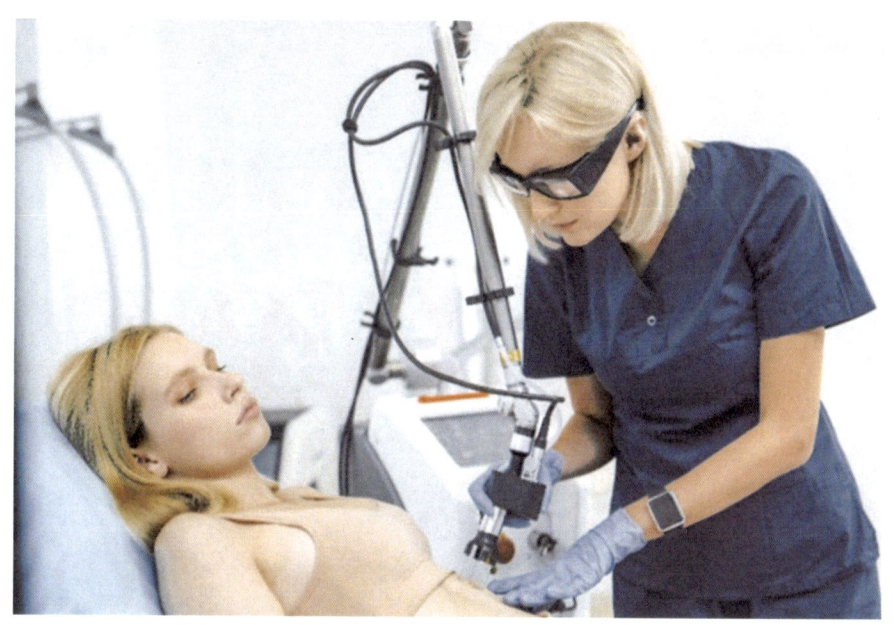

Doctor using CO2 laser

The capacity of the CO2 laser to transfer energy to the water molecules made the energy generated by the new CO2 laser suitable for tissue vapourisation and a whole new era of wrinkle removal by skin resurfacingbegan. The experiments on trying to find the 'Holy Grail' of being able to removehair by laser light followed throughout most ofthe rest of the sixties. In 1967, while Dr Chris Barnard carried out the world's first human heart transplantation at the Groote Schuur hospital in Cape Town, attempts were made by other laser scientists to reduce the potential damage to background skin by directing the light energy to individual follicles using a wire-thin fibre optic apparatus. Many of these devices were sold in the US throughout the late sixties until the FDA banned their use.

In 1968, Union Carbide commissioned a study by Dermascan (manufacturer of the Proteus thermolysis machine) of the effects of applying laser energy applied directly to each hair follicle. The results were largely unsuccessful in that the perceived depilation may have been related to a type of electrolysis effect. Today, the company is more famous for those three nights in 1984, when their chemical plant in Bhopal, India leaked the deadly gas methylisocyanate into the atmosphere, resulting in the eventual deaths of 20,000 people.

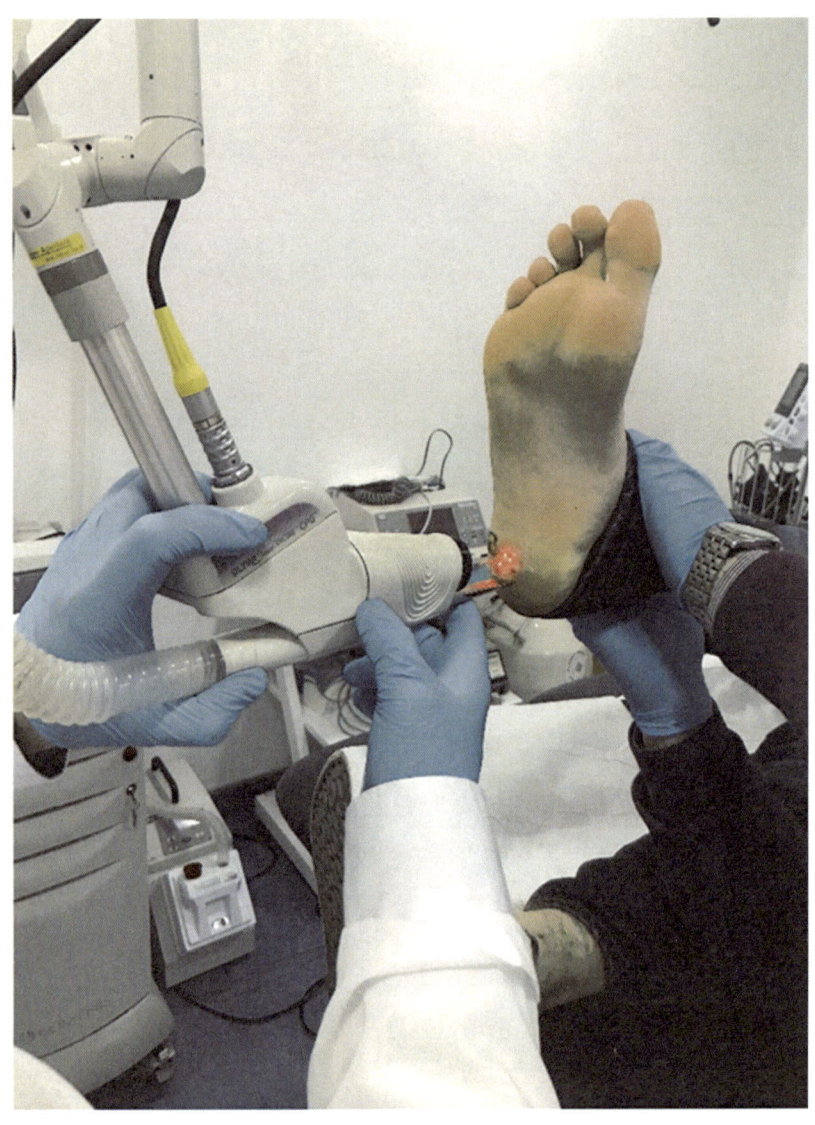

The author using a C02 laser to treat warts

During the 1970s, research into finding a means of hair removal with laser continued with Omnicron Corporation producing a photo epilator that used coherent light to epilate hair. The device never produced marketable results and things remained that way until another attempt was by Lasertron Inc. in the 1980s when they used an argon laser to direct energy at the haemoglobin surrounding individual hairs.

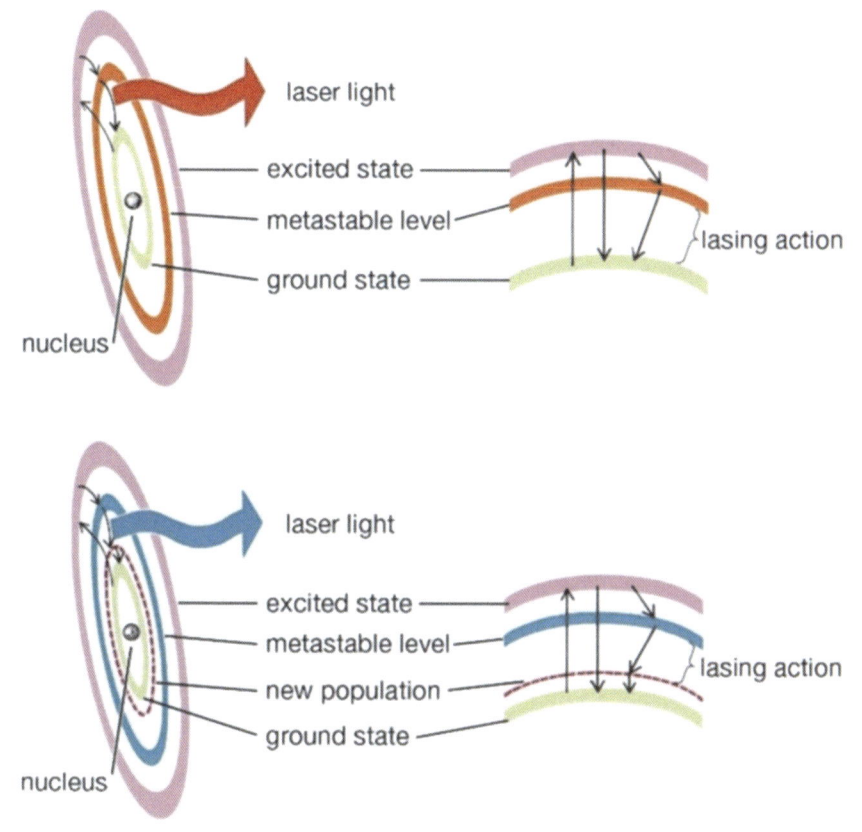

Ruby laser and helium-neon laser

The device was marketed before proper clinical tests were done to establish its efficacy and before long, patients were complaining as it proved to be unsuccessful for permanent hair removal. In 1983, Oshiro and Maruyama noted that hair follicles were damaged after pigmented nevi were treated with a ruby laser. Whenever they increased the laser power to affect the hair follicles, the epidermisbecame severely damaged.

These observations led to Anderson and Parrish developing the theory of 'selective photothermolysis'. This theory was that since a laser of wavelength and pulse duration of light could be used to target a chromophore, selectively destroying it while sparing the surrounding tissue. The space race started by the launch of Sputnik continued and, in that year, Sally Ride, the first American female astronaut returned safely to Earth aboard the Challenger space shuttle.

While tumultuous things were happening on the world stage, including the fall of the Soviet Empire, the freeing of Nelson Mandela and Saddam Hussein's fateful annexation of Kuwait, the development of laser hair technology seemed to have reached an impasse. There were some highlights when ThermoLase Corporation built and tested a low power NdYAG laser for the removal of tattoos and birthmarks.

During the mid-nineties, the quest to find the 'Holy Grail' laser seemed to quicken when a company called ThermoLase used a topical suspension of carbon particles applied to skin followed by treatment of a Q-switched variant of this NdYAG laser called the SoftLight (TM) to treat hair. The laser certainly produced some results and within a short time, it received FDA approval and became the first device for hair removal in the US. ThermoLase went all out to market the product and within a short period, they started using the device in a chain of clinics called Spa Thira. It soon became apparent that this was not the 'Holy Grail' laser as the device seemed to only delay hair regrowth by 3-4 months, but it did not provide permanent hair reduction. This led to several lawsuits against the company and in the period 1998-99, they closed most of their spas. However, all was not lost for ThermoLase because it is apparent that many clients who had unsuccessful hair removal reported improvement in their skin's texture. It appeared that the heat emitted by the laser in association with a lotion that was employed caused a form of skin resurfacing. Before long, Thermage exploited this benefit by obtaining FDA approval for SoftLight (TM) resurfacing, marketing it as a safe, fast, and effective alternative to CO_2 and erbium skin resurfacing.

The Influence of Dr Rox Anderson

Dr Anderson completed his medical residency in dermatology and research fellowship at Harvard, where he eventually became a professor in dermatology. He acquired his science degree from MIT, and his medical degree from the MIT-Harvard medical program.

1980 – Rox Anderson and John Parrish begin to investigate the application of the theory of 'Selective Photothermolysis'.

1981 – Scar-free laser tattoo removal program began in Canniesburn Plastic Surgery and Burns Unit, Glasgow, Scotland with a Q-switched Ruby.

1981 – Treatment of port wine stains begin, Boston, USA, with a pulsed dye laser by Rox Anderson and John Parrish.

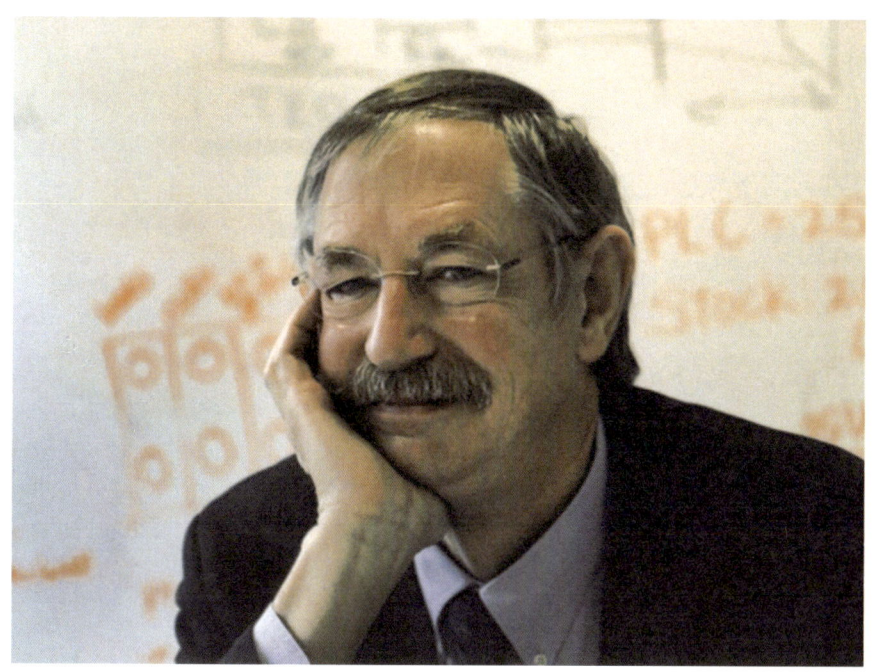

Dr Rox Anderson

1991 - First IPL device designed for vascular treatments was produced in Gothenburg, Sweden called the 'Supralite 2000', later renamed the 'Plasmalite' – launched in 1996 for hair removal 1994 - Dr Rox Anderson and Dr Grossman, first used a water-cooled delivery handpiece during epilation with a long-pulsed ruby laser. The laser was developed by Palomar at Massachusetts General Hospital and the chilled head meant that the laser did not thermally damage the surrounding skin, leaving it less irritating than other methods and relatively pain-free. This EpiLight® ruby laser is still in use in many US clinics today.

1995 – The world's first commercial IPL for the removal of hair, called the 'PhotoDerm' was launched by ESC, Dr Rox Anderson, one of Boston's most prolific researcher-entrepreneurs.

Anderson has made many contributions to aesthetics and to medical practice including laser hair removal, photodynamic therapy (use of light-activated localized drugs for cancer and macular degeneration), laser treatment of port-wine stains in children, as well as various uses of photothermolysis using pulsed dye lasers.

1998 – The Era of the Intense Pulse Light (IPL) Laser

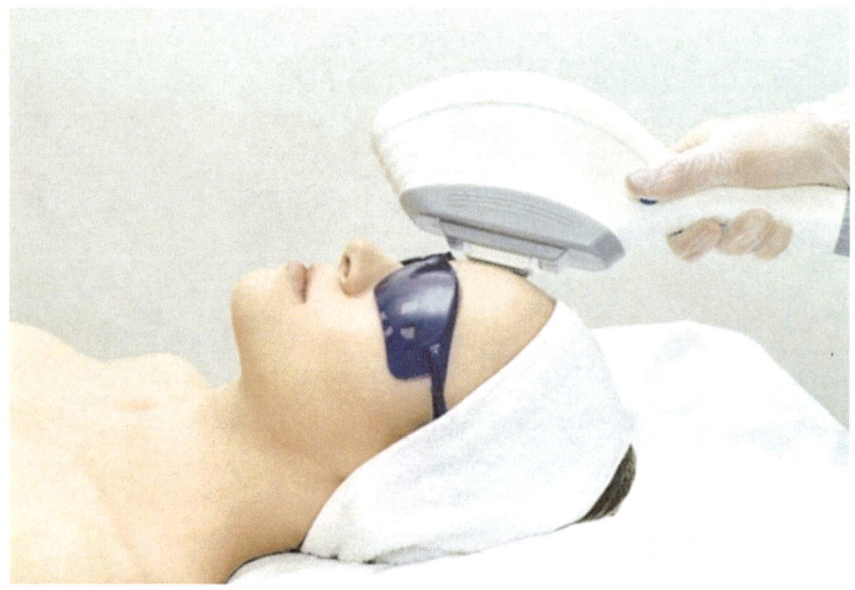

In 1995, in the small town of Los Gatos, dermatologist Patrick Bitter experimented with a new type of laser invented by Israeli, Dr Shimon Eckhouse. Eckhouse postulated that if he used a Xenon flashlight to emit broad-spectrum light made up of multiple wavelengths, he could use a cut-off filter to restrict the bandwidth to a certain range. By applying different filters, he could imitate laser action using the shorter wavelengths to clear pigment spots (lentigines) and broken vessels (telangiectasias) and the longer ones to rejuvenate and smooth the skin. Using a range of wavelengths and some clever software, a company could produce a device that could cure many ailments at once. Then, in the dying moments of the twentieth century, the new concepts of Intense Pulsed Light (IPL) and photorejuvenation were born and the world moved closer to finding the 'Holy Grail' laser. Ironically, these devices were not real lasers as they were flash lamps giving off white light, like that of a lightbulb with wavelengths in the range of 400-765 nm.

The flashgun delivered an intense, visible, broad-spectrum pulse of light, in the visible spectral range of 400 to 1200 nm. The resulting light targeted specific structures and chromophores (e.g., melanin in hair, or oxyhaemoglobin in blood vessels) that are heated to destruction and reabsorbed by the body.

The new IPL device shared some similarities with laser treatments, in that they both use light to heat and destroy their targets. But unlike lasers, which used a single wavelength (colour) of light to match only one chromophore and hence treat one condition, IPL could use interchangeable filters, allowing it to be used against several conditions, including rosacea and pigmentary lesions. The resulting light had a spectral range that targeted specific structures, which were heated to destruction and reabsorbed by the body. In 1998, ESC Sharplan announced the introduction of Vasculight® and the concept of IPL® technology for photo-rejuvenation. In the year 2000, this company became Lumenis, and they introduced the Quantum SR as the pioneer IPL of the new Type I photo-rejuvenation procedure.

By 2001, the new century had begun, and numerous Israeli companies began to produce IPL machines and market the photorejuvenation procedure. Later that year, some of the scientists who had helped form ESC/Lumenis created a new company called Syneron Medical. This was founded in 2000 by Shimon Eckhouse, after he departed from Lumenis, which he had founded in 1991.

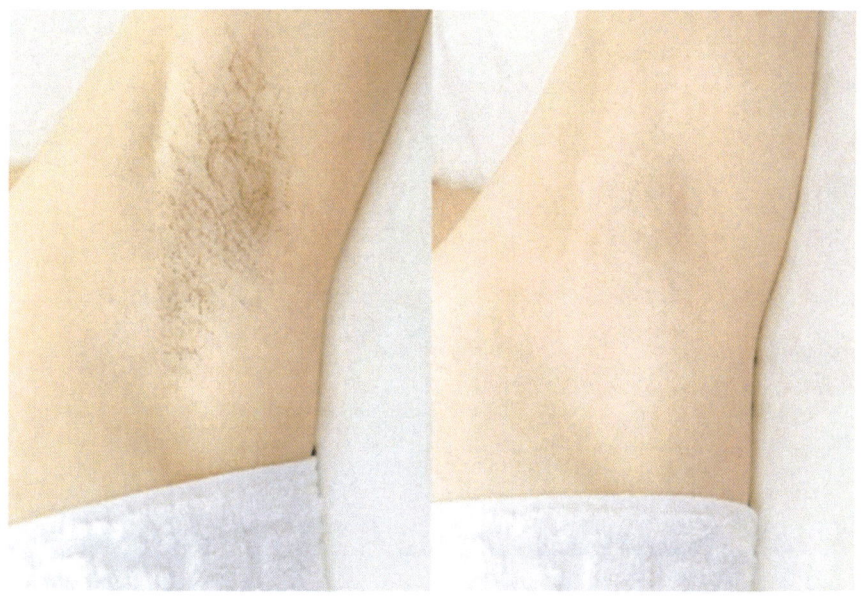

IPL laser underarm hair removal before and after shaving

2004 -The Era of Non-Ablative Radiofrequency (RF)

Non-invasive body contouring now represents the fastest growing area of aesthetic medicine. There are currently a few leading non-invasive techniques for reducing skin laxity and localised subcutaneous adipose tissue: Low Level Laser Therapy (LLLT), Cryolipolysis, radiofrequency (RF), High Intensity Focused Ultrasound (HIFU) and Radiofrequency Microneedling (RFMN). In the period 2002-2004, non-ablative radiofrequency (RF) technology came into the market and this in turn led to the development of many new devices such as the Thermage®, Syneron Polaris®, VelaShape® and Titan®.

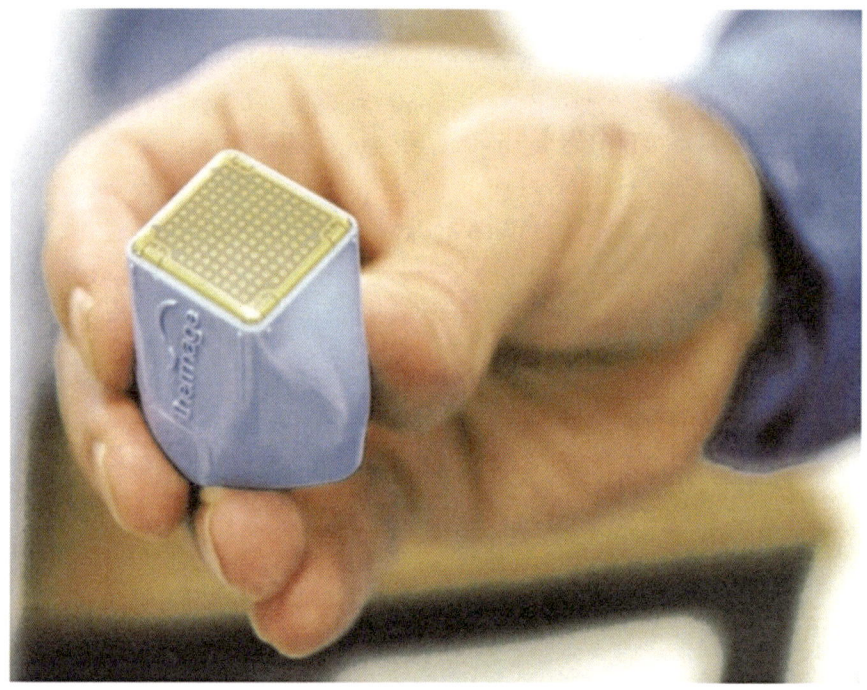

A Thermage® tip circa 2005

In 2002, Syneron announced the introduction of the Aurora RF, a new type of laser that promised to enhance photorejuvenation using the addition of RF (bipolar radiofrequency) to the pulsed light source. They also introduced the Polaris RF, using a combination of radiofrequency and 900nm laser light. Many of these devices fell into disfavour as they were initially quite low- powered and created a high level of non-responders after expensive treatments that often-required multiple painful sessions. The Syneron Polaris RF was quite powerful, but the period of its use was limited due to ongoing court cases between Lumenis and Syneron. Lumenis sued Syneron in 2002 for theft of trade secrets. This action brought both companies into the US district court, with Lumenis bringing a preliminary injunction against Syneron's sale of Aurora devices. The litigation was resolved in 2004, when Lumenis granted Syneron unlimited, non-exclusive worldwide licenses for Lumenis patents relating to the use of incoherent light in aesthetic and medical applications, including all its IPL-related patents.

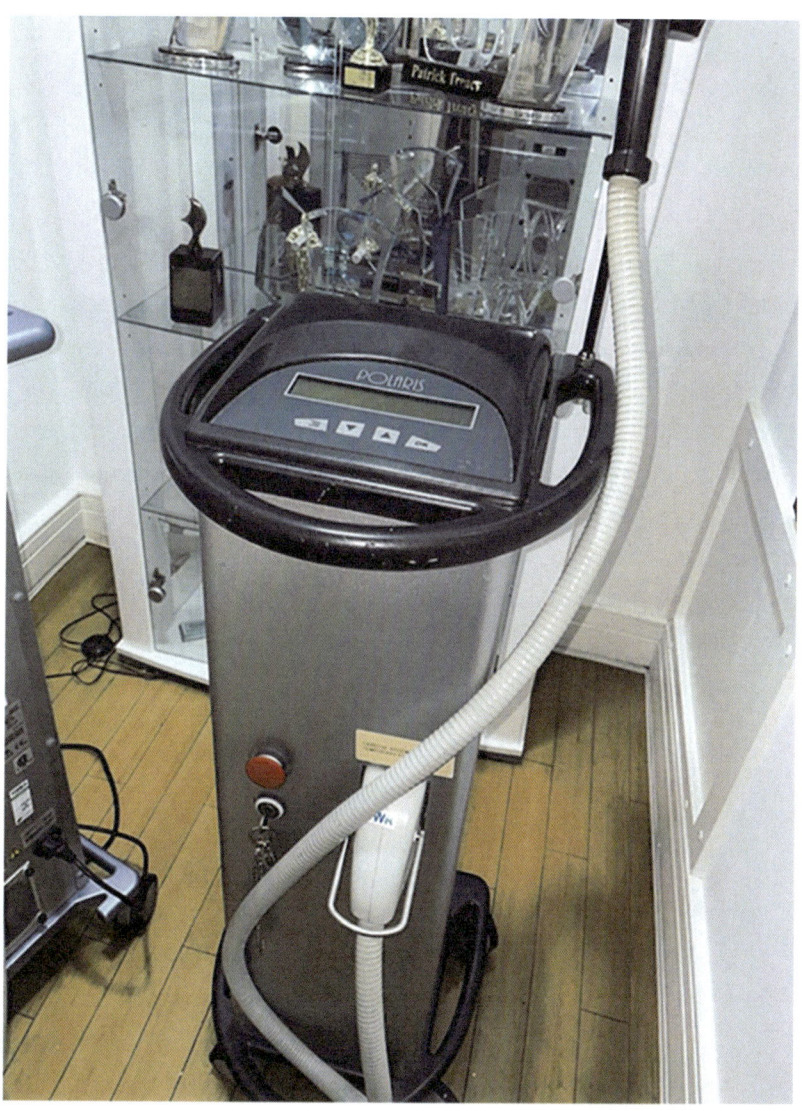

The Syneron Polaris RF

Something had to change, and it happened with the discovery of non-sequential fractionalised technology developed by Reliant Technologies Inc. (new Solta Medical) in 2004. The technology was developed from a US patent licensed from the Wellman Center for photomedicine with Prof R. Rox Anderson as the inventor, based on a concept called fractional photothermolysis. The first device was called a Fraxel, and it took advantage of the skin's regenerative process by treating it in a fractional manner. Different Fraxel systems used either an Erbium fibre laser at 1,550 nm, or a dual wavelength Erbium fibre-pumped Thulium fibre laser with both 1,550 nm and 1,927 nm, respectively, in a single device.

Non-Ablative RF improves with Ultrasound

The BTL Exilis Ultra is a new technology that uses radio frequency (RF) energy and non-focused ultrasound (US) for body and face contouring and skin tightening. It reduces fat and firms' skin in the face and body by tightening the SMAS layer and retaining ligaments. The device delivers twice the energy of the original Exilis device and offers superior results in a shorter amount of time. During an Exilis Ultra treatment, precisely controlled radio frequency energy is used to heat the deeper layers of the skin. This heat causes fat cells to shrink and contracts the skin tissue, stimulating new collagen production in the process. Device uses monopolar RF energy and non-focused ultrasound and works triggering programmed cell death via apoptosis of tissue.

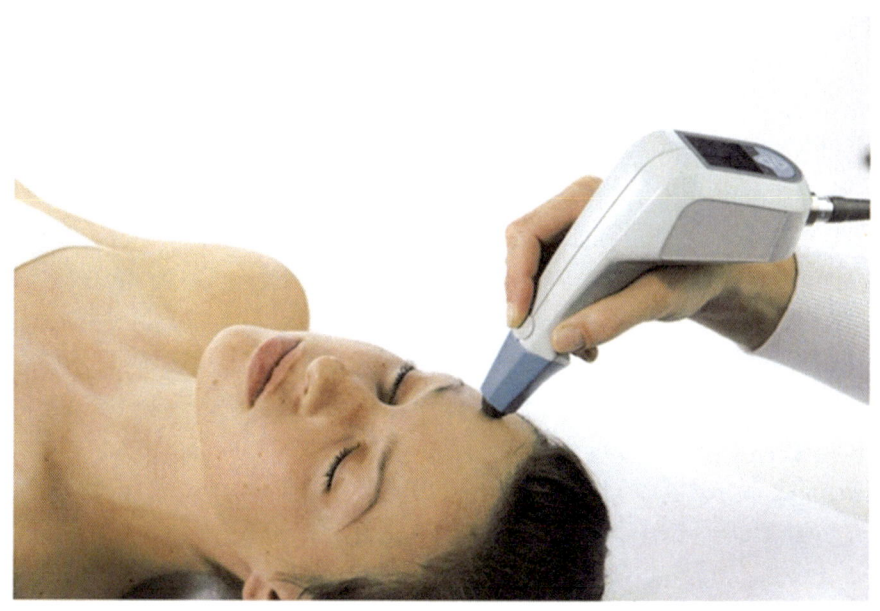

BTL Exilis Ultra

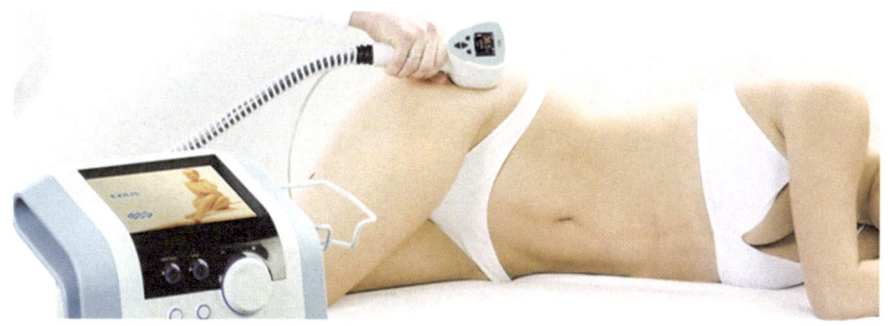

Radiofrequency combined with non-focused ultrasound

2006 – The Era of Fractionalised CO_2 Laser Skin Resurfacing(FLSR)

The CO_2 laser was one of the earliest of the laser systems to appear. It was first developed in 1964 by Patel and colleagues working Bell Labs in the United States. Itwas quickly recognised as an ideal surgical laser because of its high-water absorption, and many indications were pioneered by the late Professor Isaac Kaplan and others. The first system CO_2 laser approved for skin laser resurfacing was approved by the US Food and Drug Administration three decades earlier in 1996, the same year England beat West Germany 4-2 to win the 1966 World Cup at Wembley. Earlier laser systems used a continuous wave that were certainly effective for destroying larger skin lesions, but these lasers could not reliably ablate fine layers of tissue. This was because the prolonged time interacting with tissue produced unacceptably high rates of pigmentation problems and scarring. The short-pulsed Er: YAG laser was introduced as an alternative to the CO_2 laser and emitted light with a wavelength of 2,940 nm, which is infrared light. It quickly found a role for skin resurfacing as it minimised the patient recovery period and limited the side effects while maintaining clinical benefit. It was approved by the US FDA in 1996 for use in cutaneous resurfacing. The 2,940-nm wavelength corresponded to the 3,000-nm absorption peak of water, making it 12 to 18 times more efficiently absorbed by water than CO_2 laser light. Hence, dermatologists had a more precise ablative tool than the CO_2 laser, although its shorter pulse duration resulted in decreased thermal diffusion and less effective haemostatis. This in turn increased intraoperative bleeding, which was favoured by neither doctor nor patient.

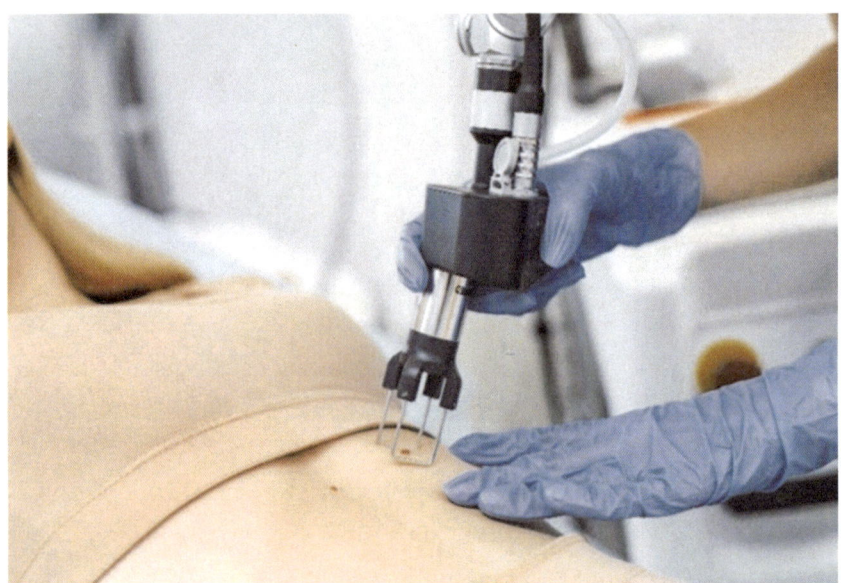

Using a CO_2 laser to remove an abdominal lesion

When I started aesthetic medicine in 1998, my first ablative laser was a Sharplan CO_2 and then I progressed to a Mediblate Er: YAG. Subsequent development of high-energy pulsed lasers made it possible to safely apply high energy densities with shorter exposure times. This meant the exposure time was shorter than the thermal relaxation time of water-containing tissue, thereby lowering the risk of thermal injury due to the capacity for the body to cool the area by blood flow.

Two of the first of these devices were made by Lumenis, one being the UltraPulse 5000, and the other was called the Silk-Touch. The UltraPulse emitted individual CO_2 pulses with variable dwell time and a peak energy, whereas the Silk-Touch was a continuous-wave CO_2 system with a microprocessor scanner. The scanner continuously moved the laser beam so that laser light did not dwell on any one area for more than 1 millisecond. Many dermatologists stated the UltraPulse CO_2 laser was the most effective modality for repairing years of skin exposure to harmful ultraviolet light and photodamaged skin. Photoaging (also known as dermatoheliosis) is a term used by dermatologists for the characteristic changes to skin induced by chronic UVA and UVB exposure. This photoaging effect is demonstrated clinically as a gradual deterioration of cutaneous structure and function. In 2004, non-sequential fractionalised technology was relatively new, its benefits of faster recovery time, more precise control of ablation depth and reduced risk of post-procedural problems were already becoming clear.

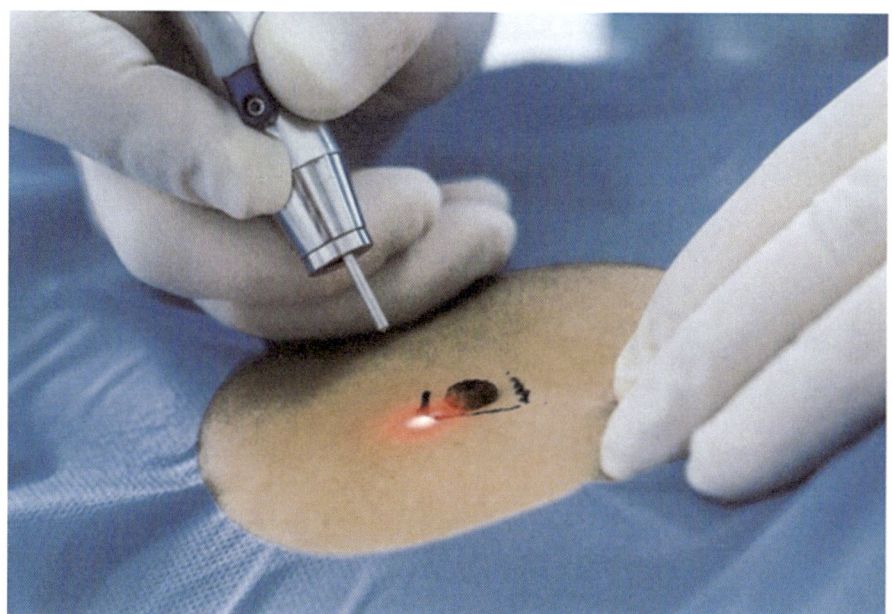

Using a CO_2 laser to remove a nevus

Damage to the outer layer of skin (epithelium) was less apparent because unlike conventional removal of skin (ablation), some of the horny outer layer (stratum corneum) remained intact during treatment and acted as a natural bandage. It immediately begged the question: could this fractional technology be married with conventional CO_2 ablative lasers? This would allow the skin to heal much faster than if the whole area were treated, as the 'healthy' untreated tissue surrounding the treated zones helps fill in the damaged area with new cells. Downtime would also be reduced, and if the erythema remained moderate, it would permit patients to apply cosmetics in a short time of five days after treatment.

In 2005, fractionated ablative CO_2 lasers arrived, and they were an immediate success as they created heated areas (microthermal zones), leaving uninjured columns of healthy tissue that certainly aided in healing. This process resulted in faster healing times and fewer adverse effects than traditional fully ablative CO_2 laser therapy. The first one I purchased was an Lumenis ActiveFx, which was an upgrade of the UltraPulse Encore with smaller spot size and a new CPG (computer pattern generator) giving a random pattern and reducing the possibility of having several adjacent spots with resultant heat accumulation. The device left intact tissue bridges between spots, which not only resulted in faster healing time but also created less thermal damage to the basal cell membrane and the melanocytes that resided there. Melanocytes contain melanin, the dark pigment primarily responsible for skin colour.

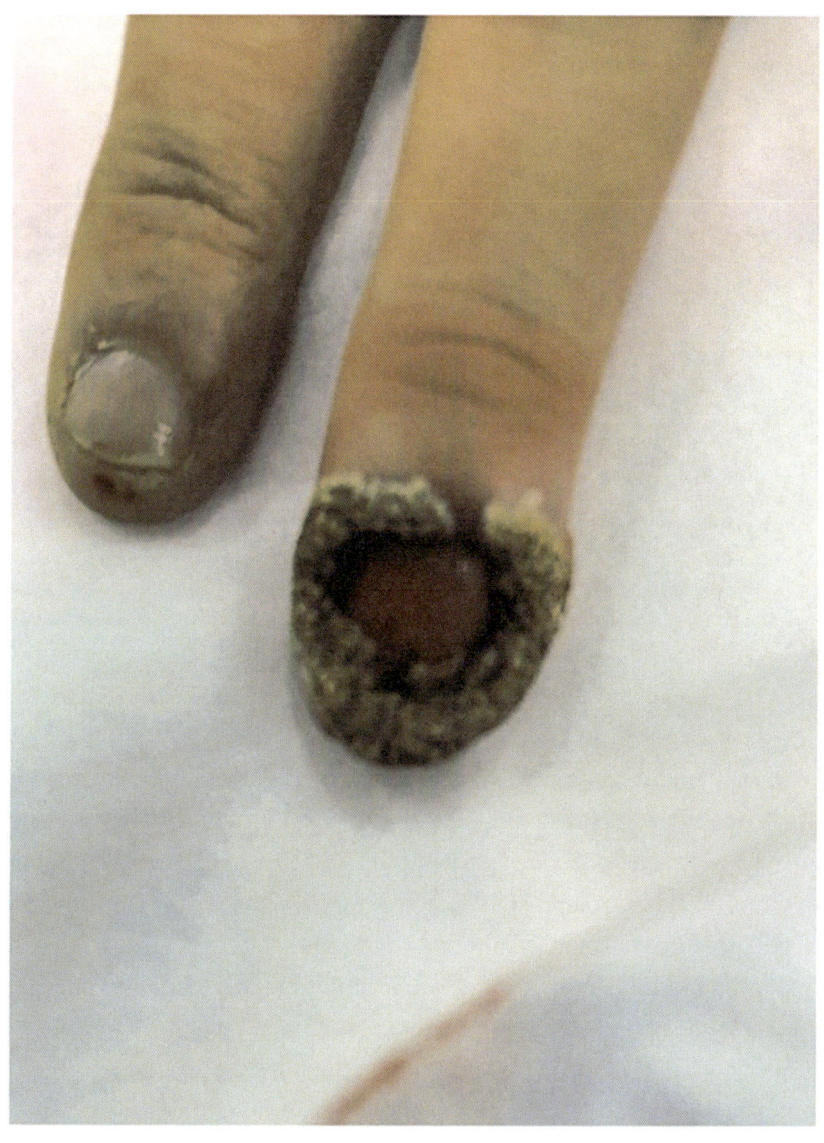

CO_2 laser treating subungal warts

Once synthesised, melanin is contained in special organelles called melanosomes that can be transported to nearby keratinocytes to induce pigmentation, which serves as protection against UV radiation.

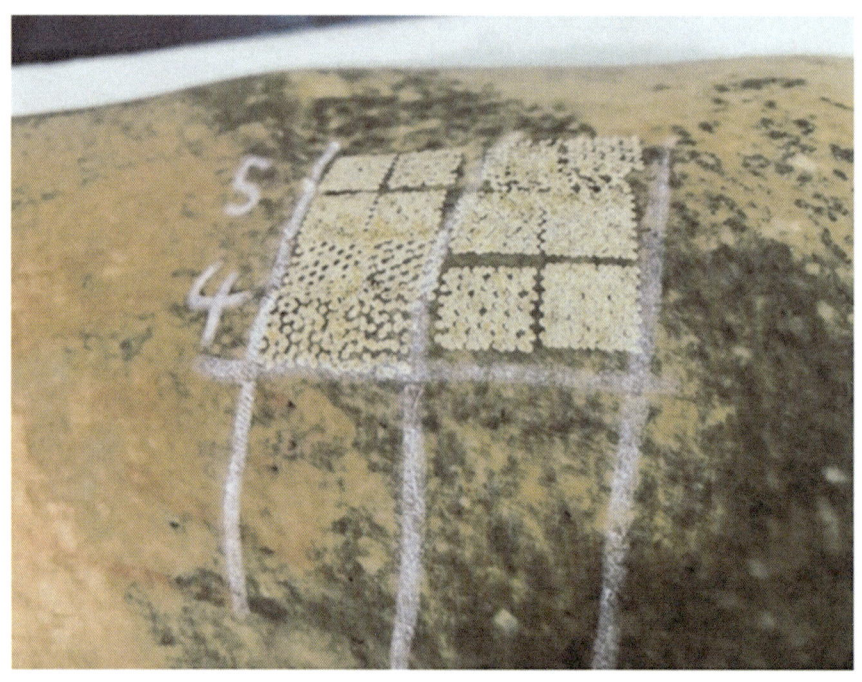

Experimenting with different densities and wattages

Laser damage to these cells could cause hypopigmentation, which could in some instances be permanent, but the skin bridges meant that there were enough melanocytes left to ensure that the possibility of this happening was minimal. The device also has a smaller spot size, resulting in less post-procedure redness (erythema) due to reduced heat build-up in these tissues. Lastly, the CPG (computer pattern generator) lays down a random series of spots rather than a sequential sequence, resulting in greater thermal relaxation time and less overheating of the treated tissue. The application of random rather than sequential beams is termed 'Cool Scan' and this feature was used with every patient in the study. I soon discovered that the new fractionalised CO_2 lasers were extremely versatile, in that they could be used for the treatment of facial rhytides, acne scars, surgical scars, melasma and photodamaged skin. Many high- energy, fractionalised carbon dioxide (CO_2) lasers became available for skin resurfacing. Although each laser system adhered to the same basic principles, there are significant differences between lasers with respect to tissue dwell time, energy output and laser beam profile. These differences resulted in variable clinical and histological tissue effects.

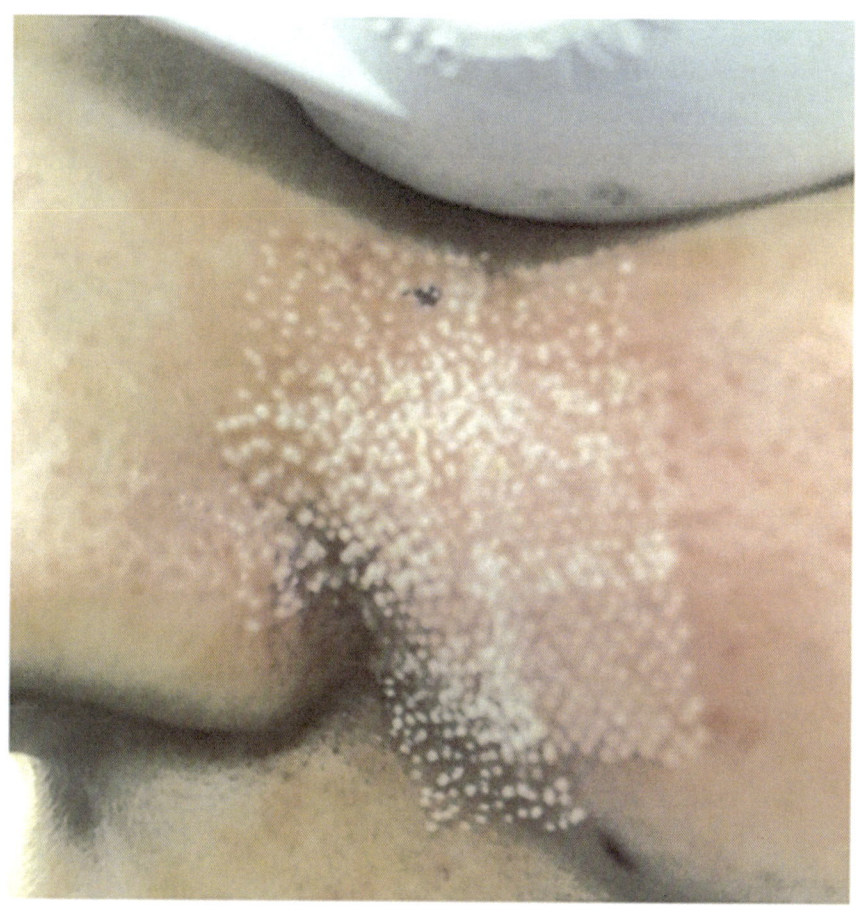

CO$_2$ treating localised acne scarring

As our clinics expanded, I also bought a 30-watt fractionated CO$_2$ laser (SmartXide, DEKA Medical Inc., San Francisco, California). This laser enabled the user to adjust power, pattern density and dwell times due to DOT (Dermal Optical Thermolysis) technology. The physician could deliver a moderate treatment requiring a few days of downtime, or a fully ablative traditional laser resurfacing treatment.

CO$_2$ casefiles from the author: Periorbital rejuvenation

My first case FLRS (2006) was a 39-year-old Irish female, who had spent some years living in the Middle East and presented with marked crow's feet (periorbital rhytids) and her brows had dropped a little (mild bilateral lateral brow ptosis). Her problems were due to a mix of chronological ageing and photoaging. After some consideration of the different non-surgical options, including HIFU and RF, it was decided that the new CO2 fractionalised laser resurfacing would give the most beneficial and long-term rejuvenation effect. I decided to give her some Botulinum toxin prior to the procedure to reduce the wrinkles, a bit like straightening out a shirt before ironing it. It also preserved the effect of the treatment for the next four and a half months.

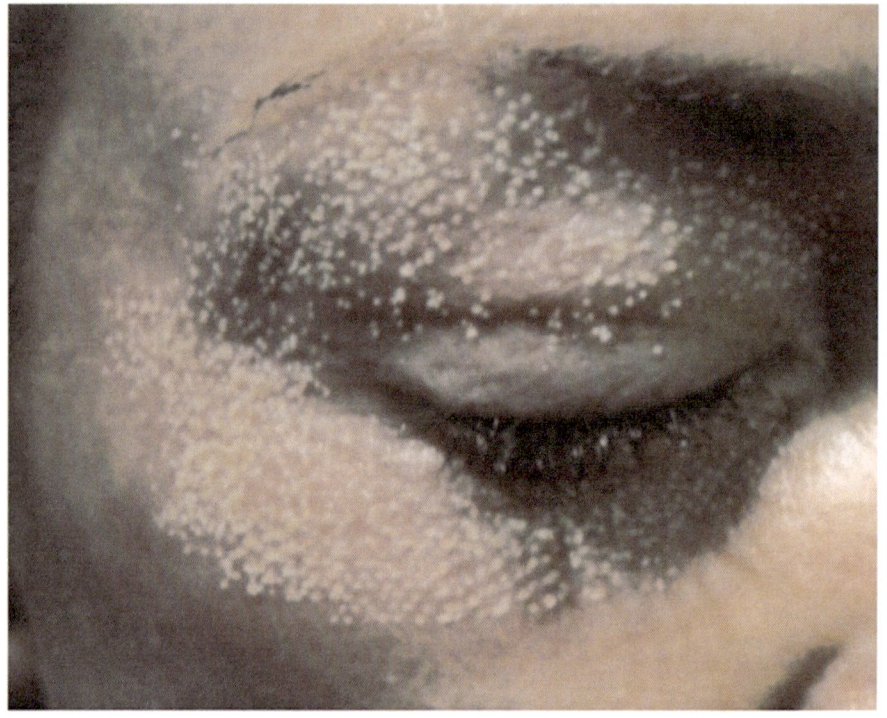

(R) eye ActiveFx (Day 1)

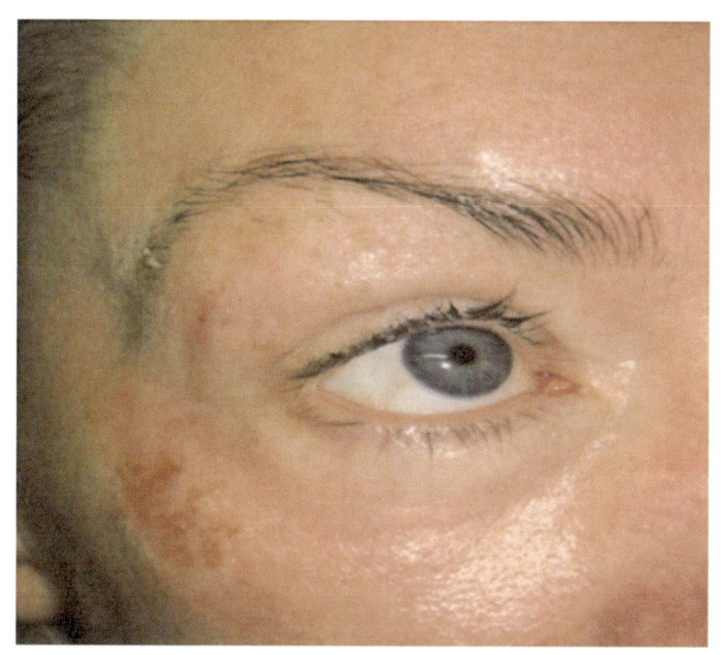

(R) eye ActiveFx (Day 3)

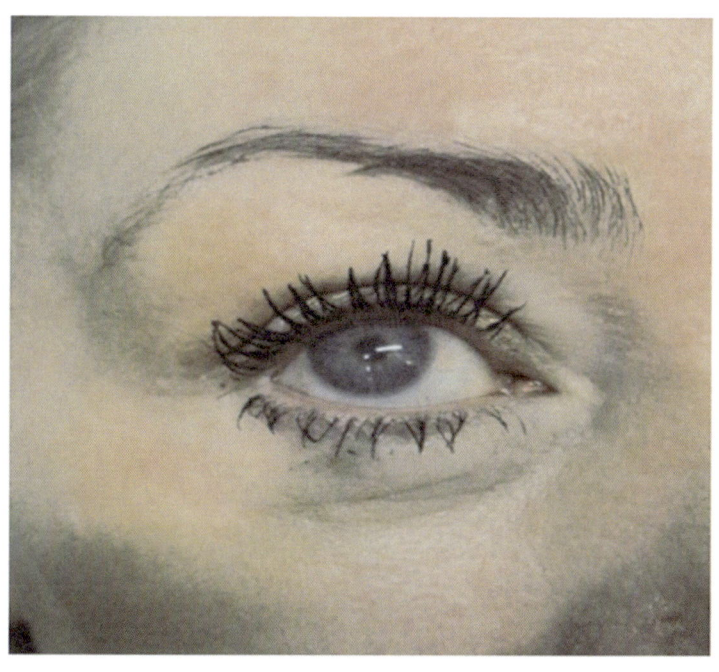

(R) eye ActiveFx (Day 30)

Histology

Histology slides of biopsy sections taken before treatment and three months after treatment. Micrographic analysis showed a 30% increase in new collagen on the CO_2 treated side.

Slides were evaluated by skin histopathologists Professor Kieran Sheahan, FRCPI, FCAP, FRCPath and Dr Tom Crotty, FRCPI, FCAP, FRCPath – consultant histopathologists, St Vincent's University Hospital, Dublin.

Image (S479/08) immediate post-procedure: ActiveFx treated (Energy) 100 mJ 9.4J/cm2 (Rate) 125 Hz 18.8W CPG 3/6/3. Laser penetration depth: 85 mm.

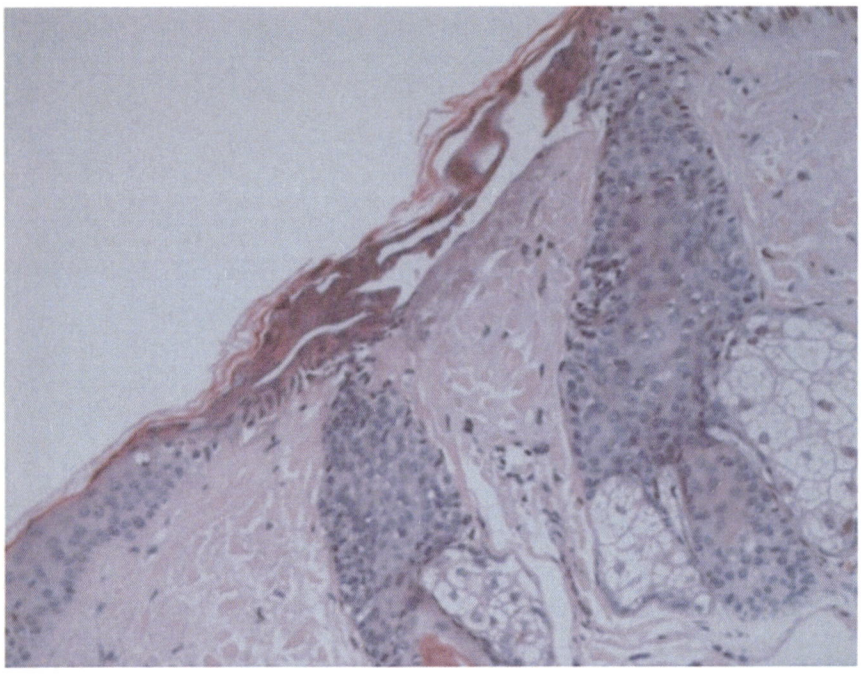

Laser penetration depth reported at 85 mm and some new collagen formation seen at this level.

Congenital Melanocytic Nevus (CGN)

In 2008, a 40-year-old male presented with a large congenital nevus covering most of his lower body. The nevus measured 35 cm x 20 cm with well-demarcated borders. Dermoscopic examination showed coarse pigment in the darker centre of the nevus and deeper pigmentation around its periphery. The patient said that over time, it had become darker with an increase in hair growth, and it had acquired a more irregular surface.

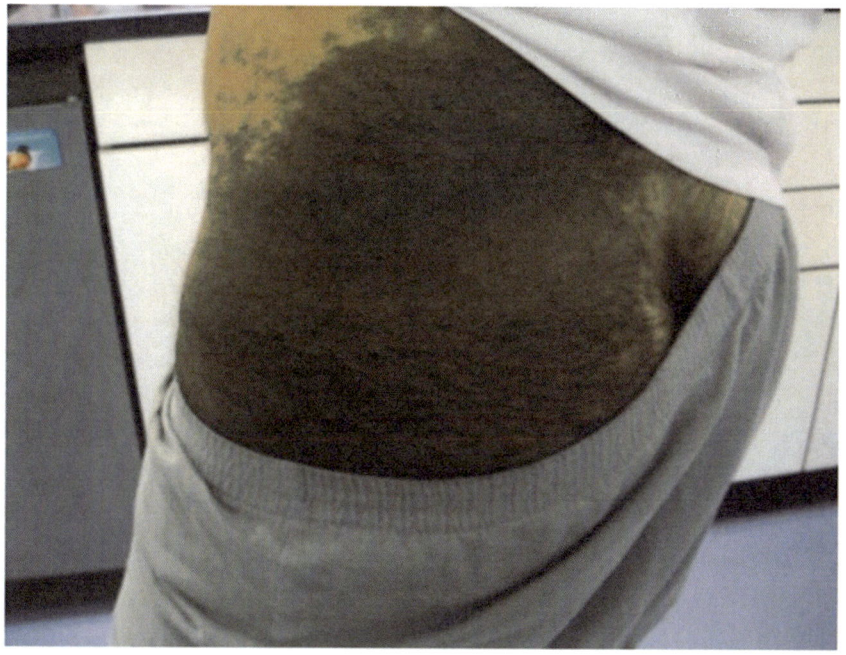

Congenital melanocytic nevus (CGN) before treatment

Congenital melanocytic nevus (CGMN) is primarily a clinical diagnosis. It is usually defined as a melanocytic lesion present at birth that will reach a diameter ≥20 cm in adulthood. Its incidence is estimated in <1:20,000 newborn. Despite its rarity, this lesion is important because it may associate with severe complications such as malignant melanoma, affect the central nervous system, and have major psychosocial impact on the patient and his family due to its unsightly appearance. It had a major psychological effect on the patient, and he felt it had prevented him finding a mate. The patient was aware of the possibility of developing melanoma within the lesion. Although the value of the incidence rate of malignancies in GCMN may still be a matter of dispute, it is estimated that for these individuals, the lifetime risk for developing melanoma is between 5% and 10%.

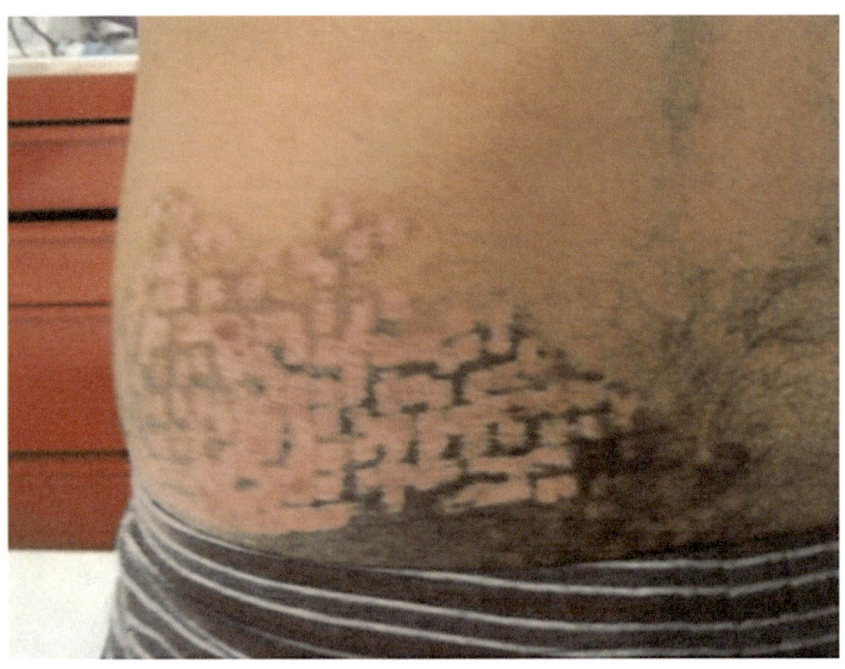

Congenital melanocytic nevus (CGN) before treatment

Congenital nevi are histologically distinguishable from acquired nevi mainly by their larger size and the fact that the nevus cells spread to the deep layers of the skin. They are also recognised as a risk factor of malignant melanoma. The issue of deciding which is the best therapeutic approach in these cases is difficult for a doctor, mainly due to the controversies surrounding the treatment of these lesions. The use of CO_2 laser in the treatment of GCMN remains controversial as there is some concern that nevus cells exposed to doses of energy may have a higher probability of malignant transformation. There is also a suspicion whether laser surgery that partially removes congenital pigmented lesions could impair or facilitate the detection of abnormalities suggestive of melanoma on the nevus. There is also the counterargument that reducing the overall number of melanocytic cells can only reduce the risk of these turning malignant. However, these effects must be balanced against the psychological impact that the lesion has on the patient as there is no doubt that CO_2 laser can dramatically improve the gross aesthetic appearance of these lesions.

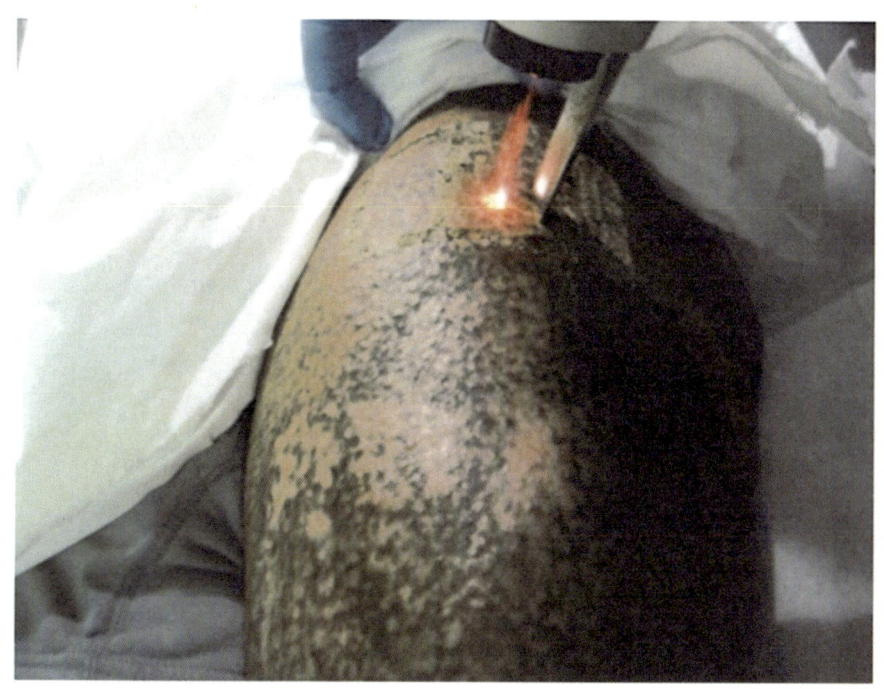

The only absolute indication for surgery in giant congenital melanocytic nevus is the development of a malignant neoplasm on the lesion. When melanoma arises in GCMN, the prognosis is poor. One of the reasons is the fact that cutaneous melanoma associated with GCMN typically grows in the dermis and this makes it more difficult to detect in clinical exams. More than half of the patients will die within three years and the median age at death is 4.5 years after detection. Prophylactic surgical excision is justified based on the assumption that melanoma may arise on the naevic lesion.

However, 50% of melanomas found in patients with GCMN occur elsewhere and the removal of the naevus does not guarantee protection against malignancy. It is assumed the reduction of melanocytic cells reduces the incidence of malignancy. The malignancy is due to expression of some genes. Eliminating the melanocytes may not eliminate the gene that causes the malignancy, just expression of melanin. However, the partial removal of GCMN by procedures such as fractionalised CO_2 laser treatment has only cosmetic purposes, since only the most superficial cells of the lesion are removed. In the end, I respected the patient's wishes and removed the bulk of the lesion.

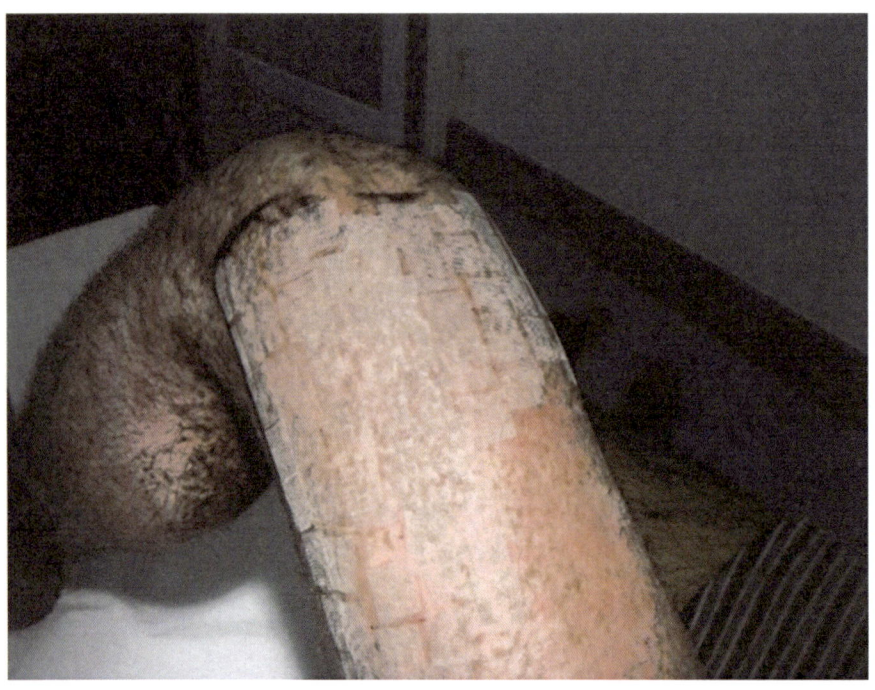

Congenital melanocytic nevus (CGN) after treatment

A variety of differing aesthetic treatments are available for non-surgical periorbital rejuvenation, but one procedure or technique alone is usually insufficient. Techniques include Botulinum injections, chemical peels, dermal fillers, plasma rich platelets, micro-needling, micro-focused high-intensity ultrasound, and radiofrequency as well as non-ablative and ablative lasers. Each of these devices have their own relative benefits as well as their own risks. Periorbital rejuvenation techniques continue to improve as new technologies become available and targeting the injury deep in the underlying tissue means no visible signs of trauma on the outside and plumper, smoother skin.

CO_2 laser skin resurfacing has long been considered by many practitioners as the 'gold standard' for the treatment of rhytids and photodamaged facial skin, although it has a longer downtime and higher risks. Its popularity was prompted by a realisation of both doctors and patients that many of the much-hyped non-ablative methods were not comparable with ablative skin resurfacing and were often subject to extravagant claims in terms of efficacy.

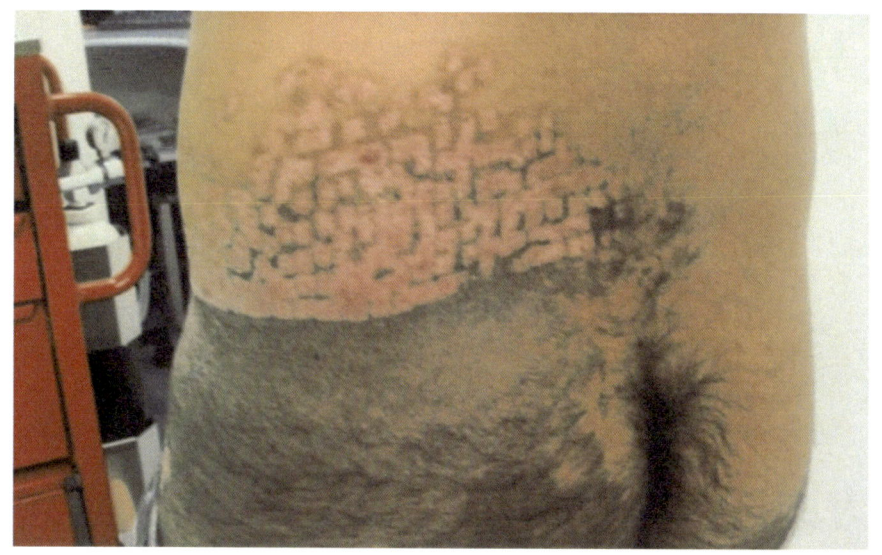

Congenital melanocytic nevus (CGN) after treatment

Photoaging is demonstrated clinically as a gradual deterioration of cutaneous structure and function. It manifests itself in the epidermis and upper papillary dermis by giving skin a roughened surface texture as well as laxity, telangiectasias, wrinkles and variable degrees of skin pigmentation.

The face, and more especially the eyes, is the area for which most patients seek cosmetic rejuvenation. The periorbital area consisting of the eyelids and surrounding areas, including the eyebrows, bony eye socket and rims, cheeks and forehead is also the first area to show signs of ageing. Periorbital ageing involves changes that are multidimensional and multifactorial.

Fractionalised CO_2 lasers are extremely versatile, in that they can be used for the treatment of facial rhytids, acne scars, surgical scars, melasma and photodamaged skin. Although non-sequential fractionalised technology is no longer considered novel, its benefits of faster recovery time, more precise control of ablation depth and reduced risk of post-procedural problems are already well established. There are presently several high-energy, fractionalised CO_2 lasers currently available for cutaneous resurfacing. Although each laser system adheres to the same basic principles, there are significant differences between lasers with respect to tissue dwell time, energy output and laser beam profile.

2018 -The Era of Fractionalised Radiofrequency Microneedling (FRMN)

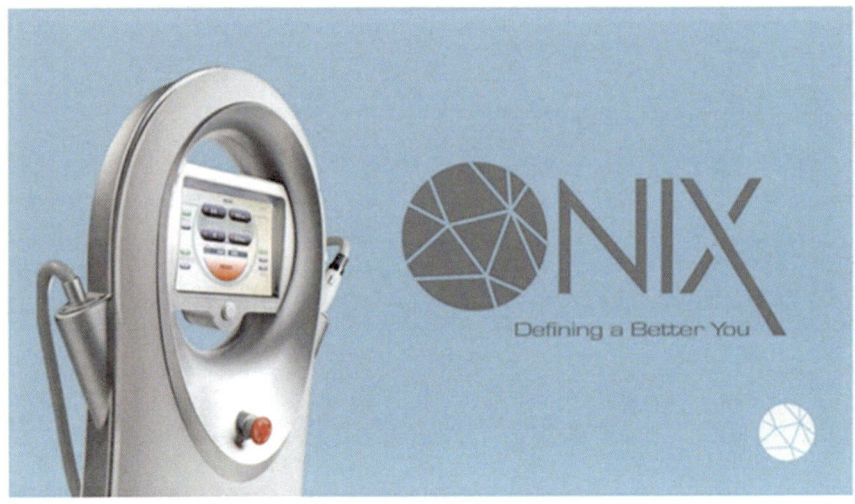

Fractional microneedle radiofrequency (FMR) devices deliver energy to the deep dermis through insulated microneedles without destroying the epidermis. Our clinic uses this minimally invasive radiofrequency options for skin tightening, acne scarring and sometimes even hyperhidrosis focusing on safety and efficacy by use of microneedle fractional RF device (Onix™, SHE Co., Korea). Our clinical experience has shown that the combination of bipolar RF and RF microneedling can achieve substantial skin tightening and collagen remodelling in patients who are not candidates or prefer to not undergo surgery. The multi-frequency fractional RF microneedling device (Onix™, SHE Co., Korea), has a disposable single-use treatment cartridge tip consisting of thirty-six golden 0.3mm non insulated 30G microneedles. These electrode pairs are contained within the area of 10 mm^2, with the exposed electrodes extending from to 6 mm below the skin surface. These bipolar electrode pins form a closed circuit through the irradiated skin, delivering between 0.5MHz- 2 MHz of conducted RF current to the skin. An adjustable RF power up to a maximum of 220 W can be delivered, in relation to the intensity (1–5) and a dwell time up to amaximum of 7 secs can be obtained. Since radiofrequency (RF) flows along the least resistance path, bipolar RF will be usually superficial and will heat the upper part of the dermis.

INSULATED NEEDLES & TECOOLING PLATE

✓ 36 Gold plated needles
✓ Needle diameter: 0.3mm (30 Gauge)
✓ Insulted Needle: 0.3 mm exposed tip
✓ Needle length: 0.5mm to 6.0mm
✓ Thermal Electric Cooling System with Peltier element

Insulated

Exposed   0.3mm

Skin Laxity and Neck Tightening

Radiofrequency microneedling (FMR) allows for subdermal adipose remodelling and skin tightening. It achieves this by thermal heating of the reticular dermis to 50 °C to 52 °C, which triggers a healing cascade stimulating the formation of new collagen and elastin fibres. The bipolar RF also tightens the skin by contraction of the underlaying reticular ligaments and fibroseptal network. This leads to induction of neocollagenesis, elastogenesis, and angiogenesis. The Onix™ device handpiece uses non-insulated gold-plated microneedles for deep dermal remodelling. Ultrasound gel is applied to all treatment areas. The handpiece is then gently applied to the treatment area to create constant, uniform coupling and circular movements were enacted to match the area of the retaining ligaments.

Three treatment areas were identified for patients:

(1) The cheek, platysma auricular fascia, nasolabial fold and masseteric cutaneous ligament
(2) The lower eyelid, zygomatic cutaneous ligament, and the area of the orbicularis retaining ligament,
(3) The jowl, neck, and submental area, and the buccomaxillary ligaments

Casefiles from the author: Facial skin laxity

Method

The treatment areas were cleansed with alcohol prior to the treatment. The treatment parameters were set as follows: treatment target temperature of 43.0°C and energy of RF 3-4. Each treatment area was heated to a temperature of 43.0°C, and maintained at that temperature for at least seven seconds.

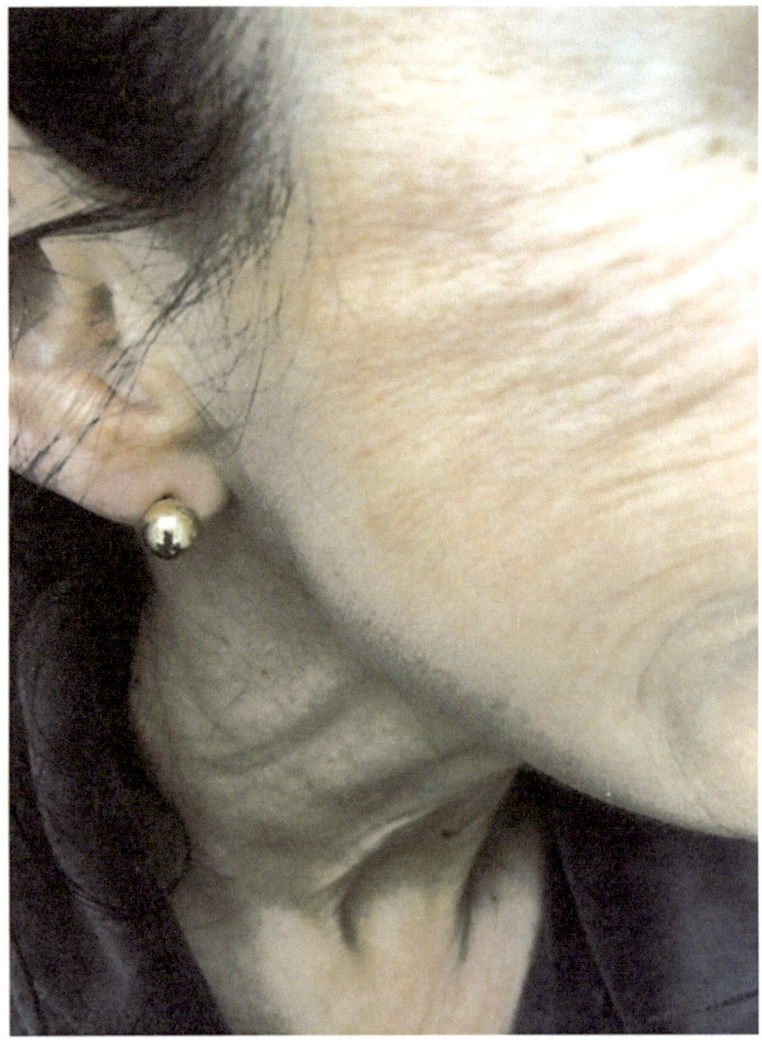

Skin Laxity Patient Face Before Needle Depth 1.5-2.5mm RF Level 3-4

The patients underwent a series of 4–6 weekly treatments with these settings. Any side effects of treatments were noted. Clinical photographs of the face and neck was taken using a digital camera before treatment and at approximately 2 weeks after the final treatment. All treatments were performed under the direction of a single research technician.

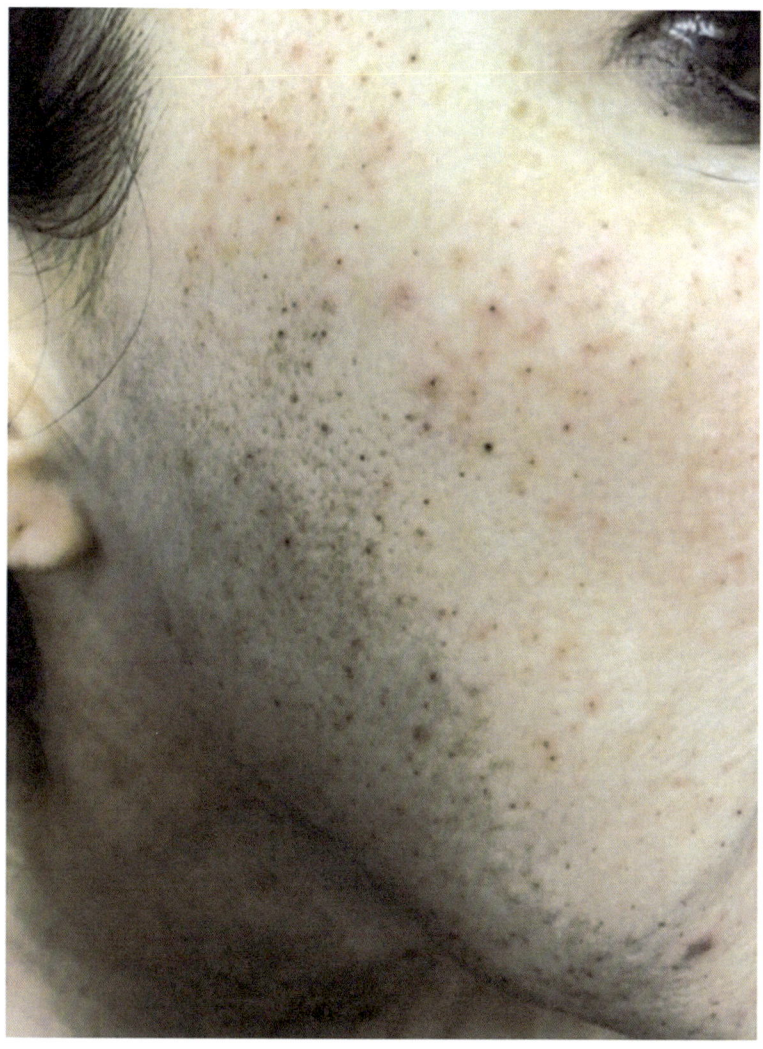

Skin Laxity Patient Face after treatment. Needle Depth 1.5-2.5mm RF Level 3-4

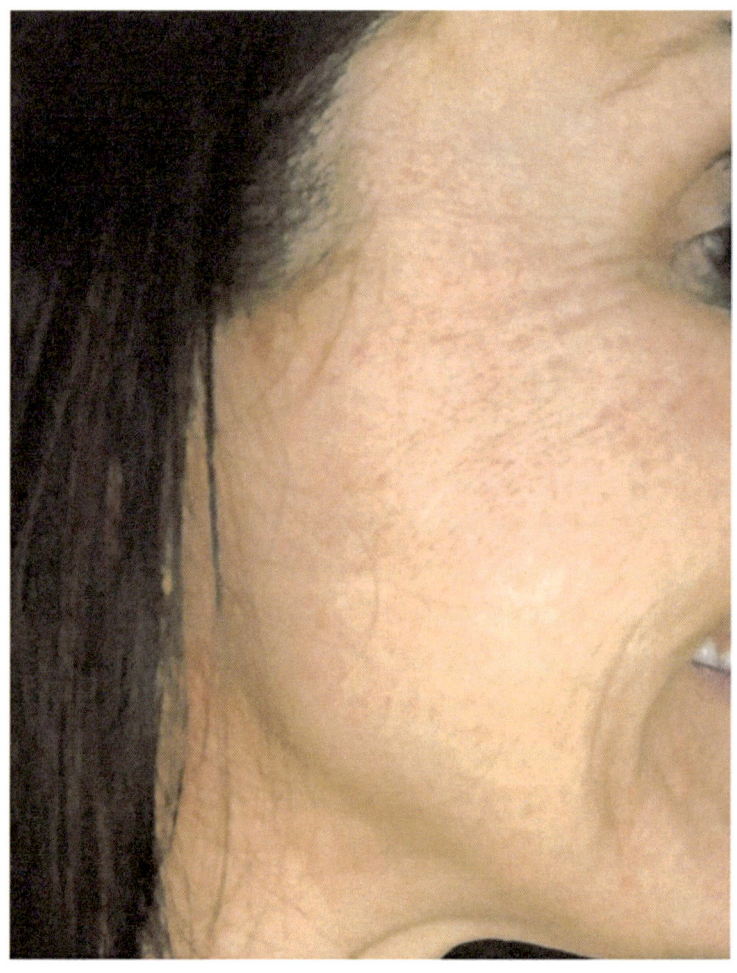

Skin Laxity Patient Face after Needle Depth 1.5-2.5mm RF Level 3-4 Week 6

Acne Scarring

Acne vulgaris is a common condition experienced by up to 80% of people between 11 and 30 years of age and by up to 5% of older adults. It is characterized by noninflammatory open or closed comedones, inflammatory papules, erythematous papulopustular lesions, cysts, which often leave behind residual scarring and pigmentation. Although a commonly encountered it remains a challenging problem to treat for the dermatologist. Laser resurfacing was introduced in the 1980s with continuous wave carbon dioxide (CO_2) lasers; however, because of a high rate of side effects, more specific lasers, including the Er:YAG lasers were developed. Ablative fractional lasers can effectively treat acne scars and enlarged pores, but cause considerable pain and downtime for patients, as well as potentially causing postinflammatory hyperpigmentation (PIH), especially in Asian skin.

The therapeutic approach to the treatment of acne scars and photoaging varies according to the type of lesion. Traditional carbon dioxide (CO_2) laser is associated with long healing times, persistent erythema, and high risk of post-inflammatory hyperpigmentation. The drive to attain cosmetic facial enhancement with minimal risk and rapid recovery has inspired the field of nonsurgical skin rejuvenation. Fractional radiofrequency (FRF) is renowned for its use in cosmetic dermatology, especially in the treatment of rhytids, striae, and cellulite but its use in acne scars has been more recent. Post-inflammatory hyperpigmentation can be managed successfully with topical agents such as azelaic acid and hydroquinone. The therapeutic approach to the treatment of acne scars and photoaging varies according to the type of lesion. Fractionated radiofrequency microneedling (RFMN) induces deep dermal heating and leaves the epidermis less affected. In my experience it gives the best results, especially with icepick scarring.

Extra exclusion Criteria of acne scarring study:

- History of keloid or abnormal scarring
- Patients with metal materials in body (including metal teeth)
- Active systemic or local infections
- Recent ablative or non-ablative laser rejuvenation procedures
- Roaccutane within the previous 6 months
- Soft tissue augmentation within the previous six months

Acne Scarring Results

After initial assessment clinically and by use of photographs, the patients were revaluated by both the patient and two clinical staff to determine clinical improvements in acne scarring. Based on the primary endpoint for efficacy of results being based on an end point of patient satisfaction, almost all the subjects were judged to have achieved significant clinical improvement four to six sessions, comparable or better than CO_2 laser and much better than micro-needling alone.

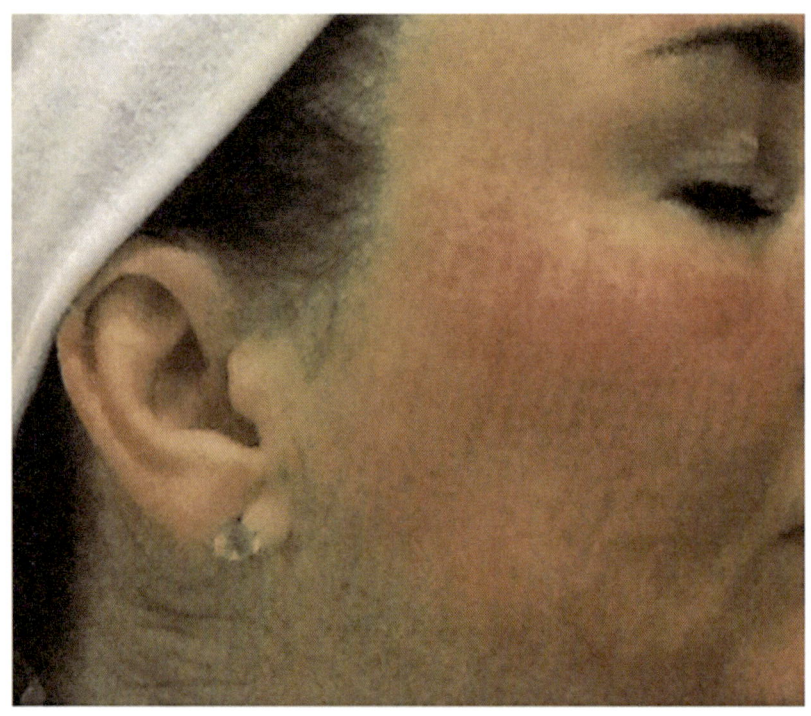

Acne Scarring Patient Needle Depth 2.5-3.0mm RF Level 4-5

Conclusion

The results with acne scarring were comparable in the author's opinion to similar cases with fractionalised CO_2 laser and a definite improvement to multiple sessions of micro-needling alone. We didn't experience any complications in any of our patients using this method and a literature search confirms this when the method is properly applied in appropriate patients. Although we only had a small number of hyperhidrosis patients, FMR treatment was effective for the treatment of PAH without significant adverse reactions due to direct volumetric heating of the lower dermis.

The influence of Dr Richard Fitzpatrick (1944- 2014)

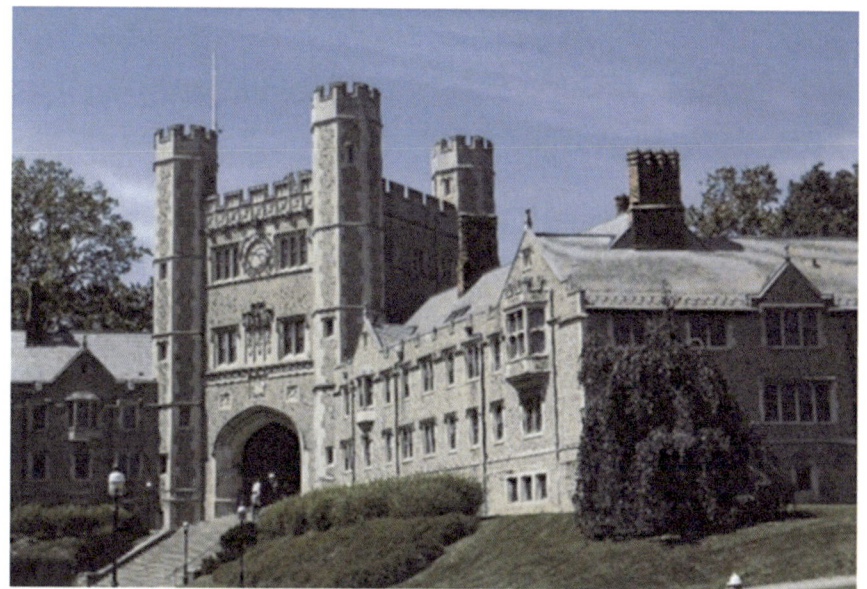

Richard Fitzpatrick graduated from Princeton

'Fitzy' as he was commonly known, was an internationally recognized dermatologist and laser surgeon. His historic discovery of skin resurfacing with lasers is among the leading advances in dermatology as he created many well-known laser procedures with the UltraPulse CO2 laser. After graduating from Princeton University in 1966, he studied medicine at Emory University, achieving membership in Alpha Omega Alpha, and completing an internship in general medicine at the University of Southern California. He entered the Navy, serving as a general medical officer achieving the rank of Commander, and completed his residency in Dermatology at UCLA in 1978. He then moved to San Diego and opened Dermatology Associates in La Jolla and Encinitas. He authored more than 130 publications, three medical textbooks and nearly sixty textbook chapters.

In 1999, Dr Fitzpatrick launched the skin care brand SkinMedica. In 2000, he received a patent for fibroblast derived growth factors used topically for antiaging. In 2001, the popular product TNS Recovery Complex® was launched, creating the first topical Growth Factors solution—pioneering the creation of the entire category.

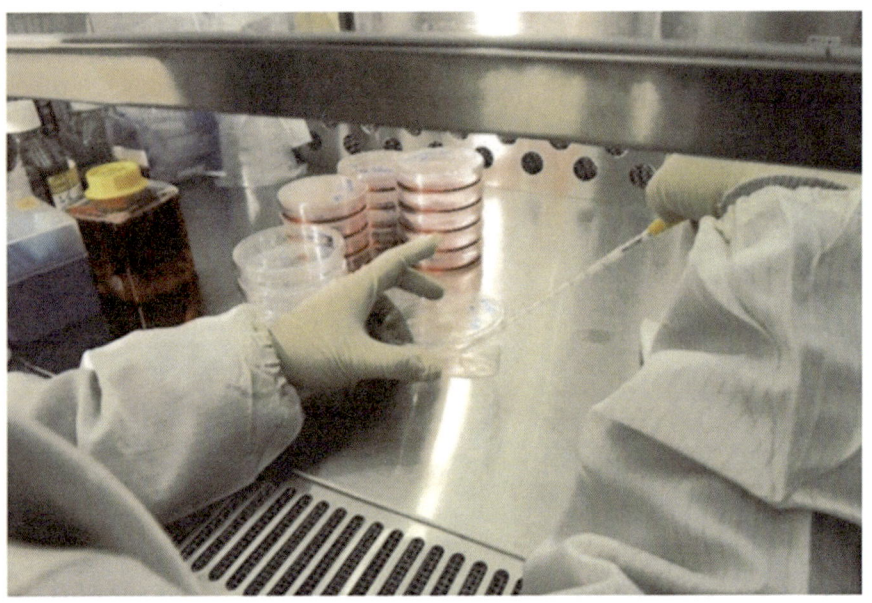

Fibroblast cells on petri dish placed into incubator

Chapter 4: Chemical Peels

A chemical peel is a technique used to improve and smooth the texture of the skin. Chemical peels are intended to remove the outermost layers of the skin. To accomplish this task, the chosen peel solution induces a controlled injury to the skin. Resulting wound healing processes begin to regenerate new tissues. The dead skin eventually peels off. The regenerated skin is usually smoother and less wrinkled than the old skin. The deeper the peel, the more complications that can arise. Professional strength chemical peels are typically administered by certified dermatologists or licensed aestheticians.

The History of Chemical Peels

It is known from detailed notes on papyrus that medical personnel were using peels formulations to treat dermatological conditions in ancient Egypt as far back as 1550 BC. This was the period just before the coming of Rameses I when the Hysos kings ruled the great land, and it is documented that like today, skin physicians were in great demand amongst the more affluent women as sun-damaged skin was a sign of lower rank in society. In those days, before Botox® and skin lasers, women used a variety of substances such as alabaster, oils and salt to improve the skin. Of interest is the fact that sour milk was highly valued as an exfoliant, most probably because it contained lactic acid, an alpha-hydroxy acid commonly used today. But time, like the sun in the sky, passes on and eventually, an Egyptian family from Luxor waged a fierce set of wars against the foreign Hysos kings and finally drove them out of Egypt forever.

Many years later, a copy of the formulations of these chemical skin cures was found between the legs of a mummy in the Assassif district of the Theben necropolis. The manuscript passed through many hands until it was eventually purchased by Edwin Smith in Luxor in 1862, and thereafter became known as the Ebers Papyrus.

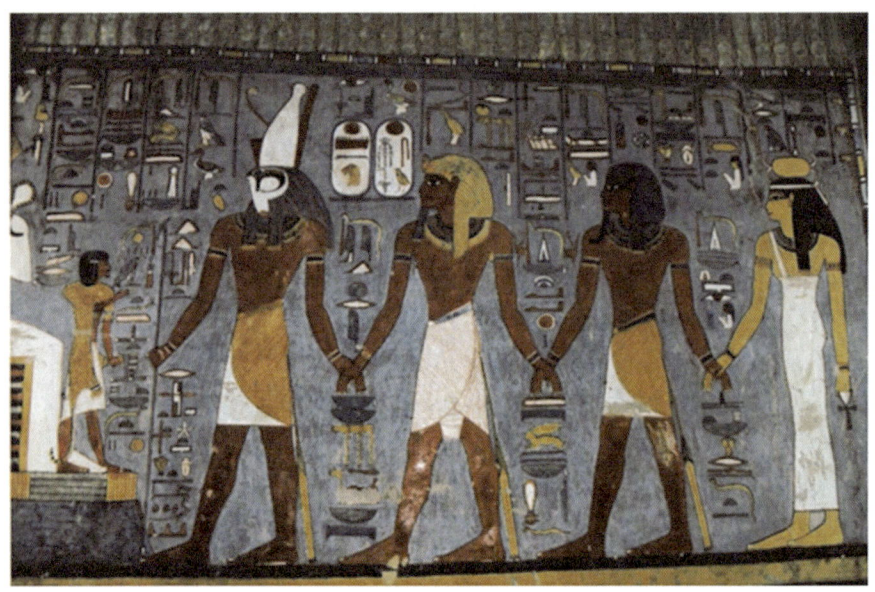

Rameses 1

In Europe that year, Otto van Bismarck became premier of Prussia, dissolved parliament and started collecting taxes for a conflict that ended with the Franco-Prussian War. The war had Bismarck's desired effect of unifying the southern Germanic states and unfortunately nearly cost the life of a young German army physician called Paul Gerson Unna. In 1871, despite serious injuries, he returned to the University of Heidelberg to continue his studies and eventually became one of Germany's greatest dermatologists. In 1881, Unna opened the *Dermatologikum* private dermatological hospital in Hamburg and the following year, he described a chemical peel composed of resorcinol, salicylic acid, phenol and trichloroacetic acid that is still in use today. His controversial doctorate on the histology of the epidermis and was controversial and eventually published in 1876. In 1886 he proposed the use of ichthyol and resorcinol against skin diseases.

The use of Phenol

Phenol was discovered in 1834 by Friedlieb Ferdinand Runge, who extracted it from coal tar. In 1841, the French chemist Auguste Laurent obtained phenol in pure form.

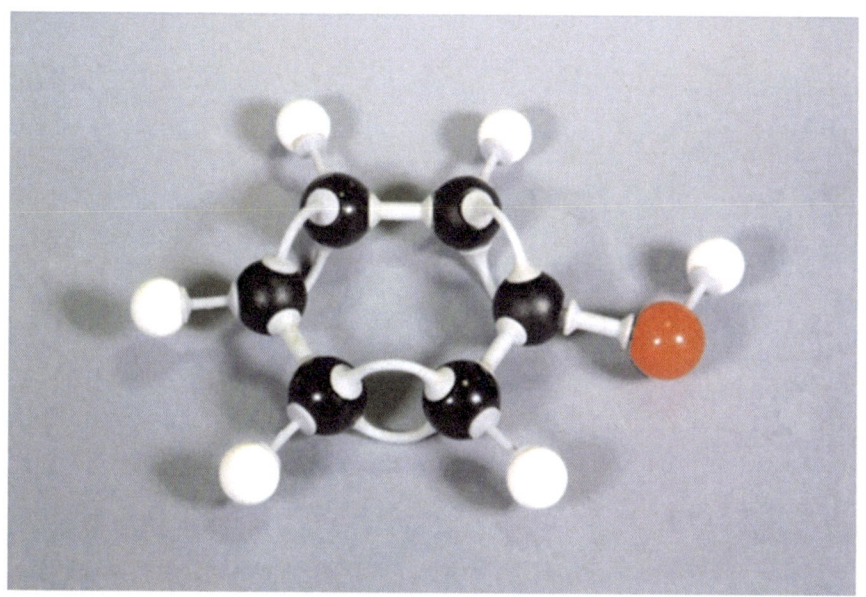

Molecule model of Phenol

The antiseptic properties of phenol were used by Sir Joseph Lister (1827–1912) in his pioneering technique of antiseptic surgery. Lister decided that the wounds themselves had to be thoroughly cleaned. He then covered the wounds with a piece of rag or lint covered in phenol, or carbolic acid as he called it. The skin irritation caused by continual exposure to phenol eventually led to its use in 1903 by the chairman of New York University dermatology society as a peel for acne scarring.

In 1919, Paul Unna became professor of dermatology at the University of Hamburg. In 1927 he described a chronic disease of the skin with seborrhea of the scalp and of the areas in the face and trunk that are rich in sebaceous follicles. It became known as Unna's disease. The phenol method of exfoliation continued to be used, and during World War I, its antiseptic properties were used for wound care, especially after the rising number of explosions burns to the face in the dirty trenches. It was during this period that a French physician called LaGasse noted the improved aesthetic outcome of wounds dressed in phenol bandages. It is not known whether any of these soldiers eventually died of cardiac toxicity, but we do know that after the war ended, his techniques were brought to America by his daughter Antoinette who then began a cosmetic practice in California.

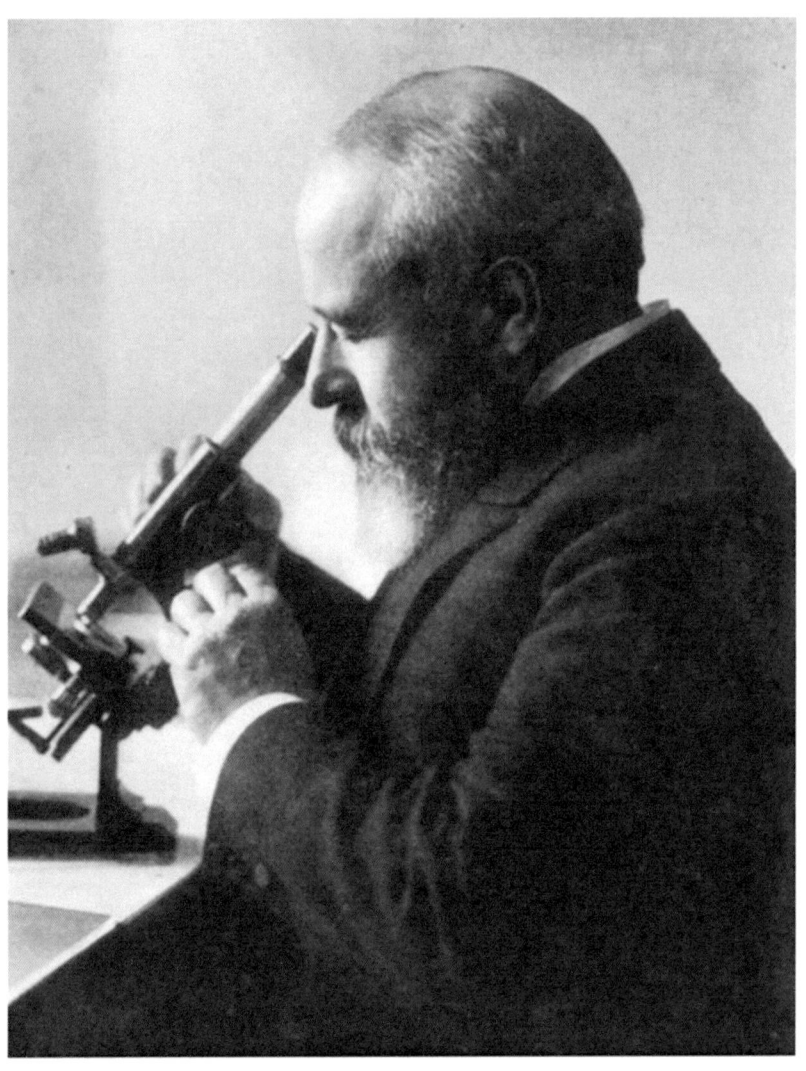

Paul Gerson Unna

The art of chemical peeling remained amongst these cosmetic practitioners until the early sixties when Litton and later, Baker and Gordon, presented patients that they had treated with some of these cosmetic formulations to their dermatological colleagues. The Baker- Gordon peel of about 50%-55% phenol is still widely in use today. It is made by combining 3mls of 88% phenol, 2cc of distilled water, 2 drops of croton oil and 8 drops of Septisol. The croton oil and Septisol are added to allow deeper penetration and more absorption of the phenol. In 1966, Baker published results of its effect on 250 patients.

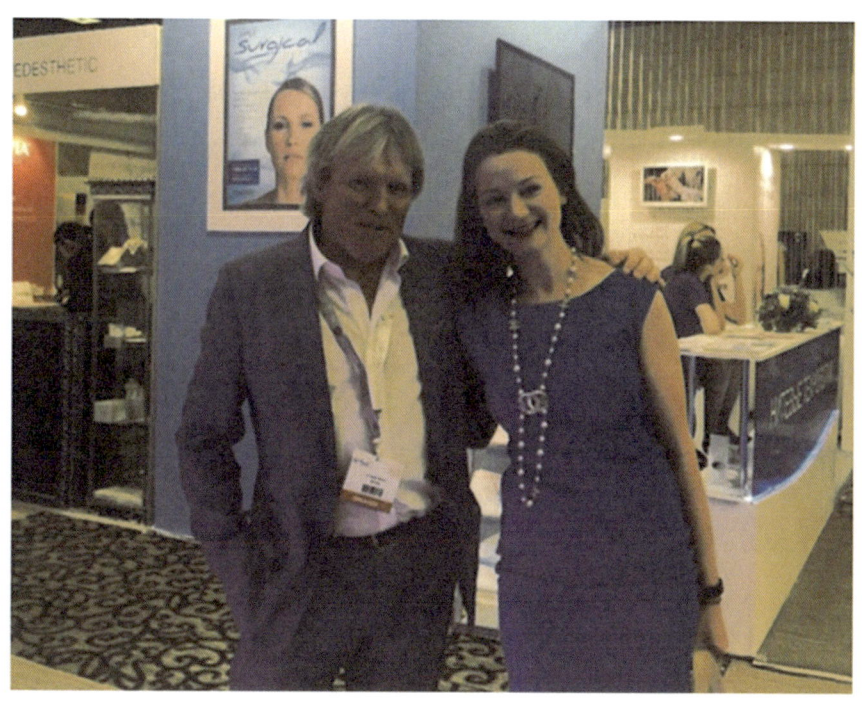

Lecturing with chemical peel expert Dr Uliana Gout East European AWMC Congress Moscow 2017

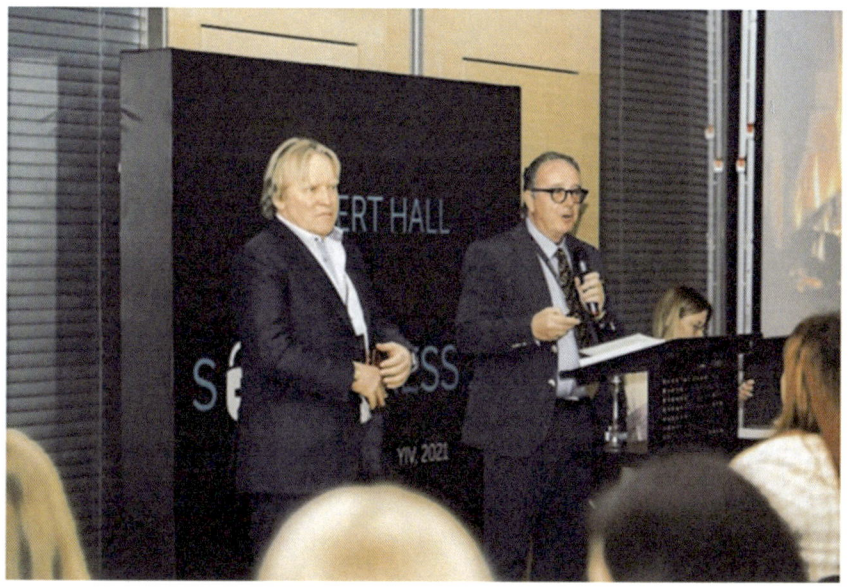

Lecturing with Prof. Torelli Lotti in Kiev 2021

Types of chemical peels

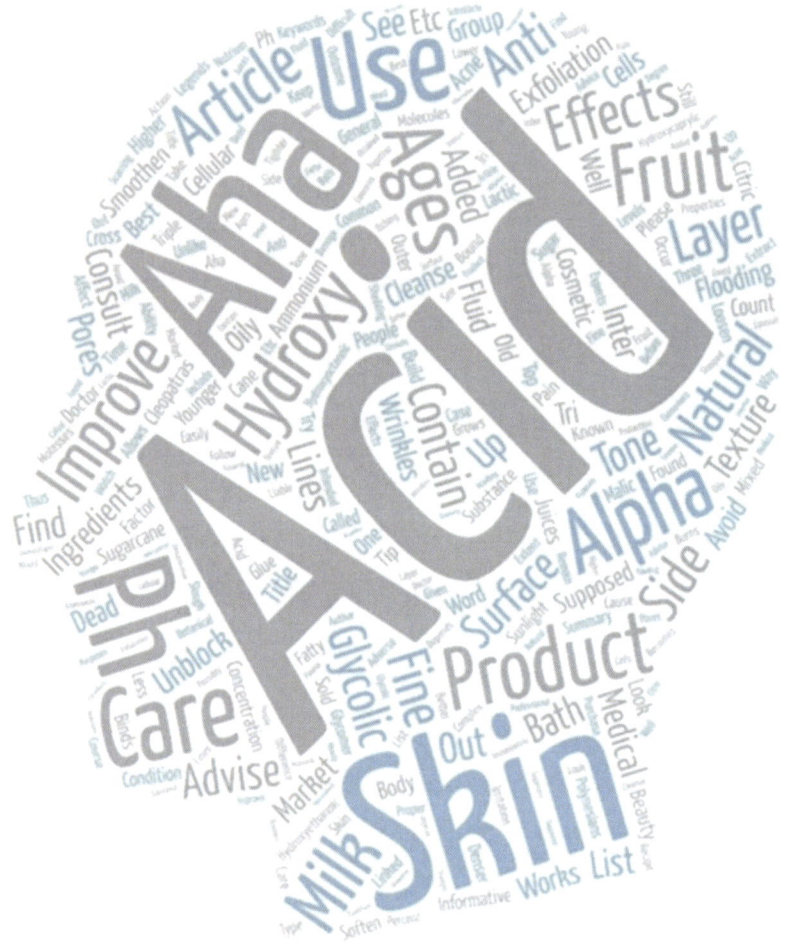

Before we look at the different types of chemical peels, we should first establish what skin problems we are trying to alleviate. In general, most peels are used to reduce the effects of chronological ageing, sun damage, scarring or pigmentary changes. These conditions occur at different levels within the skin and the type of chemical used must reflect that. Some pigmentary problems such as melasma occur in the upper epidermis and can be treated with superficial peels while other defects such as perioral wrinkles around the lip may require a deep peel, such as phenol. Either way, these chemicals will tend to result in a more youthful, smoother, less blotchy, or more even, textured skin. The cosmetic doctor must choose a peel that relates to a certain depth of injury to create a desired effect and individually balance this against potential toxicities and complications in each individual patient. In general, peels are divided into three categories: superficial, medium, and deep. The type of peel a physician uses often also has a lot to do with his personal experience and whether he has had previous problems with the various agents.

Superficial Peeling Agents

When people talk about superficial peels, they generally mean AHA (Alpha-hydroxy acids) peels involving the use of fruit acids such as glycolic acid derived from cane sugar at concentrations of 50% or higher. These peels are generally used to clear the upper layer of the skin in comedonal acne, to remove fine lines and sometimes to improve dry, flaky skin. In general, there are five main fruit acids:

- Glycolic acid peels
- Citric acid peels
- Lactic acid peels
- Tartaric acid peels
- Malic acid peels

There is something deeply humbling when we realise that most of these agents have been around since medieval times. We know that the ancient Egyptians used lactic acid in sour milk to improve the effects of sun damage. Cleopatra is said to have used asses' milk to bathe in. Asses' milk was believed to have a beneficial effect on the body, and Napoleon's sister is also reported to have used asses' milk for her skin's health care. It is known that tartaric acid from wine was popular with French ladies during the seventeenth century and if we look at the other acids – citric from lemons and limes, malic from apples – we soon get the emergent picture. These chemicals are generally safe to use, and their effect is time dependent. The milder concentrations (<10%) are often used in home kits, the medium (<25%) by beauty therapists and the higher amounts (<70%) by nurses and doctors. The use of another agent such as a pre-peel primer or MDA - microdermabrasion can be used to potentiate the effect of an AHA peel. In general, these type of AHA peels should be neutralised with an alkali after use, but because this reaction is slightly exothermic, many practitioners tend to wash them off after use.

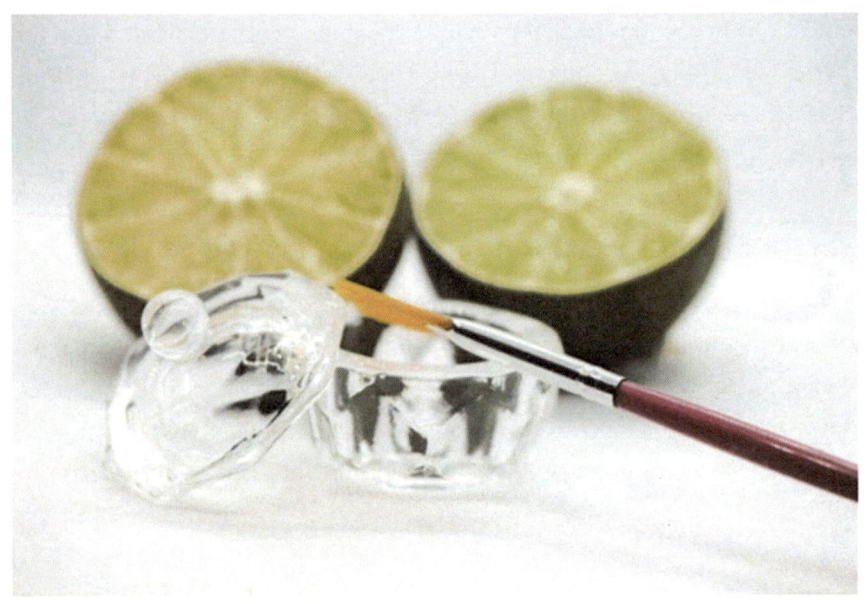

Citric peels from lemons and limes

After they are applied, the skin tends to become red, slightly swollen, and painful. When you are applying the peel, some white patches may appear, signifying some epidermal-dermal separation and if this occurs, it will tend to heal within seven to ten days. In general, we do not want frosting to occur with this type of peel as this tends to signify that the peel is coagulating with albumin in the dermis, and it has gone down too far. AHA peels usually exfoliate for about a week and new skin grows back over the area within a few weeks. If another AHA peel is required, one should wait until the skin has fully recovered. It is also preferable to use some sun protection for a limited period after their use.

Medium-Depth Peels

Medium-depth peels are mostly used for fine lines, wrinkles, superficial scars, stretch marks and to rejuvenate skin. Because of the prolonged period of downtime of about five days and the need to protect the skin from wind and sun for some months afterwards, medium peels are mostly used now in patients that cannot be fully treated with IPL and others who are not bad enough to require Erbium YAG resurfacing. There is little doubt that some patients prefer them as they tend to give a smoother texture and a more immediate effect than three to five courses of more expensive IPL treatments. Although trichloroacetic acid (TCA) is the most used medium depth peeling agent, it can also be used in combination with glycolic acids to reduce the possibility of scarring and to decrease the possibility of hyperpigmentation. TCA is different than more superficial AHA type peels in that the technique is not time-dependent and the agent does not require further neutralisation. It also produces a frost or whitening of the skin, which is dependent on the concentration used.

- Trichloroacetic acid (TCA)

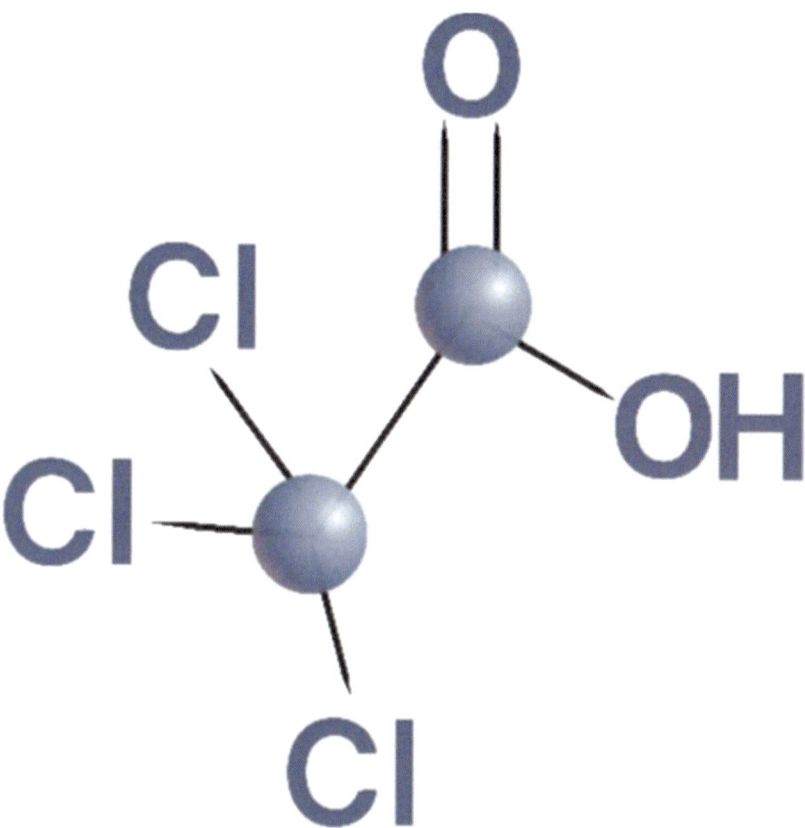

Trichloroacetic Acid (TCA)

This chemical may also be used at lower (5%-15%) concentrations as a superficial-to-medium peeling agent. It is typically used as an intermediate-to-deep peeling agent in concentrations ranging from 20%-50% and the depth of penetration is dose dependent. This peel is very safe at lower concentrations butcan reach varying levels of dosage; if not treated with caution, it can lead to scarring and other complications.

Easy TCA is one of the most popular, safe, medium peels. It is manufactured in Spain and made up to 17.5% concentration. It develops an intense frosting that usually dissipates within about 15-30 minutes after application of a cooling post-peel cream that contains anti-inflammatories. The TCA solution dissolves keratin, coagulates skin proteins, and causes precipitation of salts. It is neutralised by tissue fluids. The skin remains red for about 5 days and then turns brown and sheds like a snakeskin on the 5th or 7th day. Some practitioners rub the skin to try and get the solution to penetrate to a deeper level. This peel is usually applied with a cotton bud or a sponge and can be redone every week until the desired effect is obtained. It is sometimes useful to apply Ane-Stop topical anaesthetic or Emla after the procedure to decrease any residual burning sensation and increase patient comfort. Re-epithelialisation of the skin is normally complete within 10-14 days. TCA 50% is seldom used because of a higher risk of scarring and the availability of the combination peels.

- The Obagi Blue peel

The Obagi Blue peel has become popular in both the US and Europe. It was originally developed by Dr Zein Obagi to be used in all skin types, because this is suitable for all skin types, especially those that are prone to hyper pigmentation after peeling. Because of this, the Obagi Blue is performed in 4 different steps to prevent post inflammatory pigmentation. These stages are probably more relevant to the ethnic skin tones of New York Italians, African Americans, and Asians than they are to downtownDublin. There is also the downside of having to endure a bluish tinge to your skin for some days post procedure.

- The Jessner peel

This peel was discovered by Jewish dermatologist Max Jessner who fled Nazi persecution in Europe to live in the United States. In 1928, Jessner travelled to Buriat- Mongolia on an expedition to study syphilis and the effects of the anti-syphilitic drug Salvarsan. Salvarsan, also known as Arsphenamine was first synthesized in 1907 in Paul Ehrlich's lab by Alfred Bertheim. Its antisyphilitic properties were discovered by Sahachiro Hata in 1909 and was originally called "606" because it was the sixth in the sixth group of compounds trialled. It was a great improvement over the inorganic mercury compounds that had been used previously. After Jessner returned, the Nazi government removed his professorship, because of his Jewish background. As propaganda against Jews increased, he was forced to emigrate to Switzerland in 1934.

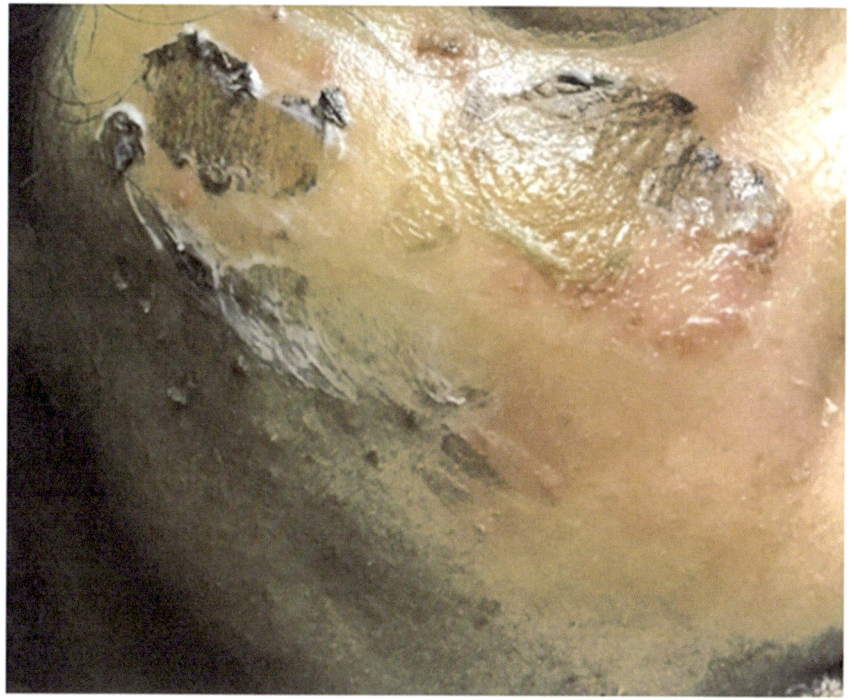

Jessner Peel

Ten years later he settled in New York, where he experimented with mixing salicylic acid, lactic acid, and resorcinol (each at 14%) to make a new chemical peel. Some practitioners use an AHA peel to prepare the face prior to peeling. The proceduralist then waits for a light frost to appear before neutralising the AHA and BHA acids with water or an alkali. Like TCA peels, the face becomes slightly painful, and a fan may be used to lessen the discomfort. The Jessner's peel frosting may take many hours to dissipate.

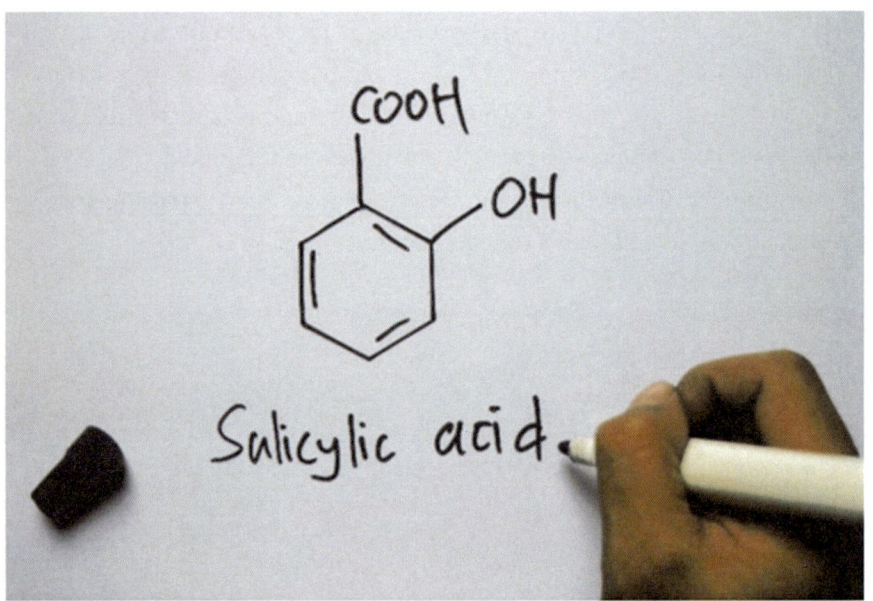

Salicylic acid

Salicylic acid (from Latin salix, willow tree) is a lipophilic monohydroxy benzoic acid, a type of phenolic acid, and a beta hydroxy acid (BHA). This colourless crystalline organic acid is widely used in organic synthesis and functions as a plant hormone. It has been used for several decades to remove the outer layer of the skin and is used to treat warts, psoriasis, ringworm, dandruff, acne, and ichthyosis. It is found in medications, such as AcneSal 2% and Whitfield's ointment at 4%. It can penetrate acne comedones better than other acids. The effects of the salicylate are like aspirin, in that it has an anti-inflammatory and analgesic effect, resulting in some decrease in the amount of redness and discomfort associated with chemical peels.

Deep Peels

Deep peels are usually done to improve moderate wrinkling of the skin. They are usually performed with 88% phenol as it provides a relatively deep and predictable injury to the dermis. Phenol is the hydroxylated form of benzene and when it is used at this full strength, it immediately coagulates the skin tissue and prevents further absorption. If phenol is diluted, a different reaction occurs with disulphide bonds in the dermis and deeper penetration of the skin is technically possible. This phenomenon becomes important if a patient's skin 'cracks' or 'tears' during a peel because deeper wrinkles may then form as the diluted phenol can cause further skin lysis. We can also use this effect to our advantage as post-peel occlusion with a zinc oxide waterproof mask will deepen the level of the peel and the amount of time required to grow new skin. Full face phenol peels are more popular in Spain and the US than in Britain or Ireland, where they tend to be used in more local applications such as the upper lip or around the eyes. Phenol peels also may be performed in various formulations, such as pure phenol (88%) or phenol mixed with soap, water, croton oil or olive oil. The names of these formulations are:

- Gradè
- Baker-Gordon
- Venner-Kellson
- Maschek-Truppman

The most popular phenol peel is the Baker-Gordon formulation as it produces the most dramatic results and is the most effective peeling agent currently used to smooth out moderate wrinkles. The solution contains phenol 88%, 2 ml water, 8 drops of liquid soap (Septisol) and 3 drops of croton oil. Because this formulation is quite dilute with irritants; it penetrates deeper than pure phenol and may permanently affect the ability of the skin to tan. This peel is like an Erbium YAG laser, in that it is reserved for the face as it can cause scarring of the neck, arms and legs. It also causes more discomfort than any of the other peels and often should be done under a regional block or general anaesthesia.

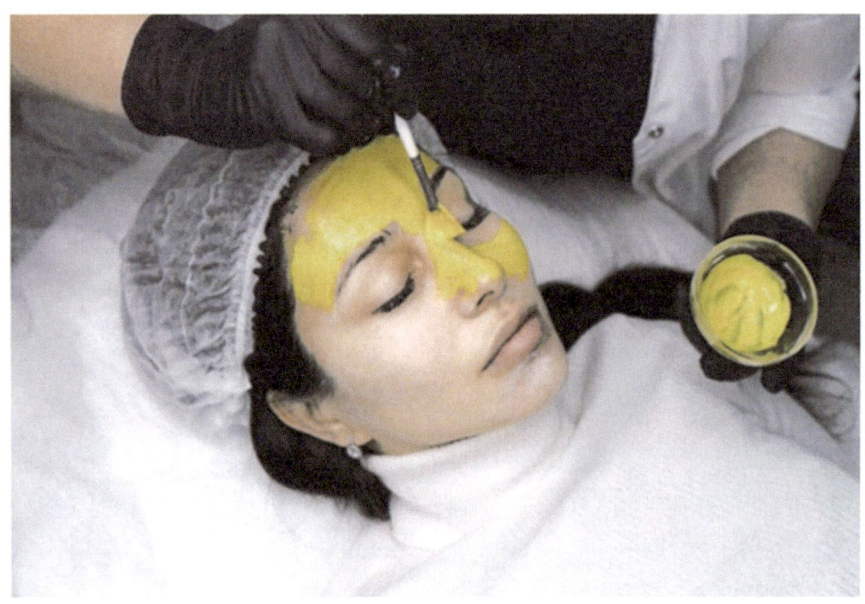

Facial brush peel retinol treatment

Patients should be aware they may require analgesia and anxiolytics for most of the first night after this peel. The biggest problem with phenol peels is their ability to cause cardiac arrhythmias. To avoid this complication, no more than 25% of the face should be peeled before a 10 to 20-minute break is taken and the entire peel should take 60 minutes or more. A patient should remain attached to a cardiac monitor during the procedure with lignocaine on standby. Having said that, I have seen better results from using full-strength phenol peels to treat wrinkles in upper lips than I have with the most modern Erbium YAG laser. Intravenous fluids should be used for hydration and renal flushing.

Patients should remember that redness after a phenol peel may last nearly six months and that they must use an extremely high sun protection factor during this period. There is also a higher risk of scarring and other pigmentary changes following this deeper peel.

I note that the skin of some patients may also appear unnaturally 'graven' or 'waxy' with a type of bluish hue, which is probably also related to damage to the skin's pigmentation system. A complete armamentarium using phenol, trichloroacetic acid, and dermabrasion allows the physician to successfully treat a variety of difficult photoaged skin problems in a consistent fashion. These three techniques have their specific indications, and patient selection is the key to a successful outcome. Historically, phenol peeling has been embraced by plastic surgeons as the method of choice for improving the appearance of coarse facial rhytides. The principal advantage of phenol peeling is its predictability: it requires no pre-treatment regime. It is important to realize that phenol, trichloroacetic acid, and dermabrasion are not exclusive of each other, but are additive in their value.

Complications of Peels

Most of the common problems with peels can be prevented by proper screening of patients. We have already mentioned that Irish patients with Fitzpatrick skin types I and II are probably the best candidates for peeling. Fitzpatrick skin types III-VI are preferably pre-treated with a bleaching agent such as 4% hydroquinone or 4% kojic acid to prevent post-inflammatory hyperpigmentation. Patients with a history of herpetic infection should be put on anti-viral medication prior to the procedure. This normally would mean taking Zovirax (acyclovir) for 3 days prior to the procedure and up to 2 weeks afterwards. I also like to use Isotrex® or Cordes Vas® (tretinoin) as part of a pre-treatment regimen as it thins the outer horny layer of the skin to allow better penetration and helps remodel new collagen in the dermis. Patients should also be aware that oral retinoids such as Roaccutane (isotretinoin) should have been discontinued for a period of twelve months prior to peeling as there is an increased risk of hypertrophic scarring.

Chapter 5: Fat Removal

A recent report from the American Society of Plastic Surgeons (ASPS) revealed that Americans spent more than $16.5 billion on cosmetic plastic surgery and minimally invasive procedures in 2018. They spent an estimated $2 billion for liposuction (258,558 procedures), a basic technique that involves inserting a narrow tube (cannula) under the skin through tiny incisions and manipulating the cannula to break up and suction out fat cells. This is not a treatment for obesity, or a substitute for proper diet and exercise, or an effective treatment for cellulite.

The History of Liposuction

The 1920s was a decade frequently referred to as the 'Roaring Twenties' or the 'Jazz Age', because of the economic boom following World War I. French speakers refer to the period as the '*Années folles*' (Crazy Years), emphasising the era's social, artistic, and cultural dynamism. Although the first known use of suction to remove fat from the body was performed by French surgeon Charles Dujarier in this period, the development of modern liposuction is credited to father and son Italian gynaecologists, Arpad, and Giorgio Fischer.

It started back in 1921 when Dujarier decided to practice the new art of liposuction to create a better shape on a young ballerina's knees. Unfortunately, his patient developed gangrene and required an amputation. It was the same year that the new Irish Free State was established. After that, many other attempts were followed with less tragic results, although several complications such as haematoma, long-term seroma, necrosis, and infections occurred. In 1972, the German physician Schrudde published a new less invasive technique to remove subcutaneous fat, using a uterine curette in a 'sharp' technique of subcutaneous surgery.

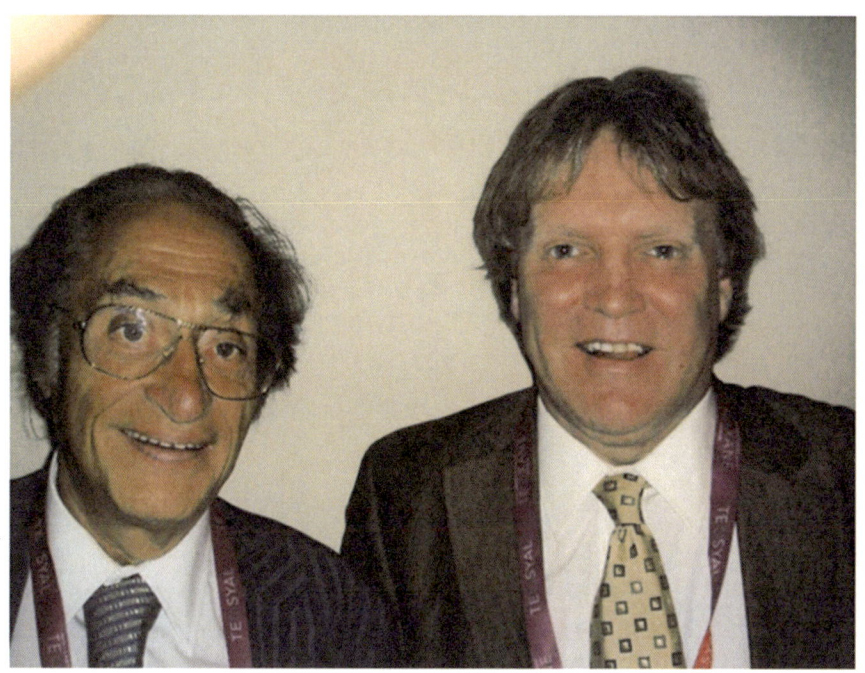

The author with the late Dr Yves-Gerard Illouz

In 1975, Italian cosmetic surgeon Arpad Fischer and his gynaecologist son, Giorgio, developed the modern technique of liposuction with the invention of an electrical, rotating scalpel encapsulated by a cannula that suctioned out dislodged cells. They were the first to introduce blunt hollow cannula attached to a suction source and the crisscross suctioning technique from multiple incision sites. This 'blunt' method allowed obtaining better and more predictable aesthetic results with much less complications. The Fischers applied their method only to outer thigh adiposity. It was the same year that Pol Pot took over the government in Cambodia.

In 1978, the technique was taken to Paris where it was refined and popularised by the French plastic surgeons, Yves-Gerard Illouz and Dr Pierre Fournier. Yves-Gérard Illouz was a co-founder of Médecins Sans Frontières (Doctors Without Borders). He was born in Oran, part of the colony of French Algeria, and studied in France, earning a bachelor's degree in arts and philosophy and in 1968, a medical degree as general surgeon from the Medical College of Paris. Illouz then developed the so-called 'wet technique' in which a solution of saline (salt water) and hyaluronidase was injected into the fat before suctioning to decrease bleeding and make suctioning easier.

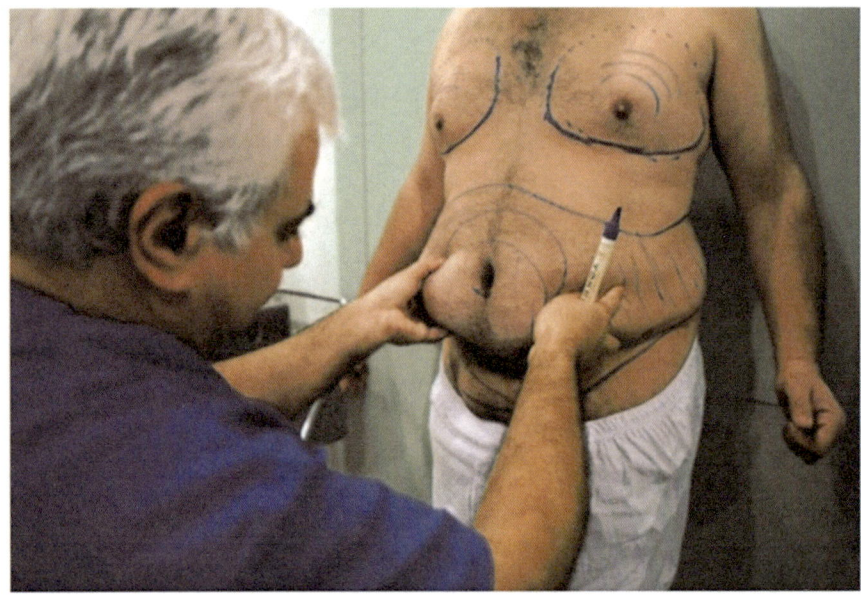

Marking before liposuction

In 1977, Illouz modified the blunt cannulas, making them of a smaller diameter to reduce the section of nerves, lymphatic vessels, and blood vessels. He introduced three different sizes depending on the area to be aspirated: the larger (10 mm) for the flanks, hips, and buttocks, the middle one for knees, ankles and abdomen and the smaller for the face. I met Yves-Gerard for the first time when we shared the platform as keynote speakers at the European Society for Laser Aesthetic Surgery (ESLAS) conference in Athens in April 2007. I was deeply sorry to hear of the passing of Yves in 2015 at the age of eighty-six. Over the next few years, I met him in Paris and visited his house with my good friend, Dr Jack Ohana, when he first became ill.

Dr Pierre F. Fournier has rightly been attributed the title of 'founder of modern aesthetics'. He began his medical career from quite humble beginnings; after serving in the French army in World War II, he opened a small clinic in the suburbs of the French capital. By offering lower prices than most other surgeons in central Paris, clients soon started to line up at his door. He met Giorgio Fischer in the early 1970s and invited him to his Parisian clinic, where he treated some

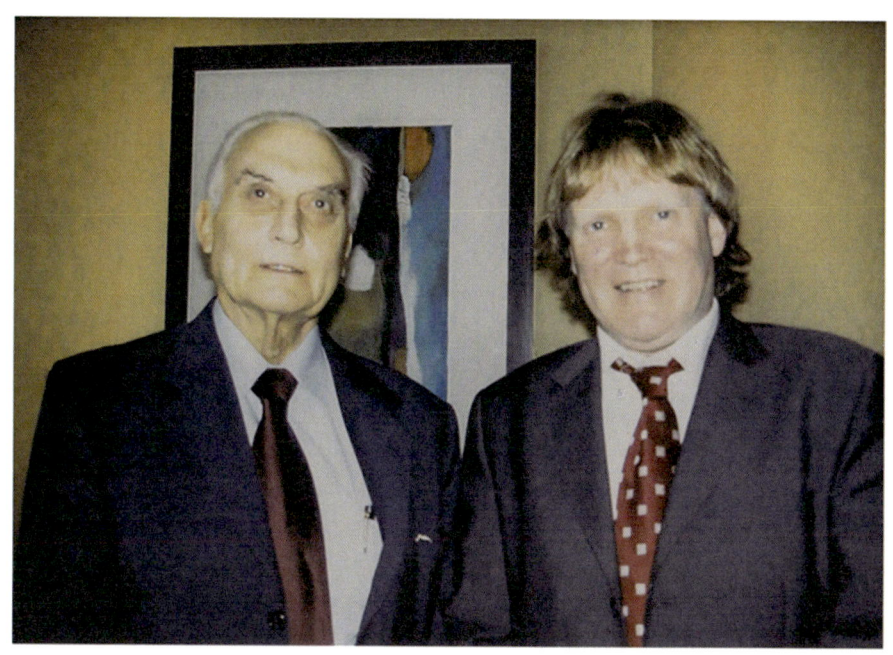

The author with Pierre F. Fournier

patients. Fischer wanted to build a factory to produce his invention, but Pierre's friend, Yves- Gérard Illouz, suggested that Giorgio should first try a suction machine used by gynaecologists for abortions, which effectively worked perfectly for the same purpose. Abortions were legal in France in that period. They presented their results at the American Congress of Plastic Surgery and started touring the world, teaching their techniques. I met Pierre for the first time in Miami in January 2004 at the American Academy of Aesthetic Medicine, having gone there to learn about thread-lifting. At the stage, he was still practising as a septuagenarian but came across as a charming gentleman; in the words of an interviewer: 'his mind and wit as sharp as the instruments he used'.

During later IMCAS conference sessions in Paris, he would often invite me to his house in Paris, where his wife gave a beautiful piano recital. He oncepresented me with an original framed copy of one of his older 1960 lectures, *TheConcept of Beauty*, which I proudly hung back on the walls of my clinic in Dublin.

LIPOSUCTION

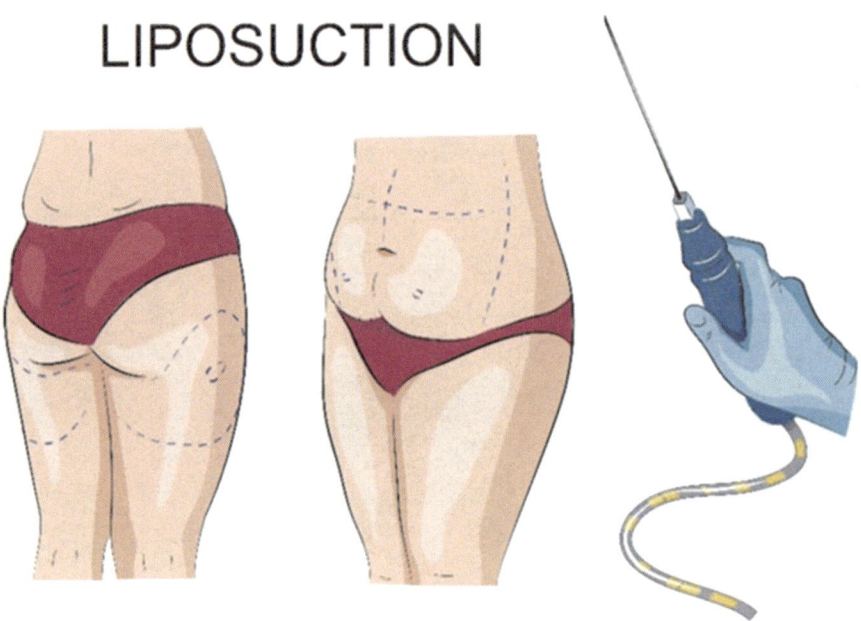

In an interview with *The Times of Malta* in 2012, he said, "Human beings do not only want to live, but they also want to live in the best physical and mental condition possible – as close as possible to perfection." Although he admits there is no true definition of beauty or perfection and that their perception varies from one culture to the other.

In 1984, Pierre introduced the use of the local anaesthetic, lidocaine, laying the groundwork for the tumescent technique used today. It was the same year that Indian Prime Minister Indira Gandhi was assassinated by two Sikh bodyguards. Both Pierre and Yves came from North Africa, and I considered both doctors to have primarily pioneered the field of medicine we are all now engaged in. Both had been true pioneers in the field of aesthetic surgery and made the procedure of removing fat safer for both doctors and patients alike. There was something humble about their approach to medicine and they were still willing to help other doctors learn their techniques. They gave generously of their time to train others. In 1982, Yves-Gerard presented a new form of lipolysis using blunt cannulas and high-vacuum suction with reproducible good results and low morbidity, and a new age of liposuction arrived. During 1984, two Swiss doctors, Kesselring and Meyer, improved cannula design and Fournier developed another technique using a syringe In 2019, I organised the Aesthetic Conference at the Royal Society of Medicine in Dublin and I invited Pierre to give the opening lecture. Currently, he was back in Morocco living with his family and now in his nineties and sadly unfit to travel. In the end, I gave the opening speech myself and recognised his great contribution to aesthetic medicine.

****

The Swiss doctors published a lot of papers on their technique. Meanwhile, liposuction crossed the Atlantic to the US but quickly fell out of favour because of increased complications and several deaths. It now appears that many of the deaths were related to American plastic surgeons combining liposuction with abdominoplasty 'tummy tucks. In 1985, a Californian dermatologist, Jeffrey Klein, invented and pioneered a new tumescent method – liposuction technique, the safest method known. He was helped in this development by a Colorado dermatologist, Patrick Lillis. In 1987, an Italian plastic surgeon, Professor Nicolo Scuderi from Rome, introduced the use of ultrasound as an emulsifying modality for fat tissue during liposuction and a new age of 'fat busting' began. This ultrasonic-assisted lipoplasty (AUL) technique was further modified when Zocchi introduced titanium ultrasonic probes and manual remodeling of the treated areas to eliminate the fluid from the burst fat cells in 1992.

Zocchi hoped that this new technique would allow liposuction to be performed without damaging nerves and veins that were often destroyed using blunt cannula liposuction. While initially embraced in South American and Europe, ultrasonic liposuction was largely rejected after many patients experienced skin peeling, burns and fluid build-up in affected areas. It was the same year that the world witnessed three days of rioting in Los Angeles after four white police officers were acquitted of criminal charges despite video evidence that they had beaten up black motorist, Rodney King.

In 1998, Californian plastic surgeon, Barry Silberg, further developed the technique using external ultrasound-assisted liposuction (XUAL). This method required traditional aspiration liposuction after high-frequency ultrasound. He lectured on the technique, as he felt that this method led to less traumatic surgery with superior clinical outcome.

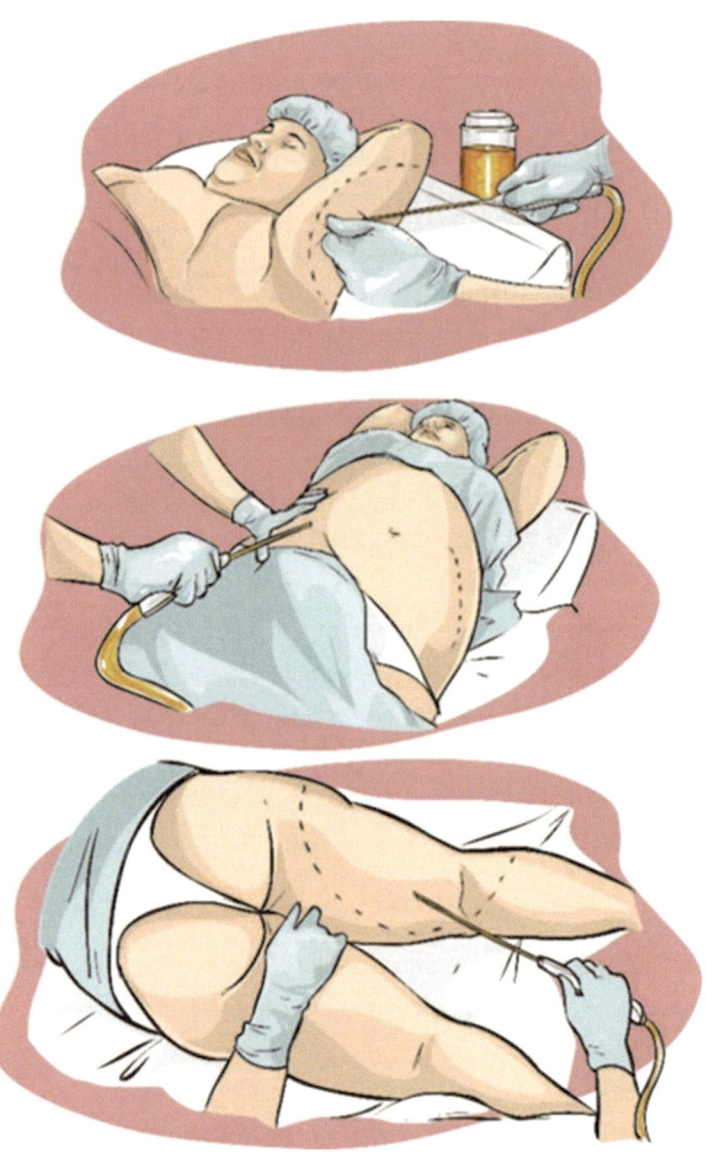

Areas to be treated with liposuction

There is little doubt that as an invasive modality, like tumescent liposuction, the technique still had many of the drawbacks that accompany invasive procedures. It was the same year that the FDA approved Viagra for erectile dysfunction.

The Era of Vaser Liposelection®

Vaser Liposelection® or high definition liposculpture is an advanced form of body contouring that improves muscular definition in the abdomen, waist, chest, and arms. The procedure used ultrasonic energy to break up fat while leaving surrounding tissue – such as nerves, blood vessels and connective tissue – relatively intact. Patients reported highly satisfactory results and low to minimal pain. Moreover, many doctors started to voice opinions that the magnitude of ultrasonic energy used to destroy the fat cells may also damage other tissue in contact with the cannula.

Many felt one of the technical drawbacks of the ultrasonic liposuction technique was that the cannula had to be inside the body. Vaser represented a significant improvement on older, traditional liposuction techniques, as clinical studies showed it could tighten skin more than basic technique.

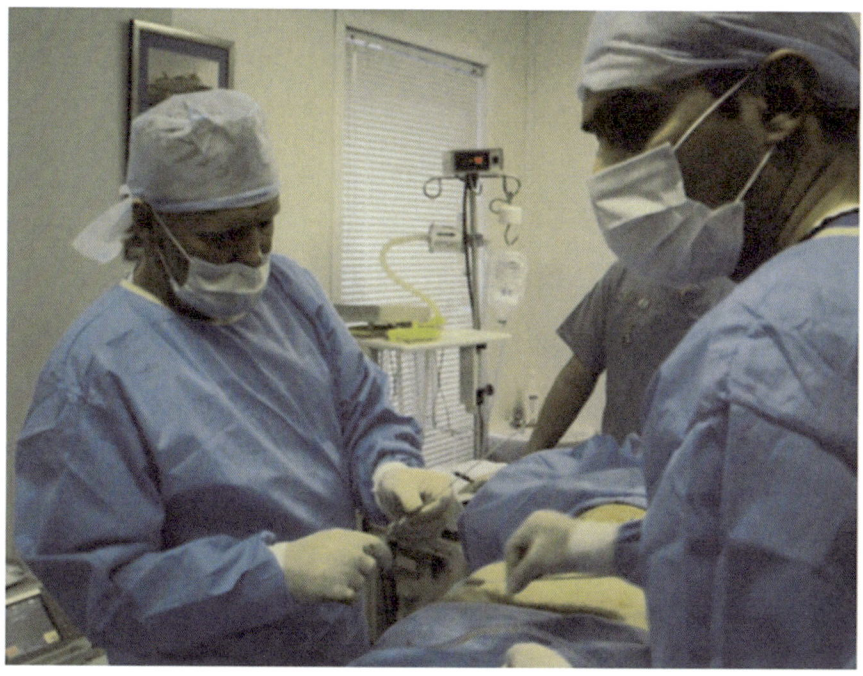

The author using Vaser Liposelection®

The Era of UltraShape® and the interesting history

behind the use of therapeutic ultrasound to remove fat.

Therapeutic ultrasound (in contrast to diagnostic and imaging modalities) has been used as a therapeutic tool in medicine for more than fifty years. The first ultrasonic machine (lithotripter) used to destroy kidney stones was produced by the German aircraft manufacturer Dornier in Munich in 1980. It was the same year that the former Beatle, John Lennon, was shot dead outside his New York apartment. In 1984, the company introduced the Dornier HM-3 (Human Model-3) and in that same year, the FDA approved the use of ESWL (extracorporeal shock wave lithotripsy) in the US for the treatment of renal calculi.

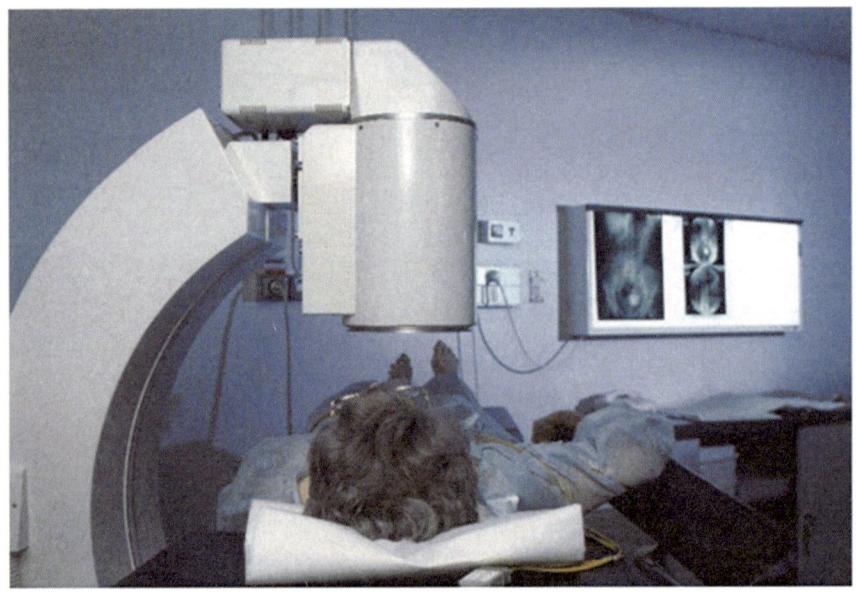

Dornier Lithotripter Device

Since that time, the HM-3, or the 'Munich Stonebuster', as the press preferred to call it, has treated over five million patients worldwide. By 1985, the technique was first applied successfully in a patient with gallbladder stones. It was the same year that the energetic Dubliner, Bob Geldof, had the idea of organising Live Aid for the starving people of Africa. In the following years, many conditions suitable for the technique of ESWL were investigated. But the story of using therapeutic ultrasound in medicine didn't really start there. In fact, it may have inadvertently started with another aircraft manufacturer because during World War II, British ophthalmic surgeon, Harold Ridley, noticed pieces of Plexiglas from the shattered canopies of Spitfire fighter planes did not cause any reaction when they became embedded in pilots 'eyes. He used this theory to use the material to implant the world's first intraocular lens at St Thomas Hospital in London on 29 November 1949. The next year, he encountered widespread criticism from his peers at a conference in the US who considered the idea of replacing the eye's natural lens with an artificial one too radical and unacceptable for the period.

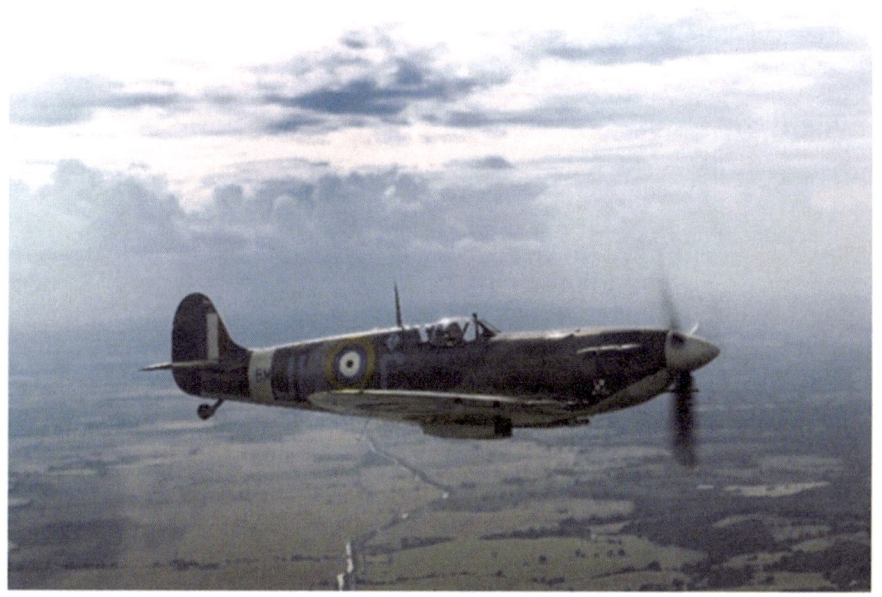

Vickers Supermarine Spitfire MK VB

Over the next twenty years, the idea of lens implants for cataracts slowly became more acceptable. In 1968, American surgeon, Charles Kelman, adapted the new technology of ESWL to remove cataracts. The procedure, later known as phacoemulsification, used a tiny probe with a vibrating tip to gently break up the cataract and wash it away. The techniques of phacoemulsification and plastic lens implant technology were combined, and the science of cataract surgery was revolutionised. In 1981, a protégé of Ridley, called Choyce, gained the first FDA approval of intraocular lenses. Today, after decades of development, modern phacoemulsification is considered one of the safest surgeries performed, with millions of successful procedures completed every year around the world. Today, the use of therapeutic ultrasound in the form of extracorporeal shock wave therapy has found its way into many other facets of medicine. However, its main use may yet prove to be the most interesting as the 'Tel Aviv Fatbuster', as the association of ultrasound with the destruction of fat cells started years before.

UltraShape® Technique

In 2001, while the rest of the world was coming to grips with the aftermath of an Al Qaeda terrorist attack on the World Trade Centre in New York, a Tel Aviv plastic surgeon called Ami Glicksman considered the possibility of using external ultrasonic waves to selectively break down fat cells without the patient having to undergo a surgical procedure. His experiments were successful, and he noted that fat lysis was selective, leaving nearby tissues intact. Further macroscopic and microscopic analyses of overlying skin noted that it also remained untouched.

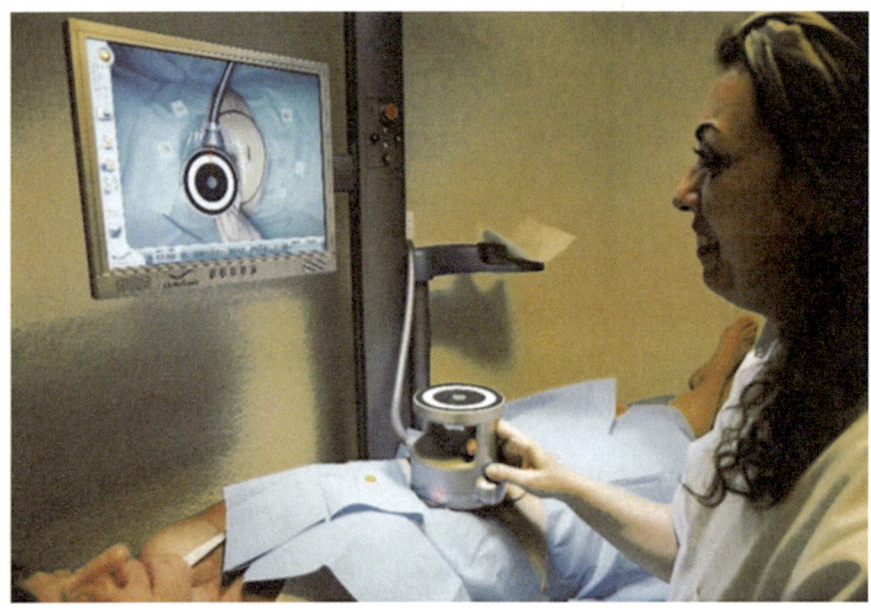

UltraShape® technique

The researchers quickly moved from the pig models and tried the external ultrasound transducer to lyse human fat from *ex vivo* tissue harvested from skin flaps excised in hospital abdominoplasty procedures. These experiments also showed that fat lysis only occurred in a specific region, leaving skin or fat outside of the focused beam intact.

The first study of twenty patients commenced in 2002, monitoring the safety and effectiveness of the treatment. Histological evaluation of all tissues excised during surgery clearly showed that the external ultrasound treatment only destroyed adipose cells, leaving blood vessels, connective tissue, nerves and epidermis intact. This new method called UltraShape® used unique G-NIUS(TM) (Guided Non-Invasive Focused Ultrasound Selective) technology to break down fat cells effectively and safely. Meanwhile, in India, 20,000 people died in a violent earthquake and further east, China was allowed into the World Trade Organisation. In 2003, the device had another competitor involving a phenomenon called 'popsicle panniculitis' – fat loss in the cheeks in children who are frequent ice- or popsicle-eaters. Basically, the idea for the new technique, called cryolipolysis, came from a long forgotten 1970 article in the *New England Journal of Medicine* that discussed how children were losing fat in their cheeks when they were sucking on popsicles.

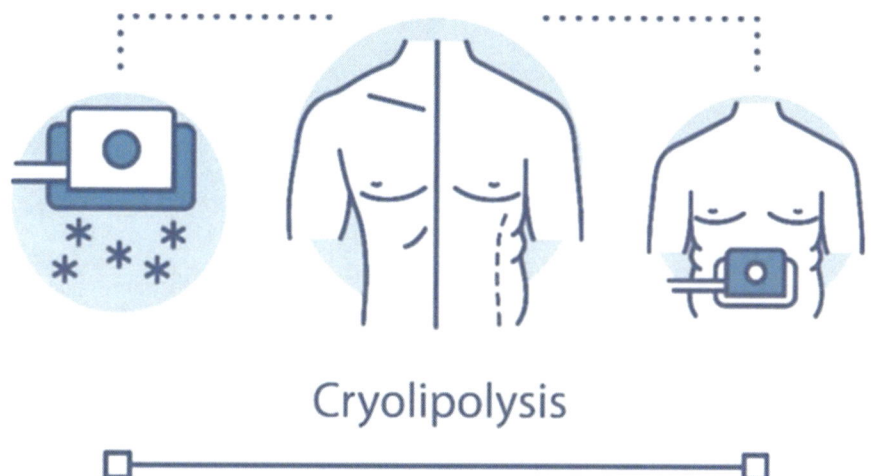

Cryolipolysis

The History of Coolsculpting®

In the Western world, during the 1960s, social progressive values such as increasing political awareness and economic liberty of women began to grow. Pop culture and politics collided at the turn of the decade, when the King of Rock 'n' Roll, Elvis Presley, visited President Richard Nixon in the White House's Oval Office. In the same period, an article written by Epstein and Oren on children and popsicles in the *New England Journal of Medicine*, went largely unnoticed until Dr Dieter Manstein and Dr R. Rox Anderson from Massachusetts General

Hospital made note of the effect and experimented fat loss in other areas of the body, using the targeted application of cold to lower the tissue temperature to about 40 degrees. Their research was also based on a somewhat bizarre but documented story, about a woman who rode a horse naked in very cold weather and claimed that she had lost fat on her inner thighs as a result.

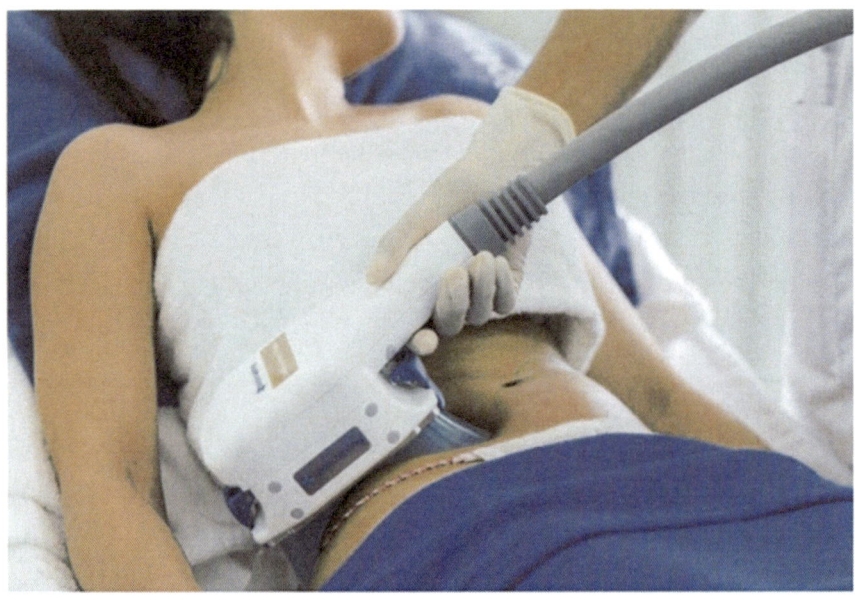

CoolSculpting®, Cryolipolysis session, non-invasive method of permanent reduction of localized fat.

The common theme in both instances was the use of extremely cold temperatures. Based on this, the doctors worked together to prove the theory that the application of extreme cold on fat tissue could, in fact, result in a reduction of fat cells. Thus, the concept of cryolipolysis was born. The CoolSculpting® procedure is not for everyone. You should not have the procedure if you suffer from cryoglobulinemia, cold agglutinin disease or paroxysmal cold haemoglobinuria. Be careful if you have any medical conditions including recent surgery, pre-existing hernia and any known sensitivities or allergies.

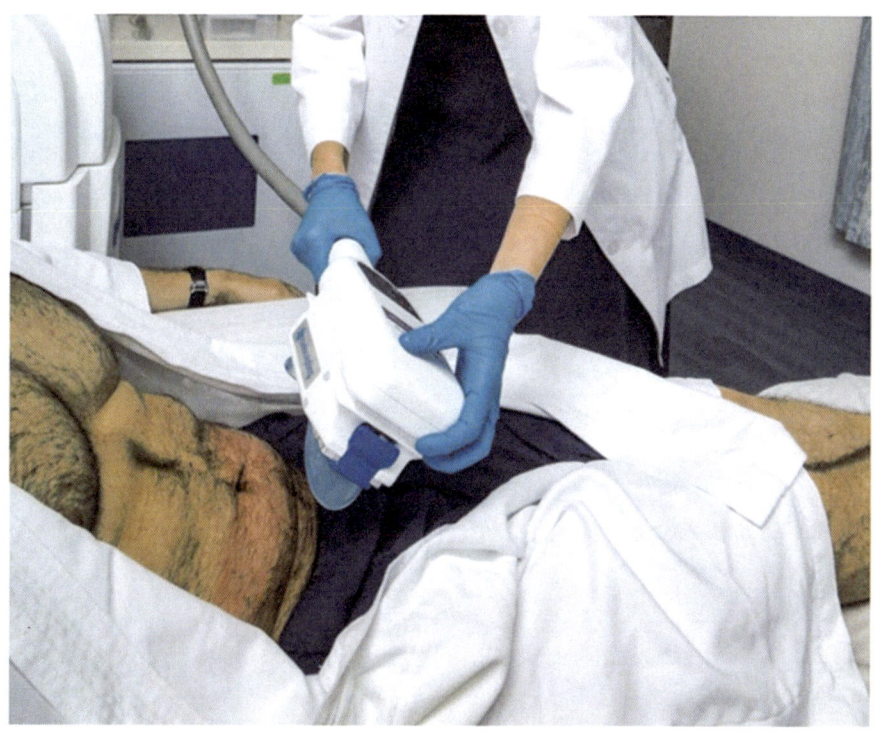

CoolSculpting®, Cryolipolysis session, non-invasive method of permanent reduction of localized fat.

The contribution of Dr R. Rox Anderson

There are few physicians in the cosmetic dermatology world that garner as much respect as Dr R. Rox Anderson. The Lancer-Endowed Chair of Dermatology, professor of dermatology at Harvard Medical School and director of Wellman Centre for Photomedicine at Massachusetts General Hospital. The effect was quite dramatic as freezing caused the fat cells of interest to die without harming nearby organs or skin. People were initially quite sceptical about it because they thought that it seemed too good to be true.

Chapter 6: Hair Transplant

Hair transplantation is a surgical technique that removes hair follicles from one part of the body, called the 'donor site', to a bald or balding part of the body, known as the 'recipient site'. The technique is primarily used to treat male pattern baldness. In this minimally invasive procedure, grafts containing hair follicles that are genetically resistant to balding (like the back of the head) are transplanted to the bald scalp. Hair transplantation can also be used to restore eyelashes, eyebrows, beard hair, chest hair, pubic hair and to fill in scars caused by accidents or surgery such as facelifts and previous hair transplants. While several surgical treatment options (plug grafts, scalp reductions, transposition flaps) have been used historically to treat androgenic alopecia, we outline the two most common techniques of HT based on the follicular unit-principle; namely, the follicular unit transplantation (FUT) and the follicular unit excision (FUE).

The History of Hair Transplant

Modern cosmetic hair transplant surgery for male pattern baldness dates from the work of New York dermatologist, Norman Orentreich, in 1952. It was the same year Princess Elizabeth of Britain was coronated queen upon the death of her father, King George VI. The technique was in fact much older than this and Japanese dermatologists Sasagawa, Okuda, Tamura and Fujita were using small autografts containing hair follicles for the correction of scars and cicatricial alopecia long before the onset of World War II. Orentreich had difficulty getting a journal to publish his paper until the Annual New York Academy of Science took it in 1959, the same year Alaska and Hawaii admitted to the Union as the 49th and 50th states.

Dr Orentreich coined the term 'donor dominance' to explain the basic principle of hair transplantation, which says that transplanted hair continues to display the same characteristics of the hair from where it was taken.

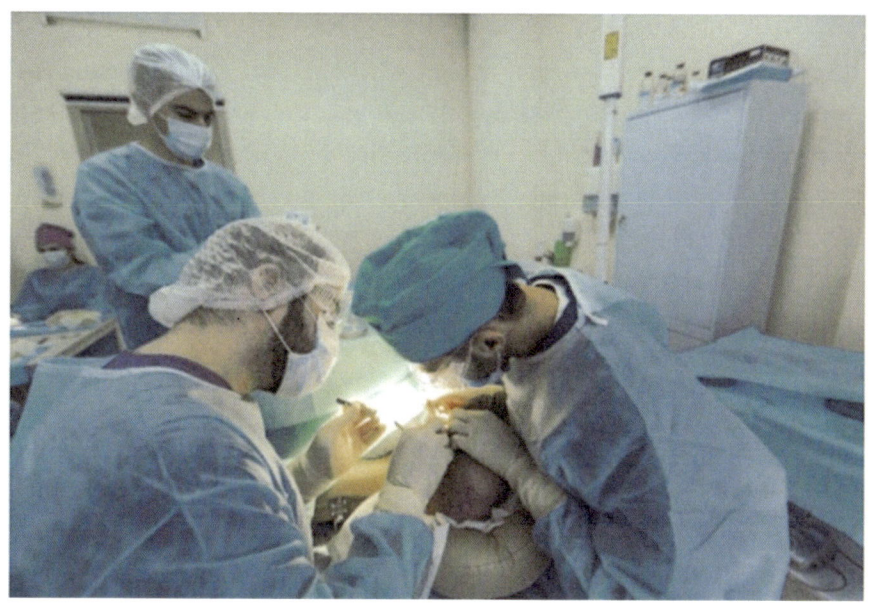

Hair transplant surgeons at work

He used the term to explain why hair tissue from the donor zone successfully regenerates new hair. Since the transplanted scalp tissue is producing healthy hairs in an area that could no longer grow hair, it is assumed that the physical traits of hair follicles from the donor zone are dominant over the physical traits of the original scalp tissue. In other words, healthy hair that is harvested from the back or side of the scalp (the permanent zone) will continue to grow as if it were still in its original location.

Donor dominance explains why hair in the donor area, which is resistant to balding, continues to grow after it is transplanted to the thinning or bald areas of the scalp. There have been some challenges to the theory of donor dominance in recent years. Dr O'Tar Norwood – the same doctor responsible for the Hamilton/Norwood hair loss charts – was the first hair doctor to officially challenge this theory after he noticed that a transplanted hair took on the same characteristics as the recipient site. While following up with one of his patients, Dr Norwood observed that a hair follicle unit that was not wavy to begin with soon adopted a wavy texture after it was transplanted into a bald spot that had once produced wavy hairs.

According to the principles of donor dominance, the donor hair should have retained all its characteristics and continued to grow in its original fashion.

The main difference between FUT and FUE hair transplants is that in FUT, the surgeon removes a strip of donor skin from which to extract. In FUT, the donor strip is removed from the mid-portion of the permanent zone, whereas in FUE, follicular units are harvested from a much broader region to obtain enough grafts. This makes it more likely that, in FUE, some of the follicular units may be lost to the balding process over time. Both FUT and FUE have their own advantages and disadvantages. You need to select in which factor you can compromise and which advantage you want.

Dr Norwood felt the transplanted hair conformed to the texture of native hairs that previously grew in the recipient site. Both theories have their devotees until this day. Many medical historians feel it is regrettable that the work of Dr Hajime Tamura of Japan was not more widely known in the West as his papers were written in Japanese. They were published in the *Japanese Journal of Dermatology and Venereology* in 1943, at the height of the Pacific War. It was also the year Adolf Hitler ordered German troops at Stalingrad to fight to the death.

While today we tend to use 0.7-mm punch grafts, and certainly ones less than 1.0 mm, Orentreich's 4.0-mm punch graft method remained the basic procedure until 1975. Although many hair transplant doctors felt this punch size was too large, the technology of the period meant that the unreliable quality of the smaller biopsy punch ensured that they never gained popularity. The result was the 'hair plugs' of the period, where graft recipients walked around with scalps that looked like a doll's head. In 1984, 'mini-grafting', the technique of using smaller grafts cut from a strip of donor tissue rather than punched out directly from the back of the scalp, was introduced to the field of hair restoration.

In 1987, Dr Bob Limmer of Texas commenced strip dissection under stereoscopic microscopes. This method of dissection used to obtain follicular units from a donor strip dramatically improved outcomes but averaged only about 150-200 grafts per hour and greatly increased the number of staff members required for each procedure. It also gave the operator an unprecedented view of the excised scalp tissue and the individual hair follicles. It was the same year that Reagan and Gorbachev met in Washington during the campaigns for Glasnost and Perestroika.

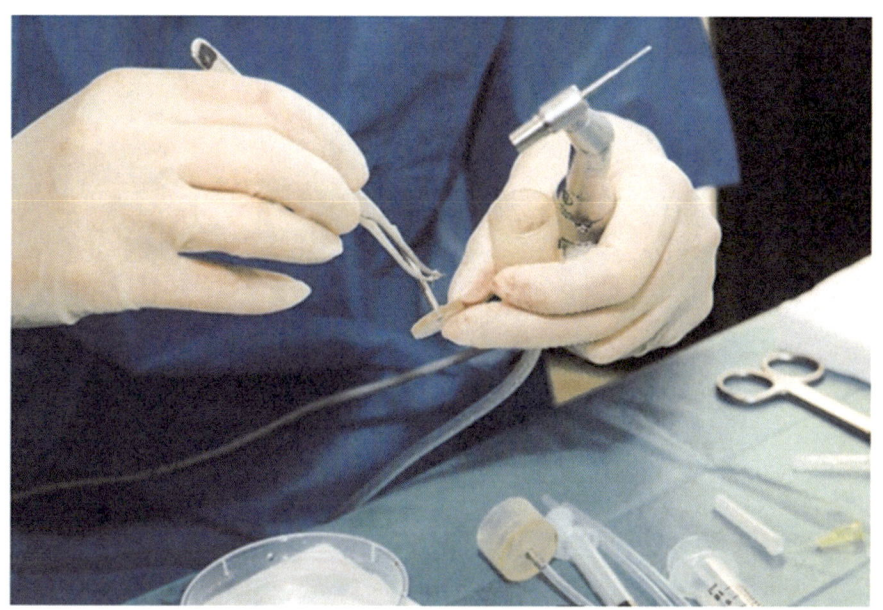

Using mini-grafting techniques

Physicians began using 'micro-grafts', even smaller grafts of 1-2 hairs, to soften the frontal hairline. The procedure that used mini-grafts at the centre of the scalp with micro-grafts placed around them to make them look more natural was called 'mini-micro grafting'. Mini-micro grafting procedures gradually supplanted the plug technique and became the main form of hair restoration surgery over the next 20 years. Other methods of hair restoration surgery, such as scalp reductions and flaps, similarly resulted in unnatural-looking results. The use of exceptionally large numbers of mini-micro grafts – a technique called 'Mega-sessions' – gained popularity in the mid-1990s.

To increase the size of the hair transplant sessions was a logical extension of the mini-micrografting technique, as it required basically the same skills of the smaller sessions. The problem with mini-micro grafting was that the grafts sizes were arbitrary and did not mimic that which occurred in nature. Mini grafts can look a bit pluggy and micro-grafted areas can appear too thin. In addition, in the mini-micro grafting technique, the skin between follicular units was not trimmed away, necessitating larger than necessary recipient sites, larger wounds and more variable healing and graft growth.

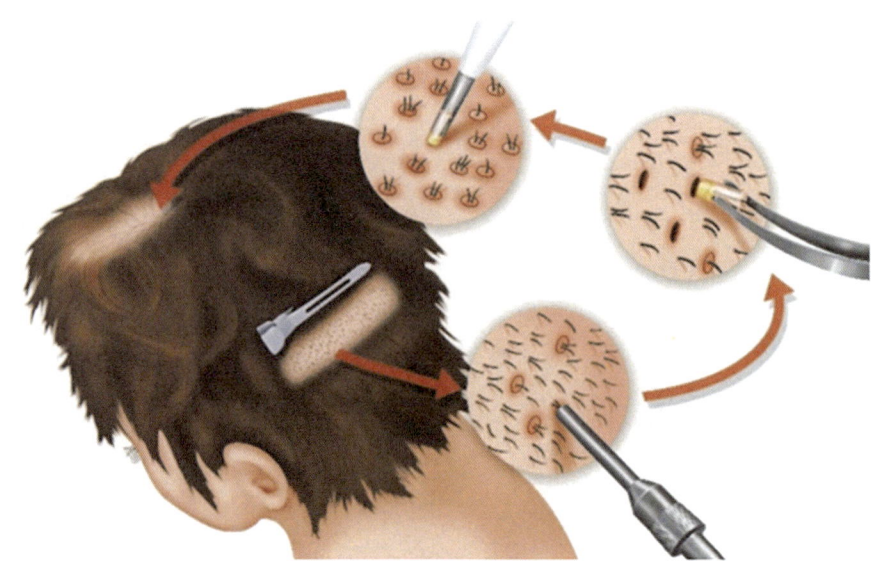

Donor dominance

Introduction of FUT hair transplantation

In 1992, Dr William Rassman started experimenting with (FUT) techniques to improve hair transplant technology, to enable surgeons to perform hair transplants with large numbers of exceedingly small grafts in single surgeries. He studied at the Medical College of Virginia and later the University of Minnesota, doing a cardiovascular fellowship under Dr C.W. Lillehei, an American surgeon who pioneered open-heart surgery as well as numerous prostheses for cardiothoracic surgery.

In 1944, Alfred Blalock at Johns Hopkins University Hospital had begun successfully performing surgery on the great vessels around the heart to relieve the symptoms of tetralogy of Fallot, demonstrating that heart surgery could be possible. Lillehei participated in the first successful surgical repair of the heart on 2 September 1952. That historic operation, using hypothermia, was led by his long-time friend and colleague, F. John Lewis. Lillehei was a professor in the department of surgery at the University of Minnesota from 1951 to 1967.

FUT: The first big advantage is that a full shaving of the head is unnecessary, as only the donor and recipient area requires exposure. This means the rest of your scalp does not need to be touched and can be covered post procedure with a baseball-type cap. In FUT, you will be left with a permanent scar, which will always be visible if you ever shave your head.

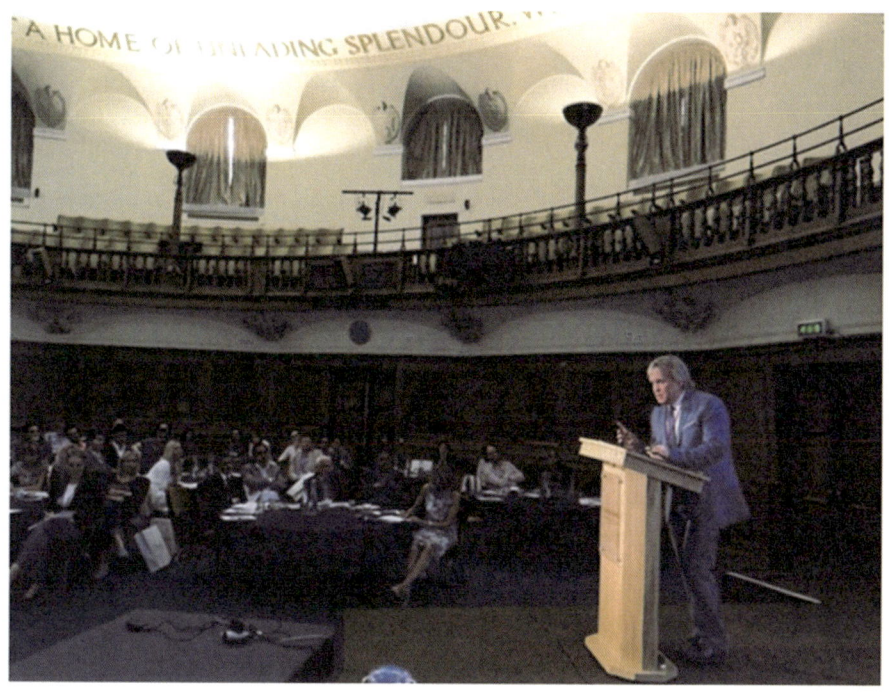

The author lecturing on aesthetic techniques in London

With FUT, transplantation of hair in naturally occurring individual follicular units was established. In 1995, he published a paper with colleague, Robert M. Bernstein, defining a new hair restoration technique. In their landmark publication, *Follicular Transplantation*, Bernstein and Rassman state that hair transplantation should be performed using only naturally occurring, individual follicular units. The paper introduces the term 'Follicular Unit' to the field and describes both the technique and planning needed to get the best long-term aesthetic results.

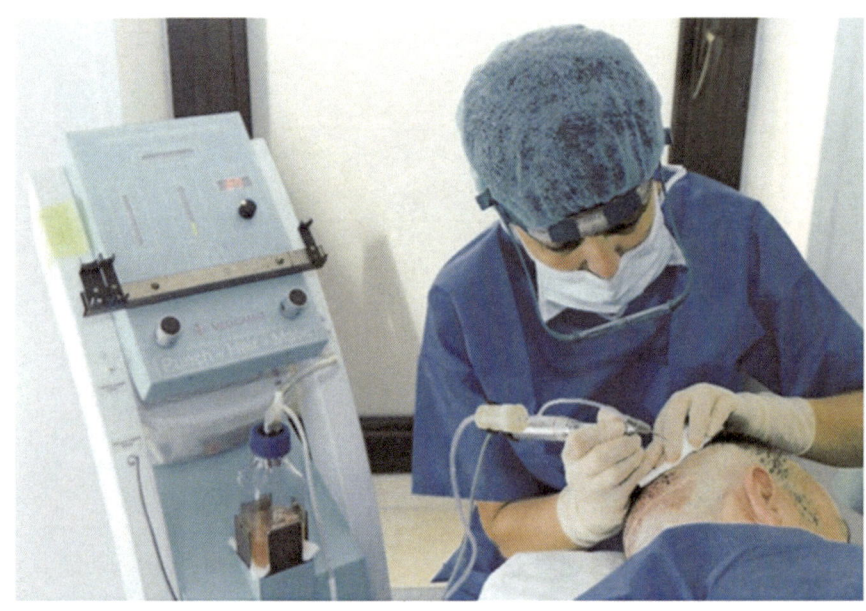

FUT hair transplantation

Follicular unit transplantation (FUT) hair stages

As FUE deals with individual follicles, this cannot happen. It is debatable whether FUE or FUT can give more follicles as I have seen as many as 6,000 being transplanted in a FUE session. It is accepted that in general, FUT can give more follicles from an area than the FUE technique. If you have Grade 5 baldness and a dense donor area, then I would favour FUT. FUT is a little more technical and may cost more. In both, there is minimal pain during the procedure. In 1996, Dr Bernstein presented the theory behind follicular transplantation at the International Society of Hair Restoration Surgery and showed results of this technique to physicians at the international meeting. In these methods, donor harvesting was done by single-strip method with elliptical excision of donor, followed by suturing. The significant disadvantage of single-strip harvesting was the resultant linear donor scar. Though it is possible to provide an exceptionally fine linear scar with the newly described trichophytic closure. This posed a cosmetic problem for patients who wished to wear their hair short.

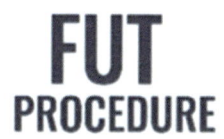

FUT
PROCEDURE

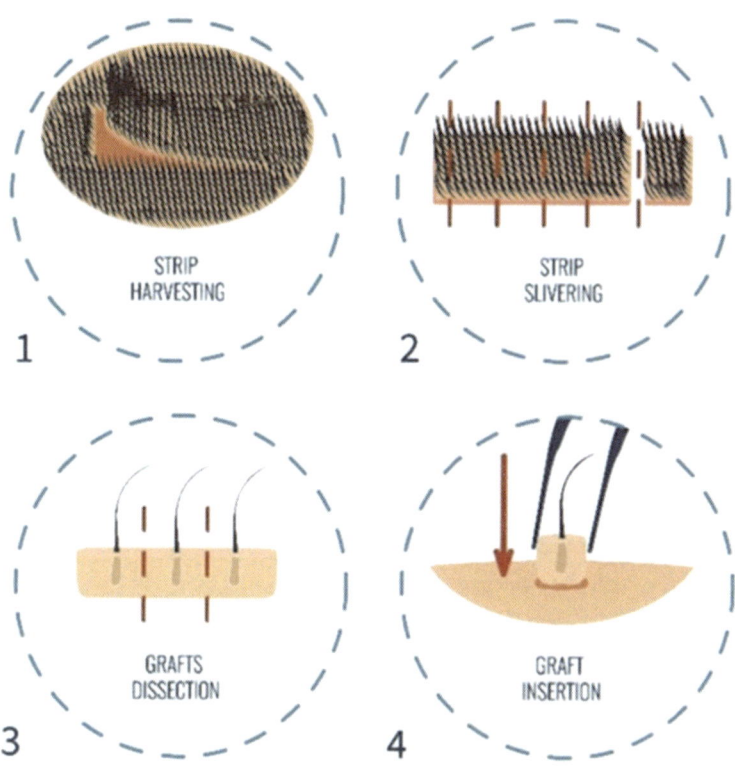

Rassman claims his greatest accomplishment was commercialising the intra-aortic balloon pump, a device now used as the standard heart assist pump worldwide. In 2003, he received the most prestigious award in the field of hair replacement, the Golden Follicle Award. He was named the most outstanding hair transplant surgeon worldwide by the International Society for Hair Transplant Surgeons. It was the same year US forces defeated the Iraqi Army and the Iraqi Republican Guard in the Battle of Baghdad.

The American Board of Surgery certified Dr Rassman in 1976. He pioneered the large session hair transplants as he was the first to perform 2,000, 3,000 and 4,000 grafts in a single session. Rassman claims both Follicular Unit Transplant (FUT) (1995) and the Follicular Unit Extraction technology (2002) was pioneered by him. His idea was to only transplant grafts of naturally occurring units of one to four hairs called follicular units.

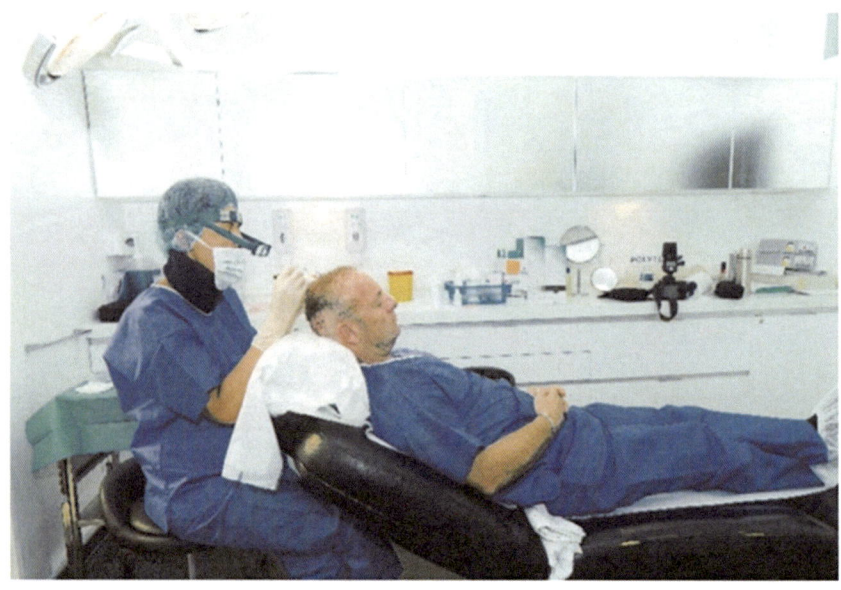

FUE hair transplantation

Introduction of FUE hair transplantation

Since physicians had become accustomed to performing follicular unit-based hair transplants, an Australian doctor began to investigate the idea of removing these naturally occurring units directly from the donor area, using a very tiny punch. The idea gained popularity in the US when Bernstein and Rassman worked on this technique and introduced FUE to the medical literature in their 2002 publication, *Follicular Unit Extraction: Minimally Invasive Surgery for Hair Transplantation*.

In FUE, an instrument is used to make a small, circular incision in the skin around a follicular unit, separating it from the surrounding tissue. The follicular unit is then pulled, or extracted, from the scalp, leaving a tiny hole (which heals in a few days). This process is repeated until enough follicles are obtained. Like FUT, FUE also faced initial resistance due to a new set of surgical skills required of the surgeon and staff. And since FUE requires a special device to extract whole follicular units, the race to develop the optimal instrument was on.

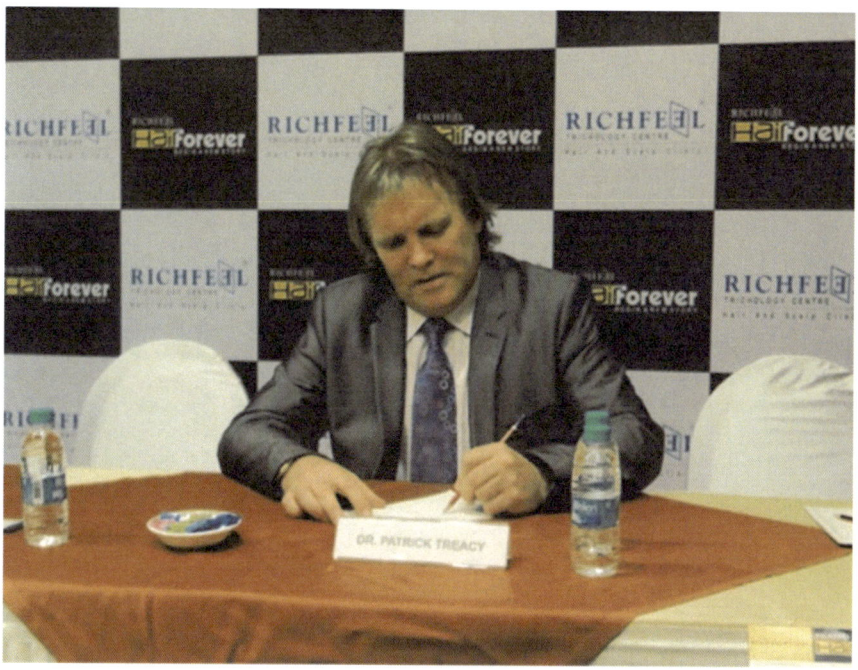

The author bringing Ailesbury FUE Hair Transplant techniques to Richfeel Hair Clinics in India, 2012

Despite these hurdles, patient demand for a hair transplant procedure that did not leave a linear scar in the donor area began to grow. FUE hair transplants gained further momentum with Harris' paper in 2005, in which the concept of a two-step sharp/dull punch instrument for FUE was introduced. The two-step procedure uses a sharp-tipped instrument to first cut part of the way into the skin and then a second punch with a blunt tip to cut deeper into the dermis.

In FUE, the extraction of intact follicular unit is dependent on the principle that the area of attachment of arrector muscle to the follicular unit is the tightest zone. Once this is made loose and separated from the surrounding dermis, the inferior segment can be extracted easily.

FUE
PROCEDURE

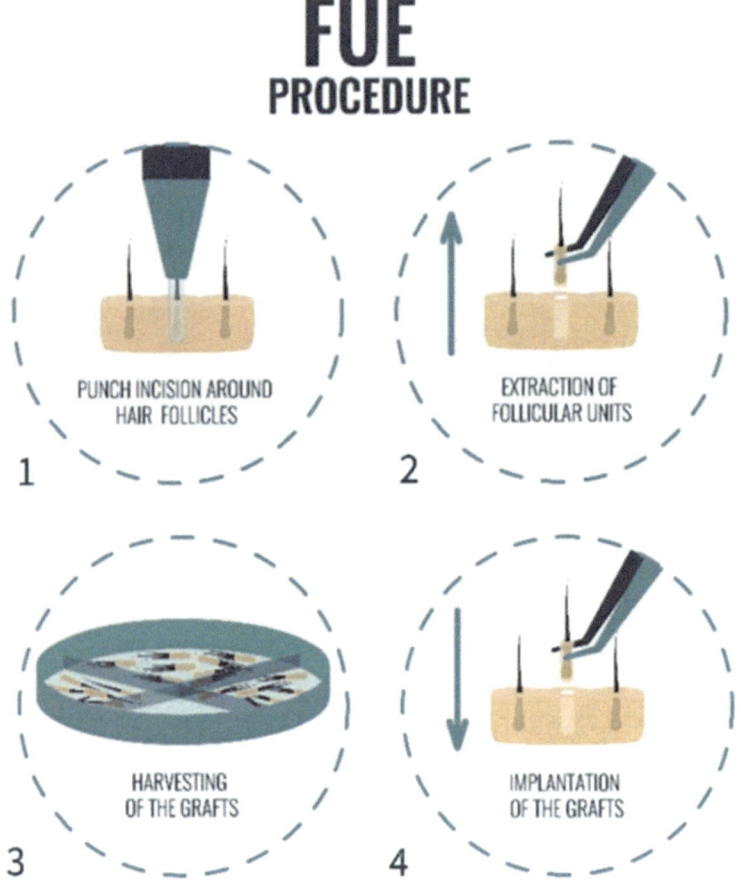

PUNCH INCISION AROUND HAIR FOLLICLES	EXTRACTION OF FOLLICULAR UNITS
1	2
HARVESTING OF THE GRAFTS	IMPLANTATION OF THE GRAFTS
3	4

Follicular unit extraction (FUE) hair transplantation stages

Because the follicular unit is narrowest at the surface, one needs to use small micro punches of size 0.6-0.8 mm and therefore, the resulting scar is too small to be recognised. This has proven to be important in minimising the damage to the follicular units during extraction. Despite the advantages of the two-step procedure, some FUE tools such as the NeoGraft® and SmartGraft® systems still use only a sharp punch. Several commonly used FUE instruments, such as the SAFE System and the ARTAS Robotic Hair Transplant System, use a sharp/blunt dual punch mechanism.

FUE: The popularity of FUE hair transplantation has exploded in recent years, although FUT is still widely performed. Both procedures have their advantages and limitations for different types of patients, so the ability to offer both procedures are seen by many practitioners as essential to providing patients with the best surgical options. The main anatomical limitation of the technique is that it is not possible to identify the bulge of the hair from outside and hence the procedure is blind. Also, since the hairs with intact unit splay at the lower end and diverge in different directions, the process of extraction can result in a higher transection rate.

The procedure is also slow as each unit must be pulled out slowly. However, with experience, the hand-eye coordination and speed of the surgeon, transection rate can be improved. The question of which procedure should be performed for a patient is largely determined by factors such as the looseness of the scalp, the length of hair worn by the patient and the volume of hair desired in the hair restoration. See FUE versus FUT: comparison.

One of the main advantages is that it is easier to learn and nearly every hair transplant surgeon offers this type of technique. In this method, there is no permanent visible linear scar, but you may need to shave off most of your head to get the bet result. It is less expensive than FUT and has become immensely popular in medical tourist countries, especially Turkey and Greece. One of the main advantages is that it is easier to learn and nearly every hair transplant surgeon offers this type of technique.

In this method, there is no permanent visible linear scar, but you may need to shave off most of your head to get the bet result. It is less expensive than FUT and has become immensely popular in medical tourist countries, especially Turkey and Greece. Robert M. Bernstein, clinical professor of dermatology at the College of Physicians and Surgeons of Columbia University in New York must be recognised for his pioneering work in FUT and FUE. He is the recipient of the Platinum Follicle Award for outstanding achievement in scientific and clinical research in hair restoration. This is the highest honour awarded by the International Society of Hair Restoration Surgery. Dr Bernstein received his dermatologic training at the Albert Einstein College of Medicine in New York, where he served as chief resident. He graduated with honours from Tulane University, achieving the status of Tulane Scholar. He received the degree of Doctor of Medicine at the University of Medicine and Dentistry of NJ, where he was the recipient of the Dr Bleiberg Award for 'Excellence in Dermatology'.

In 2000, Bernstein cautioned on the excessive use of adrenaline in hair transplants in the paper, *Limiting Epinephrine in Large Hair Transplant Sessions*. He warned that remarkably high concentrations of epinephrine to control bleeding during a large follicular unit hair transplant may be dangerous.

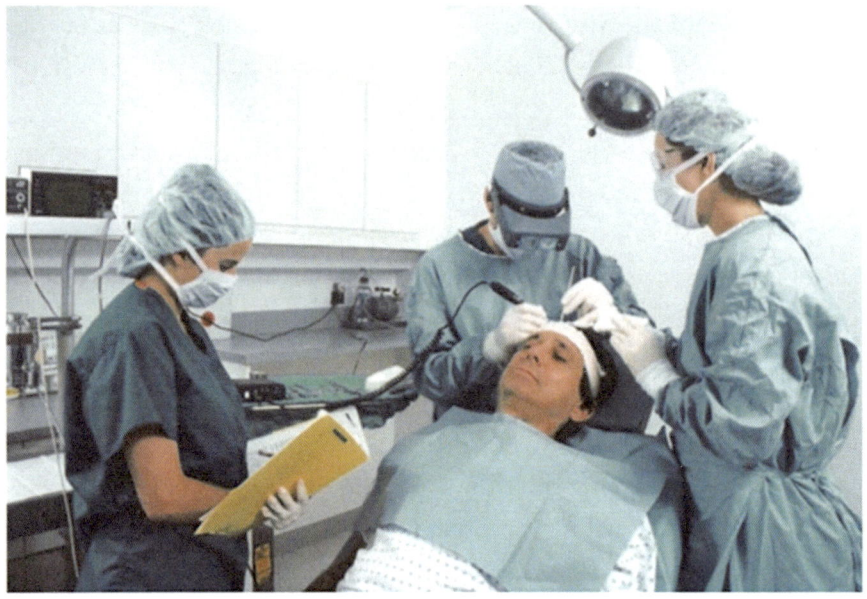

He described other ways to control bleeding in hair transplant procedures of up to 2,400 grafts without the need for these high concentrations of epinephrine, which he claimed may cause palpitations, anxiety, irregular heart rhythms and increase the risk of the hair restoration surgery. In 2005, he presented 'New Instrumentation for Follicular Unit Extraction' at the 13th Annual Scientific Meeting of the International Society of Hair Restoration Surgery in Sydney, Australia. His specially designed instrument minimised trauma to hair follicles, a major limitation in FUE. The research was published the following year in *Hair Transplant Forum International*. In this year, Ailesbury Clinic introduced FUE hair transplant to both its Dublin and Cork clinics.

More recently, Rassman has experimented using a robot for hair transplantation (now the commercial ARTAS System). This Robotic Follicular Unit Extraction (R-FUE) is a surgical hair restoration procedure in which a physician-controlled, computerised device uses a precision three-dimensional optical system to locate and harvest follicular units directly from the donor area. Restoration Robotics Inc. introduced robotic hair transplantation to the field of hair restoration in 2011 when it launched the first ARTAS robot. During the nineties, Bernstein completed many papers in FUT. Rassman in later years developed the FOX procedure, heralding a new surgical hair restoration procedure without strip harvesting.

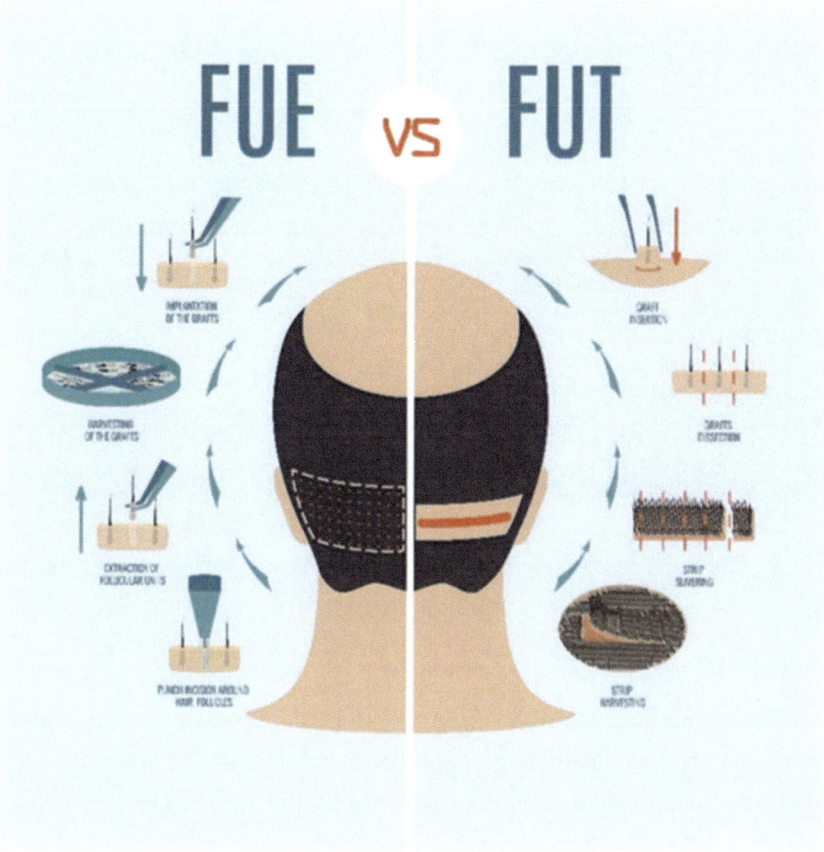

Follicular unit extraction (FUE) and follicular unit transplantation (FUT) comparison

The FOX procedure, also known as FUE (Follicular Unit Extraction), FUSE (Follicular Unit Separation Extraction) method. Dr Orentreich's idea of harvesting grafts directly from the back of the scalp, rather than harvesting from a donor strip, never fully dissipated even though FUT was the procedure of choice for most patients.

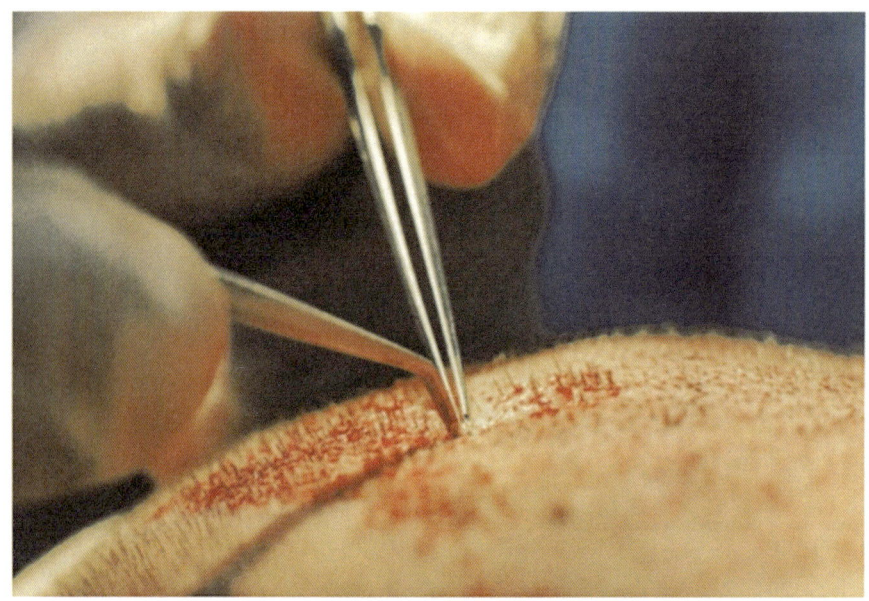

Transplanting individual follicles

ARTAS® Robotic Hair System

Follicular Unit Extraction (R-FUE) is a surgical hair restoration procedure in which a physician-controlled, computerised device uses a precision three-dimensional optical system to locate and harvest follicular units directly from the donor area. Restoration Robotics Inc. introduced robotic hair transplantation to the field of hair restoration in 2011 when it launched the first ARTAS robot. The ARTAS robot is now probably the most advanced technology in hair restoration aids the physician in the extraction of grafts and the creation of recipient sites with precision and consistency that surpasses manual techniques. An image-guided robotic arm deploys the dual-needle punch, ensuring accuracy in each harvest. The robot can be used in patients with different hair characteristics, from different ethnic backgrounds and from different parts of their scalp. Although only approved for use in men, it is effective for patients of both sexes. Dr Bernstein was an early adopter of robotic technology, and his hair restoration facility became one of the first hair restoration facilities in the world to use robotic technology for hair restoration.

Dr Bernstein has worked with Restoration Robotics on enhancements to the ARTAS robot and development of new capabilities since it became commercially available. Bernstein Medical serves as a beta-test site for developments and upgrades to the robotic system. In2013, Restoration Robotics, in conjunction with Dr Bernstein, launched the recipient site creation capability of the ARTAS robot. This feature allowed the robot to perform one more key step in the hair transplant procedure, the creation of recipient sites in the balding areas where follicular unit grafts are placed. Dr Bernstein discussed robotic recipient site creation in his 2014 publication in Hair Transplant Forum International, *Robotic Recipient Site Creation in Hair Transplantation*. In this process, the physician programs the robot with the specific angle and direction of the incisions, the site depth, average density, and total number. The robot then executes this plan while the computer keeps track of the total number of sites.

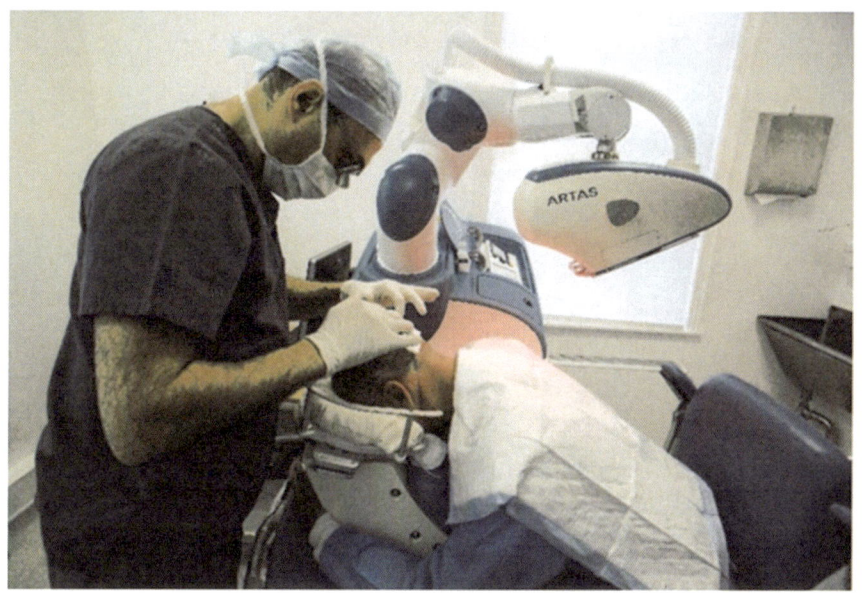

ARTAS robotic hair transplant machine being used at Farjo Hair Institute

He also introduced the Long-Hair Robotic FUE technique in 2015 to solve the short-term cosmetic problem of having to shave the patient's entire donor area for an FUE procedure. In Long-Hair FUE, the physician harvests follicular units from a patient's donor area with longer hair by taping the long hair up and shaving one or more strips in the back and sides of the scalp. After harvesting follicular units from those shaved strips, the remaining hair can be lowered, completely covering, and camouflaging the post-operative site. Long-Hair FUE, the physician harvests follicular units from a patient's donor area with longer hair by taping the long hair up and shaving one or more strips in the back and sides of the scalp. After harvesting follicular units from those shaved strips, the remaining hair can be lowered, completely covering, and camouflaging the post-operative site.

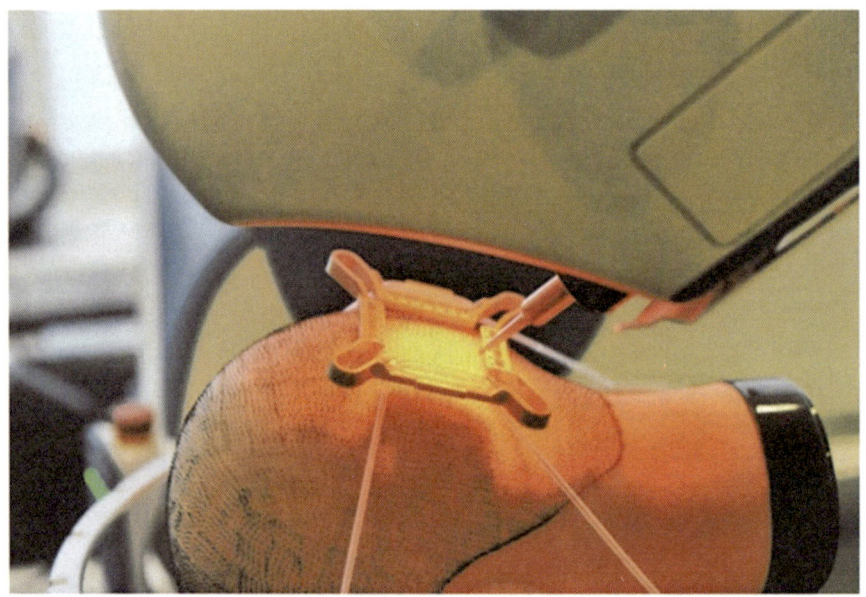

ARTAS® robotic procedure

In 2016, Dr Bernstein published a paper on his concept of Robotic Follicular Unit Graft Selection. He also developed an algorithm by which the ARTAS system can automatically select follicular units for harvesting based on the number of hairs they contain. By adding this capability, robotic procedures can harvest more hair while minimising wounding. As a result of robotic graft selection, robotic FUE can produce greater hair density while leaving fewer scars in the donor area. Restoration Robotics released another milestone upgrade to the ARTAS system in 2017 with ARTAS 9x. The system includes hardware and software modifications such as a robotic base extender, more comfortable headrest and halo, white light LED, colour camera and tensioner, 20-gauge harvesting needle, improved scar detection, faster harvesting and improved ARTAS Hair Studio software.

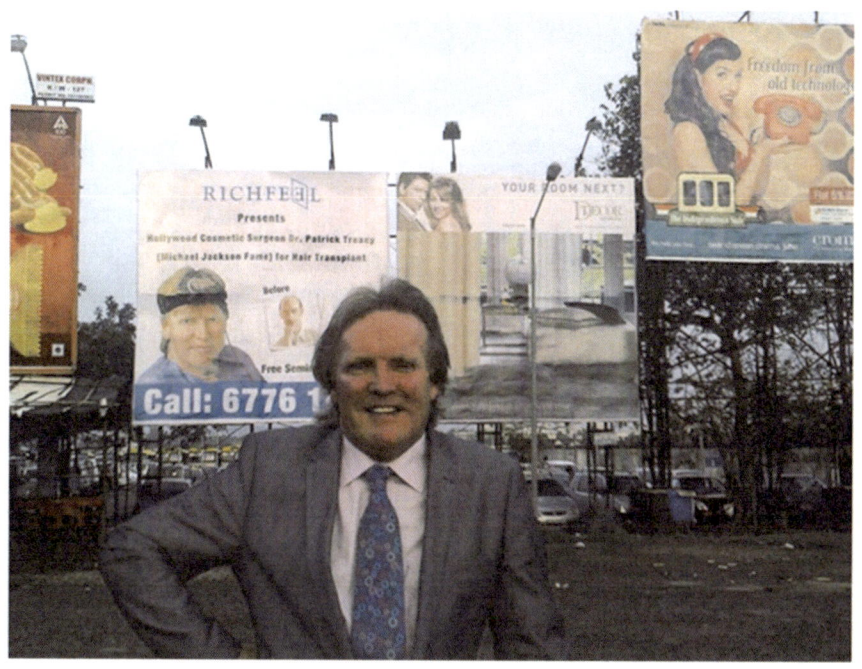

The author demonstrating Ailesbury FUE transplant techniques in Mumbai, India(2012)

The ARTAS 9x software has scar detection capability that can detect areas with low (or no) hair density and block out those areas from harvesting. This step was done manually with other versions of the robot. The ARTAS 9x robot was modified to use a white LED light instead of a red light as it was easier to look at. By switching to the white light, dissected follicular units can be removed from the scalp while the robot is working. These, along with many other components of the robotic system, aim to improve yield and minimise transection, leading to increasingly better outcomes.

The SMART® Hair Transplant Technique

The SMART® Hair Transplant is an award-winning multi procedure hair restoration technique developed by the author that combines PRP stem cell technology, motorised micro punch extraction, anabolic nutrition and LLLT red light phototherapy to shorten the time required for complete hair growth and increase follicular graft survival. I have been testing the use of platelet rich plasma (PRP) in hair transplant surgery since 2009 when Carlos Uebel from Brazil and Joseph Greco from Florida reported improved healing and graft survival with use of this method. Platelets, key players in the body's wound healing mechanism are activated to release various hair growth factors that stimulate the healing process. These factors stimulate new blood vessels to form (angiogenesis) and collagen to be produced. Cells are stimulated to divide and go into action surrounding the wound. PRP reduces infection and offers a minimally invasive surgical procedure that benefits from a shortened recovery time, increased graft survival and reduced risk of complications.

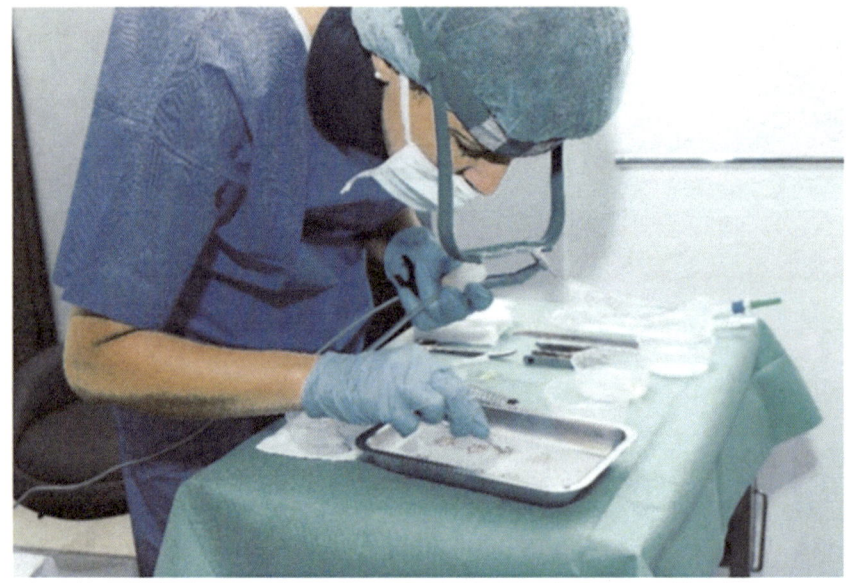

Harvesting the grafts in FUE

Motorised micro punch extraction

The SMART® Hair Implant surgeon uses a small punch (a sort of a special needle) (0,72 mm diameter) with a motorised drill to remove individual follicular units, eliminating the need for excision of skin from the back of the head. Punch gauges can vary. Typical ranges are .75mm to 1.0mm. Small punches are great for minimizing scarring but are not suitable for larger 2,3 and 4-hair grafts. Using a .75mm punch to extract a triple-hair graft could result in partial or full transection of the graft. Something like a .9mm gauge would be more suited.

Respectively, using a larger gauge can preserve yield levels but also create scars larger than desired and damage surrounding follicles. One size does not fit all.

Anabolic nutrition

Hair is made from nutrients in the body, and nutritional deficiencies can cause hair damage and hair loss. For example, biotin deficiencies have been linked to hair loss and skin disorders, and sufficient levels of the B vitamins are necessary for hair health and growth. Many Western diets are lacking in nutrients, and a poor diet may contribute to early onset of hair loss symptoms in people genetically prone to hair loss. Ailesbury Clinic uses Help Hair™ Shake which contains nutrients and herbs specifically selected for their positive effects on hair, including Niacin (vitamin B-3), Folate, Vitamin B-12, Biotin, Zinc, Manganese, Foti Root (Ho Shou Wu or Polygonum multiflorum) - a popular Chinese herb traditionally used to darken pre-mature gray hair, Kudzo Root - Chinese herb, Pumpkin Seed to help regulate testosterone levels. PABA, Chlorophyll to remove sebum, which carries DHT. As part of an overall hair loss program, Ailesbury Clinics put patients on a low anabolic profile by telling them to consider eliminating or reducing certain supplements in their diet. This includes using the SHAPIRO Chart and monitoring the use of anabolic steroids, creatine, Growth Hormone, Androstenedione, HCG diet or Whey Protein Isolate often found in body building additives.

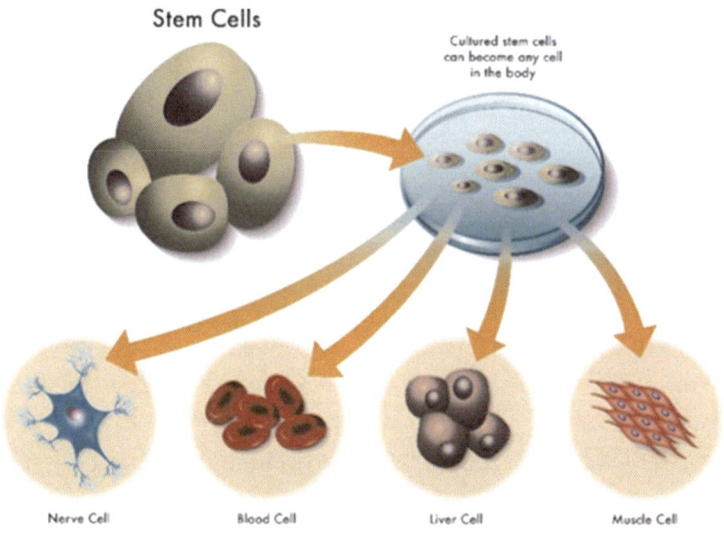

Stem Cell Technology

Red Light Phototherapy

The technique uses wavelengths with red light therapy in the range of 630 to 670 nanometres (nm) immediately post FUE procedure. Visible red light is capable of being absorbed by the molecules of the hair follicle and can stimulate the growth or re-growth of the hair following a natural biological reaction.

Red light is absorbed is because of an intracellular enzyme called cytochrome c, which is responsible for stimulating the hair follicle by sending it certain signals. Those signals promote gene activity and lower apoptosis (cell death regulated by the genes) as well as other reactions. This has been known since 1967 when it was accidentally discovered by a Hungarian scientist who noticed that exposed, shaved mice experience faster hair re-growth.

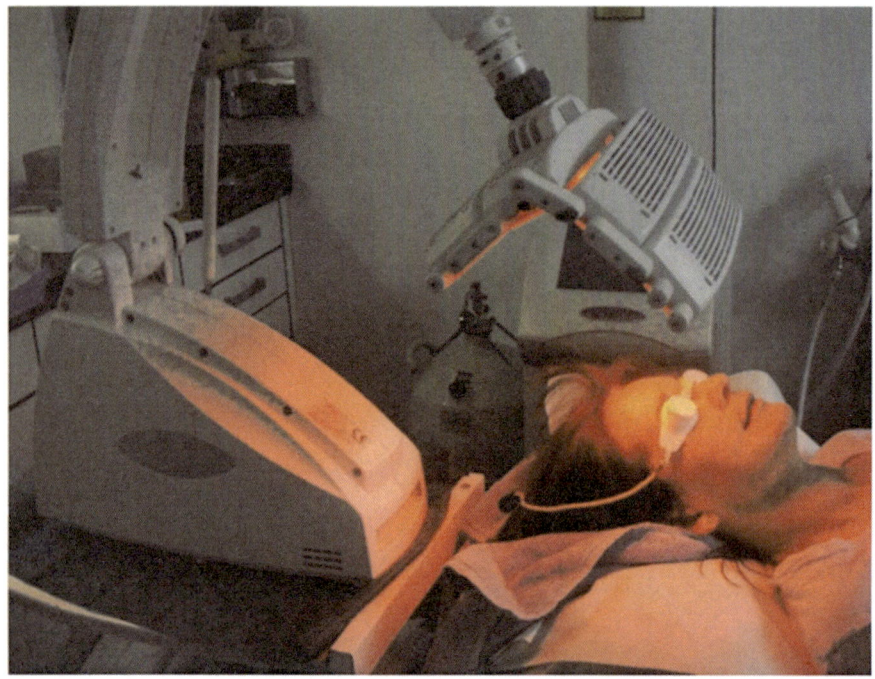

Transfer Method

Follicular Transfer is a modern hair restoration technique where hairs are transplanted in groups of 1-4 hairs - exactly as they grow in nature. It is a major advance over the older hair transplantation procedures that used larger grafts and often produced a pluggy, unnatural look. FT technique is a two-step procedure. where the aesthetic results mimic the way that hair grows in nature and will be undetectable as a hair transplant. During the first step, also called FUE

(Follicular Unit Extraction), direct extraction of selected individual follicular units from the patient's donor area is performed. allowing the surgeon to control the potential problem of visibly lower donor area density after the procedure. The Second part of the procedure is the Follicular Implantation, during which the surgeon implants the grafts with a predetermined density, pattern, andangle in a realistic hair pattern.

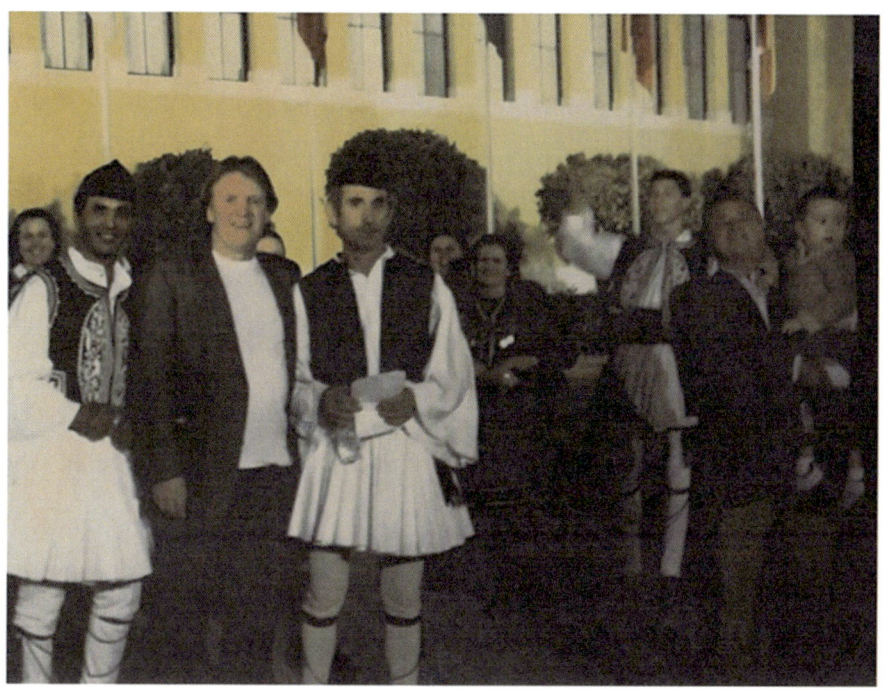

The author with Mr Kostas Giotis (CEO DHI) at the Aegean Hair Transplant conference (Athens 2007)

Chapter 7: Facial Threads

The barbed polypropylene suture is a versatile, easy-to-use means of facial soft tissue remodeling and repositioning that is effective in the malar and submalar areas when used alone or as a component of more extensive facial rejuvenation. This suspension technique may be combined with other soft tissue augmentation modalities, such as malar implants or soft tissue fillers, and with ancillary procedures such as chemical peeling or laser resurfacing. When used as the sole method of tissue repositioning, surgical and recovery time is short.

The History of Facial Threads

Modern barbed suture can trace its origins to Dr John H. Alcamo, who submitted his idea to the US patent office on 13 August 1956 and was issued US patent number 3,123,077 on 3 March 1964 for "… a suture so formed that it prevents slippage in sutured incisions or wounds…" It was the same year that Egypt seized the Suez Canal; Britain and France responded with force. Although Dr Alcamo described the design for this suture, it was not until 1967 that a practical medical use was found for them. It was the same year that Apollo 1: US astronauts Gus Grissom, Ed White and Roger Chaffee were killed when fire broke out in their Apollo spacecraft during a launchpad test. In that year, Dr A.R. McKenzie reported using barbed sutures in vitro in human cadavers and in vivo in dogs for the repair of long flexor tendons. Between 1967 and 1994, many patents were filed for their use and application in various fields of medicine.

In 1999, Dr Harry J. Buncke received a US patent for "several surgical procedures for binding together living tissue using one-way sutures having barbs on their exterior surfaces and a needle on one or both ends". It was the same year that NATO began Operation Allied Force, launching air strikes against Belgrade for 78 consecutive days until the president of Serbia, Slobodan Milošević, decided enough was enough and relented.

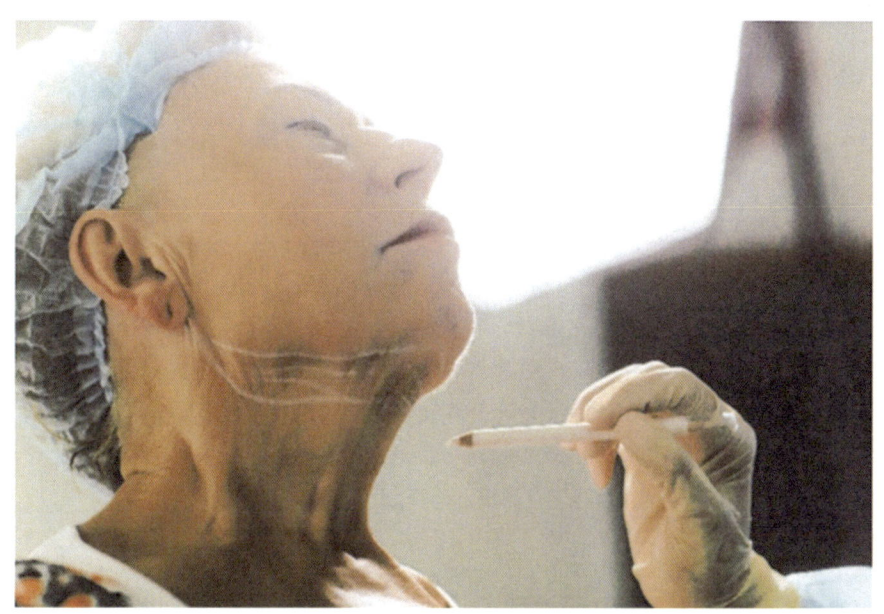

Marking out for a Thread lift

Buncke, who has been called the 'Father of Microsurgery' for his contributions to reconstructive microsurgical procedures, was an American plastic surgeon and served as a clinical professor of surgery at Stanford University. He also was a past president of the American Society for Surgery of the Hand, the International Society of Reconstructive Microsurgery, and the American Association of Plastic Surgery. His patents were acquired by Quill Medical in 2002, the same year that Tamil Tigers and the Sri Lankan government signed a ceasefire agreement, ending 19 years of civil war. Quill Medical was acquired by Angiotech Pharmaceuticals in 2006 and, with Dr Gregory Ruff, produced the Quill™ Knotless Tissue-Closure Device.

Meanwhile, in 2002, two doctors, Russian Marlen Sulamanidze and French Pierre Fournier, published a sentinel paper in *Journal of Dermatological Surgery* on introducing a new type of facelift using barbed threads, entitled *Removal of facial soft tissue ptosis with special threads*. They followed it three years later with another publication in *Otolaryngologic Clinics of North America* entitled *Facial lifting with 'APTOS' threads*. I am sure the name cleverly came from 'Anti Ptosis'

Marlen Sulamanidze, was born in Georgia in 1947. In 1972 he graduated from the Irkutsk Medical University. From 1974 to 1984 his specialization was maxillofacial surgery and later he started specializing in plastic and aesthetic surgery first in Georgia and from 1993 in Moscow. These events were witnessed in Singapore by plastic surgeon Dr Woffles Wu, who felt that the APTOS procedure gave more of a face-firming than a face-lifting effect. He was critical about the short-barbed sutures with no stable fixation point and decided to develop his own. His bidirectional barbed sutures were effectively a type of sling that was folded on itself and had a stable fixation point in the deep temporal fascia. He claimed this method conferred greater lifting power as it had a higher pull tension, and it was more logical to suspend the loose facial tissues to the dense and immovable fibrous temporal fascia. He called it the WAPTOS (Woffles-APTOS) procedure in acknowledgment of Sulamanidze's APTOS procedure.

Wu was born in Singapore, but he grew up in London. He once told me in Paris that his mother affectionately nicknamed him 'Woffles' after a rabbit from the novel *The Magic Faraway Tree* by Enid Blyton. Thankfully, he grew to accept this nickname. Wu is a Fellow of the Royal College of Surgeons of Edinburgh and has worked under Prof S T Lee, a cleft palate surgeon. In 1990, he won the Young Surgeon of the Year Award for his research on nasal anatomy. Woffles says that Sulamanidze saw him present the WAPTOS procedure at the International Confederation of Plastic and Reconstructive Surgery (IPRAS) meeting in Sydney, Australia, in 2003 and he encouraged him to call it the 'Woffles Lift' because the technique was different from his APTOS technique. Interestingly, it is said that Nicanor G. Isse from Newport Beach, California, was also in the audience and he was inspired to make his own version of a monodirectional barbed thread anchored at the temple via a surgical approach and to use it in conjunction with the endoscopic face-lift technique he had developed. Wu and Isse subsequently presented their results in a panel discussion at the Annual American Society of Aesthetic Plastic Surgeons (AASPS) meeting in Vancouver, 2004. In 2005, Isse presented his results to the *Journal of Aesthetic Surgery* in a paper titled *Elevating the midface with barbed polypropylene sutures*. His thread design was later acquired by the Contour Thread Company. These were the first thread sutures that I used.

With the Woffles Lift Version 1, the loop of the sling was in the distal face and the two free ends were tied together at the temple.

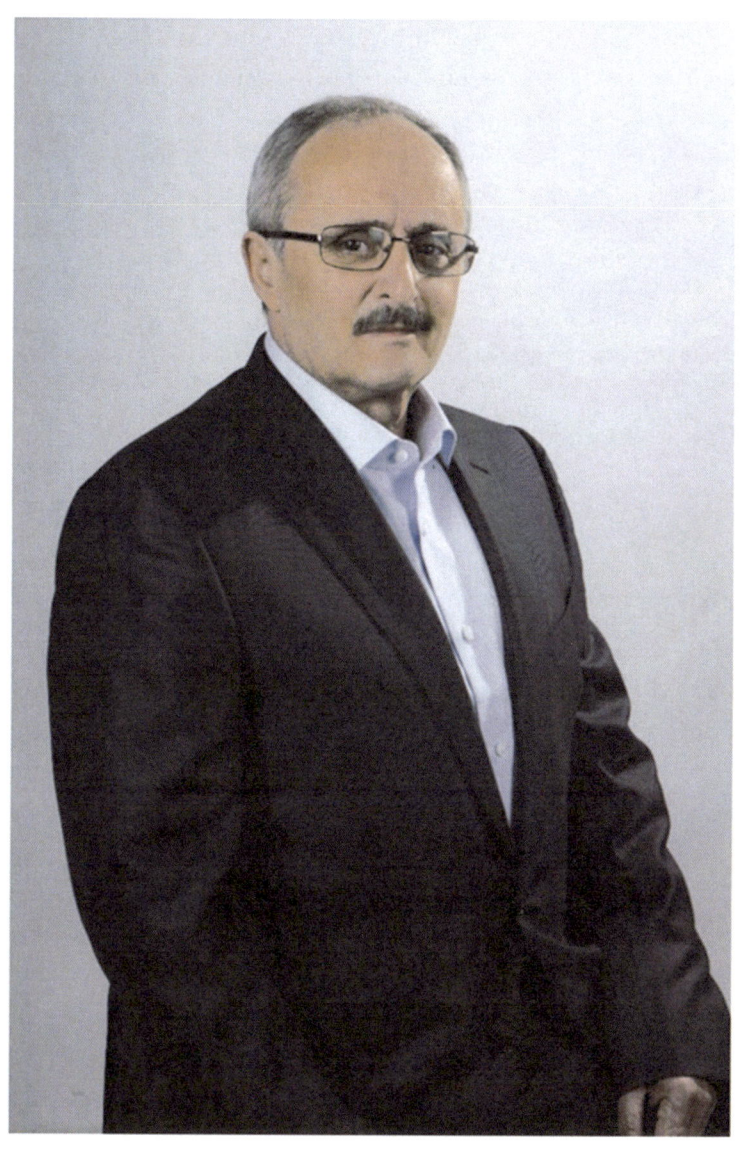

Dr Marlen Sulamanidze, inventor of Aptos technique

This occasionally gave rise to knot palpability or extrusion so he decided to invert the suture slings such that the loop of the sling would be embedded superiorly in the temporal fascia, with the free ends of the thread oriented distally. This conferred better lifting of the soft tissues in the lower face and avoided the need to tie any knots and had a lower complication rate (~2%).

He claims that he has not encountered any problems of granuloma, infection, or thread extrusion since then. In 2009, Covidien introduced V-Loc™ (Covidien Healthcare, Mansfield, MA) unidirectional barbed suture with a fixed loop, and in 2013, both Angiotech Pharmaceuticals and Ethicon Endo-

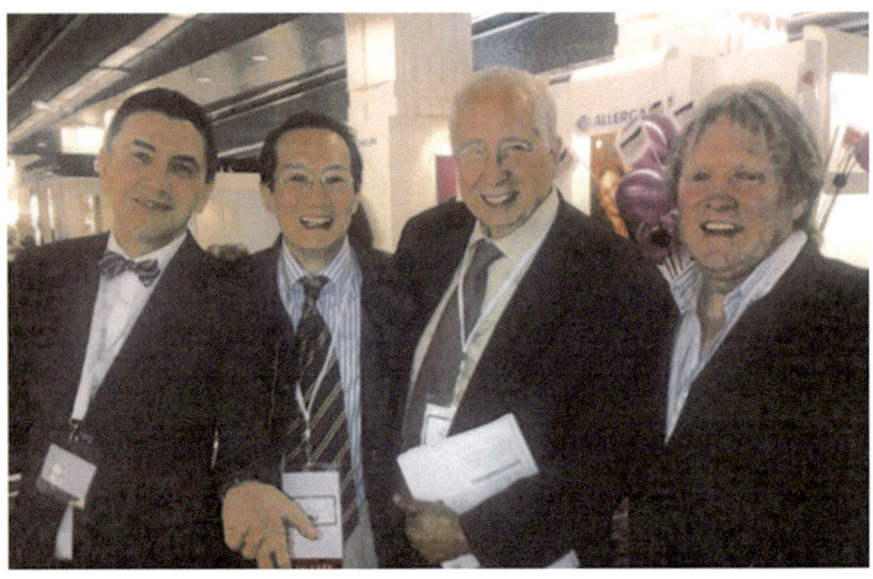

Dr Woffles Wu (Singapore), Dr Michael Scheflan (Tel Aviv), Dr Patrick Treacy (Dublin) IMCAS Congress Paris 2018

Surgery (Cincinnati, OH) introduced unidirectional barbed sutures with a variable loop at the end for facilitated fixation. Over the past decade, Marlen Sulamanidze and his sons developed different thread and techniques, including microscopic barbed (Aptos Thread), double-pointed needles (Aptos Needle) elastic needles (Aptos Spring), and more recently (Aptos Nano visage) threads. They have contributed to the history of threads, sufficiently lifting ptosis of the face and neck with minimal cuts or with tiny cutaneous incisions.

In 2010, Silhouette Soft® thread lifting was introduced. This was a non-surgical facelift with a unique double lifting and regenerating effect. This new concept in facial rejuvenation is a 30-minute procedure that results in a refined, lifted, and natural appearance restoring the 'triangle of youth' without resorting to surgery. Silhouette Soft gave immediate results by redefining and adding volume, and to continue to restore shapeliness for 18 -24 months.

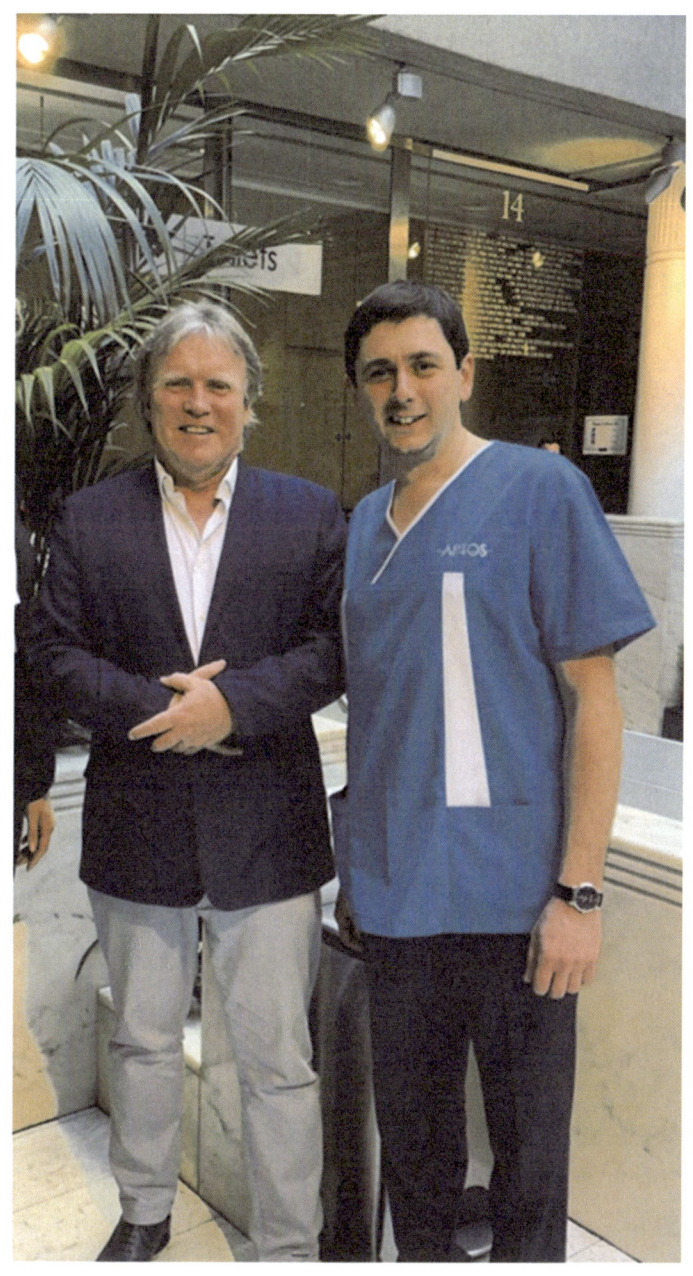

The author with Dr Gorgio Sulamanidze (London)

At the 2019 Royal Society of Medicine Aesthetic Medicine conference, I had a special section on threads. The innovators of the APTOS® technique, Mr George Sulamanidze and his wife, Dr Albina Kajaia, from Tbilisi, gave a live demonstration of a non-surgical facelift – threads versus fillers – and Dr Kwon, the President, International Association of Aesthetic and Antiaging Medicine (South Korea) and inventor of the Ultra-V PCL Thread Lifting Technique provided a workshop on thread lifting for face and for nose procedure Associate Professor Ivor Lim, plastic surgeon and group chief medical officer, Cell Research Corporation, Singapore, gave a talk on the latest trends in stem cells research. To complete the day, my research on the PLEASE Technique won the Royal Society of Medicine Aesthetic 11 Conference Poster Award 2019.

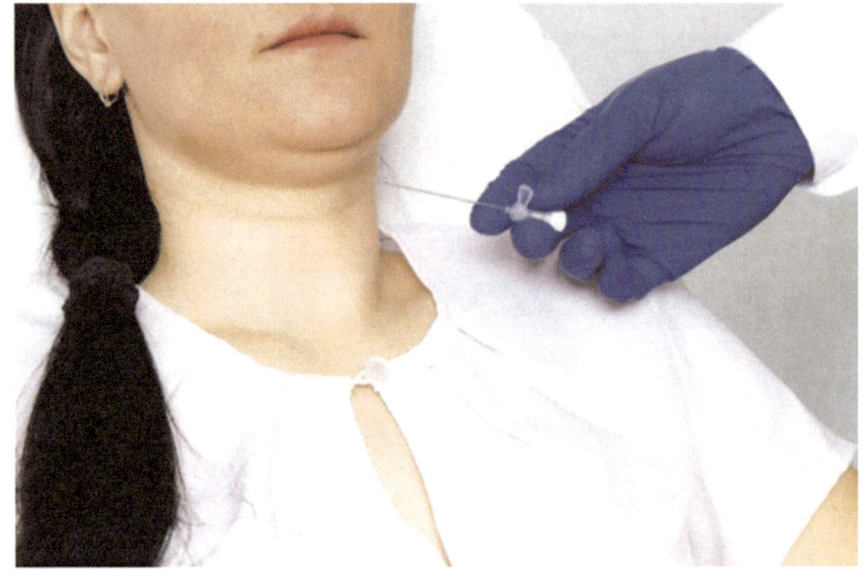

Placing Silhouette Soft® Threads

'Lifting Lateral Brow Ptosis with Contour® Threads'

A female presented with a left sagging of the upper eyelid (lateral brow ptosis) following a brain surgery procedure (minifrontal craniotomy) for an aneurysm repair. This procedure had resulted in sagging of the upper eyelid caused her to have an aged, sad, and tired appearance to her face. She denied any headaches or ocular fatigue, although she did describe a small deficit in her visual field. Otherwise, everything was normal.

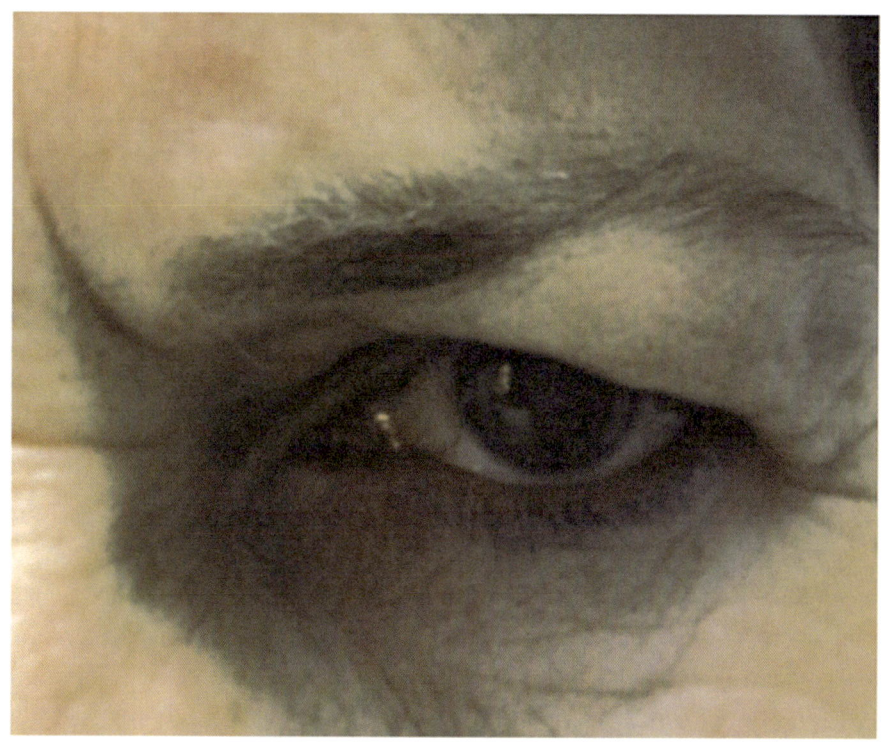

Patient with sagging of the upper eyelid (lateral brow ptosis) post-surgery

There was no loss of sensation in the resultant scar as the supratrochlear and supraorbital sensory nerves innervate the central and lateral forehead as well as portions of the anterior scalp. On examination it was obvious that the resultant damage to part of her facial nerve had cause marked descent of the periorbital soft tissues of the brow with a moderate degree of upper eyelid dermatochalasis, a medical condition, defined as an excess of skin in the upper or lower eyelid, also known as "baggy eyes." It may be either an acquired or a congenital condition. Her cranial examination including facial nerve function showed an inability to elevate her left eyebrow and the absence of Bell's phenomenon. It was evident she had post procedure damage to the frontal branch of the facial nerve causing inability to control the frontalis muscle. The procedure was performed with the patient under local anaesthesia and no sedation was required. A thorough past medical and facial surgical history was obtained. The patient's visual acuity, hairline position and brow symmetry were noted. We also noted skin quality and rhytid depth in the medial and lateral forehead. The residual motor function was noted prior to the procedure. Document the motor. The patient's face was marked preoperatively to determine the appropriate vector of the thread and its end fixation points. The presence of prominent dynamic and static rhytides in the patient's forehead was noted and influenced incision placement. The location of the hairline was noted. The superior border of the thread was placed above the hairline and exited at the level of the lateral brow. The sutures were trimmed, and the proximal ends were secured on the deep temporal fascia reinforced with Vicryl interrupted sutures.

Discussion

The main etiologic factors in brow ptosis are gravity and age. The aging face undergoes a loss of tone from a diminution in the amount of elastin and collagen in the skin. Because the lateral brow has fewer attachments to the periosteum and has no underlying frontalis muscle, it usually descends more than the medial brow. *Brow ptosis* can happen secondary to paralysis of the frontalis muscle as in this case, but also because of Bell's palsy, acoustic neuroma or even birth trauma. Medical causes include conditions such as myasthenia gravis, myotonic and oculopharyngeal dystrophy. Since the invention of the first barbed (short) suture by Sulamanidze in the late 1990s, different techniques have been described including Woffles (long) thread lifting, Waptos suture lifting, Isse unidirectional barbed threads lifting, and silhouette lifting. However, essentially, there are two types of barbed threads which are available. These are:

a. Bi-directional threads, with no anchoring points, inserted within a hollow needle and placed in such a manner that the thread cannot move either way because of the two-way direction of barbs fixing it nicely. Examples are the APTOS® threads.

b. Uni-directional barbed threads, which are anchored at a higher-level fixation point. Examples are the Contour® and Silhouette® threads. Barbs along the thread act as cogs to grasp lift and suspend a relaxed facial area. The barbs open like an umbrella to form a support structure that lifts the sagging tissue. This creates tension in the thread, and the tension lifts the skin tissue. Collagen formation occurs around the threads and their cogs or barbs, producing an increasing effect.

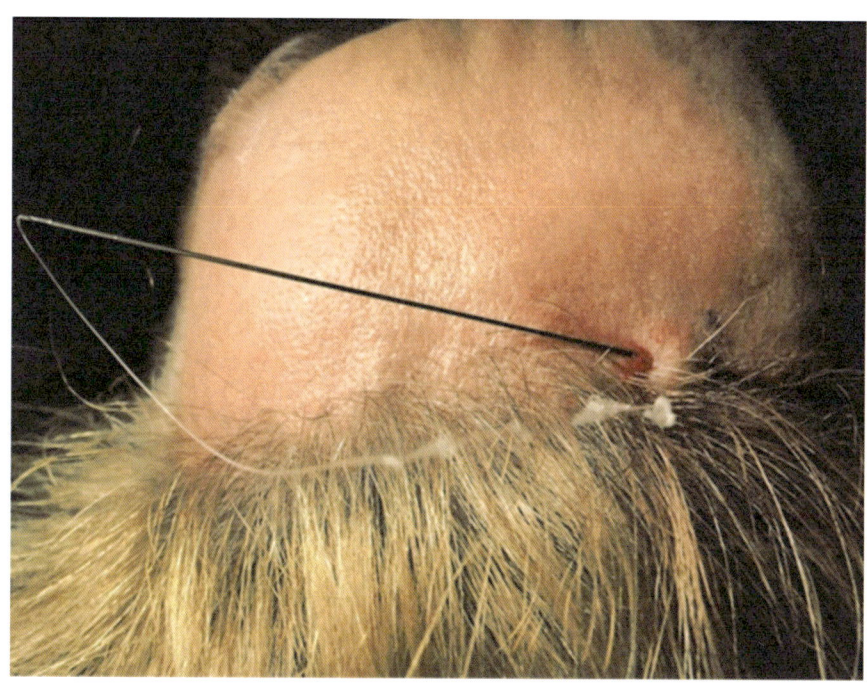

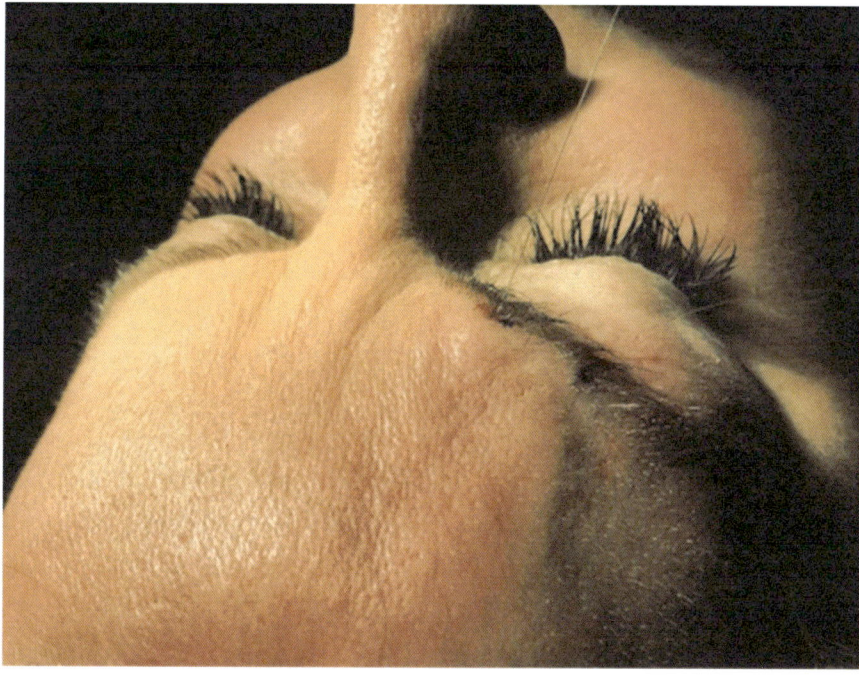

Chapter 8: Cosmeceuticals

Cosmeceuticals are products that have both cosmetic and therapeutic (medical or drug-like) effects and are intended to have a beneficial effect on skin health and beauty. Like cosmetics, they are applied topically as creams or lotions but contain active ingredients that influence skin cell function. The word describes a product that is a cross between a cosmetic and a pharmaceutical. A cosmeceutical is essentially a skincare product that contains a biologically active compound that is thought to have pharmaceutical effects on the skin.

A cosmeceutical is essentially a skincare product that contains a biologically active compound that is thought to have pharmaceutical effects on the skin. Both pharmaceutical and cosmeceutical grade skin care products actively effect skin at a cellular level, whereas cosmetic products have a shorter-term effect. They are usually used by doctors to restore pH, remove pigmentation, or restore the skin barrier. Cosmeceuticals must scientifically verify the claims stated on their packaging; as it is accepted that these formulations are backed by science, clinical studies, and rigorous testing. The main areas of concerns that these formulations address are ageing skin, sensitive/sensitized skin, sun damaged skin, acne/oily skin, loss of tone and elasticity, as well as superficial lines & wrinkles to encourage rapid cellular turnover that will renew and re-texturize the skin.

Peptides composed of chains of amino acids give proteins their structure, and transport nutrients and signal messengers to other cells. A peptide is a short chain made up of two or more amino acids. The amino acids are linked by a chemical bond called a peptide bond. When organized in complex structures (typically consisting of 50 or more amino acids), peptides then become proteins.

Proteins make up much of the body's tissues, organs, including skin. One of the most important skin proteins in collagen. 75% of our skin is made up of collagen protein.

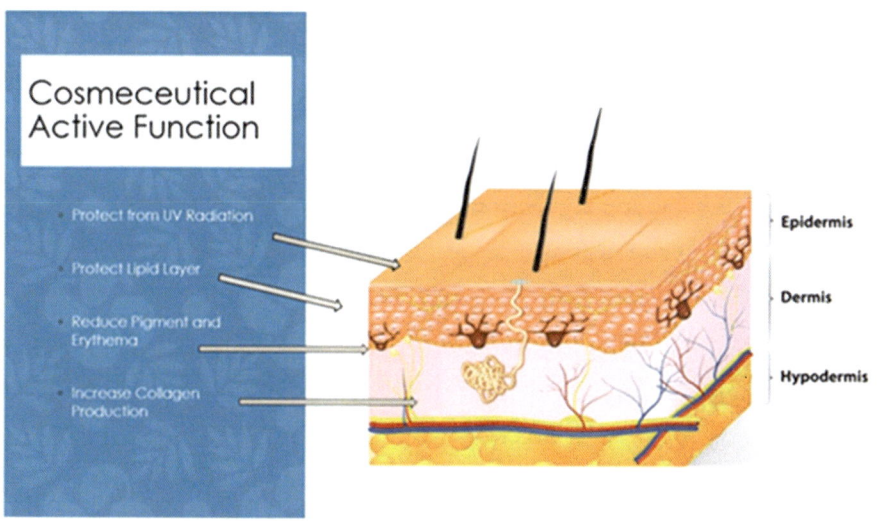

Types of Cosmeceutical Ingredients

- o Antioxidant
- o Anti-Inflammatory
- o Ascorbic Acid
- o Defensin
- o DNA Repair Enzymes
- o Growth Factors
- o Heparin Sulphate
- o Hyaluronic Acid
- o Niacinamide
- o Peptides
- o Retinoids
- o Stem Cells

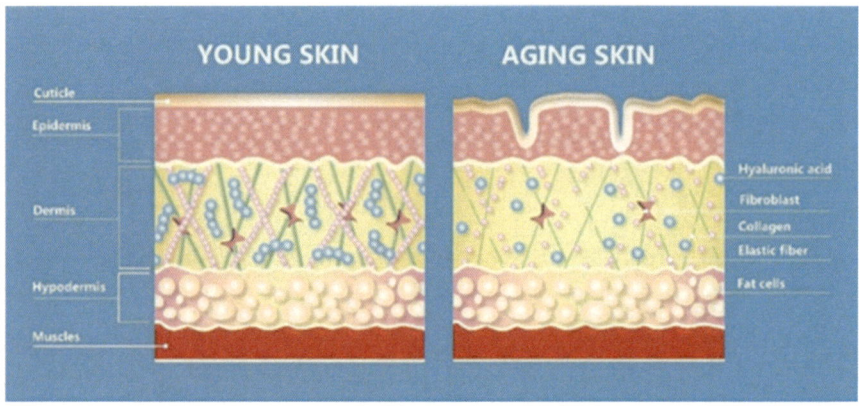

When targeting the above skin concerns, cosmeceuticals should improve skin rejuvenation, increase the firmness and the elasticity of skin, as well as improve skin complexion, and prevention and improve wrinkles. They also revive dull, tired looking skin, improve skin tone and elasticity, especially in the face, neck, and décolletage area. It is important to note that the producers of modern top-level skincare are now looking at the use of plant technology, fruit-based products and extracts as well as marine based formulations, these innovative formulations will give products an organic, green, healthy feel while still being performance driven. The aesthetic industry thrives on innovation and thanks to increased curiosity among men and women of all ages about what exactly goes into our skincare products as we look for cleaner scientifically proven plant-based technology that is result driven.

To train your skin and achieve skin health your cellular function requires a good workout, and your skin will feel it through desquamation, a gentle tingle and occasionally some patients may experience some redness, but this does not last for long. Change is simply happening to your skin. It is normal and part of the restorative powers of the skincare products that contain highly active ingredients to create performance driven formulations. Always follow the advice of your skincare professional and start your cosmeceutical skincare regimen slowly.

Key Cosmeceutical Ingredients

Below is a brief outline of key ingredients included in cosmeceutical, medical grade, top level advanced skincare that bring positive change to your skin when used correctly.

Glycolic acid
Citric acid
Lactic acid

AHAs

Malic acid
Tartaric acid
Mandelic acid

Alpha-Hydroxy acids (AHAs)

Products containing alpha-hydroxy acids have become increasingly popular in recent years. Skincare products with alpha-hydroxy acids help with fine lines and wrinkles, irregular pigmentation, sun damage, oil control, desquamation while also helping to shrink enlarged pores. Side effects of alpha-hydroxy acids include mild irritation and sun sensitivity. To avoid susceptibility to the sun, sunscreen should be applied in the morning. To help avoid skin irritation, start with a product with a maximum concentration of 10% to 15% AHA. To allow your skin to get used to alpha-hydroxy acids, you should initially apply the skin care product every other day, gradually working up to daily application.

Poly-Hydroxy acids

Polyhydroxy acids have a similar effect to alpha-hydroxy acids but are less likely to cause any irritation resulting in them being better option for those with rosacea, sensitive and reactive skin types. PHA's are chemical exfoliants – The most common being Gluconolactone and Lactobionic Acid. Again, like AHA's, poly-hydroxy acids help skincare penetrate deeper into the lower layers of the skin, exfoliating dead skin cells on the surface of the skin resulting in a more even skin tone and improved skin texture. PHA's also fight glycation which is a process that takes place when digested sugar permanently attaches to the collagen in your skin and can weaken it, along with elastin levels.

Beta-Hydroxy acid (Salicylic Acid)

Salicylic acid removes dead skin and improves the texture and colour of sun-damaged skin. It penetrates oil-laden hair follicle openings and, as a result, greatly helps with oily and acne prone skin types. Once salicylic acid is put to work on the skin, it penetrates the pores and dissolves the bonds between surface skin cells. It is this process that unclogs pores and makes it a great fighter against blemishes due to its antibacterial properties. Salicylic Acid is a deep cleaning ingredient that mops up excess oil and dirt of the skin and it is due to the exfoliating properties that makes it stand out on the skincare spectrum.

Hydroquinone

Skin care products containing hydroquinone are often called lightening agents. These skin care products are used to lighten hyperpigmentation, such as age spots and dark spots related to pregnancy or hormone therapy (melasma or chloasma). Your doctor can also prescribe a cream with a higher concentration of hydroquinone if your skin does not respond to over-the-counter treatments. Hydroquinone treatment goes hand in hand and is combined with sunscreen because sun exposure causes skin hyperpigmentation – the concern that hydroquinone is working on and creating solutions within the skin. It is best to test hydroquinone-containing products in a small area first to ensure there are no adverse reactions as some people are allergic to it. If you are allergic to hydroquinone you may benefit from use of products containing kojic acid.

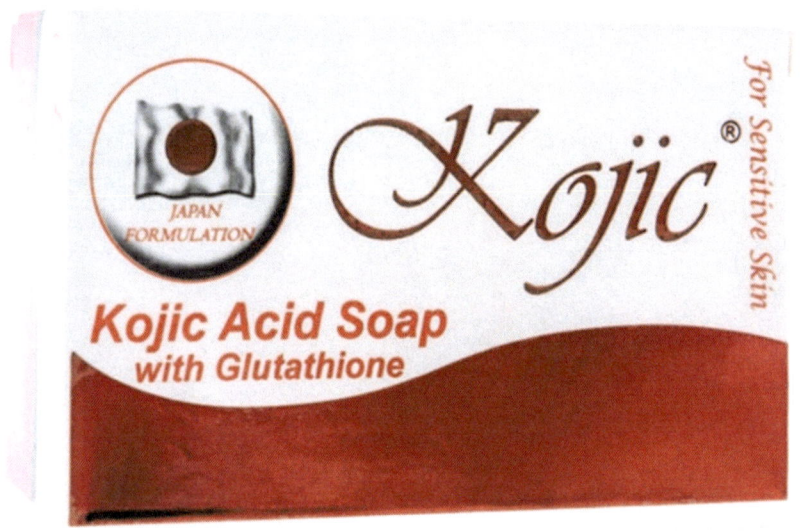

Kojic Acid

Kojic acid is also a remedy and solution for the treatment of pigment problems and age spots. Discovered in 1989, kojic acid works similarly to hydroquinone and is derived from a fungus, studies have shown that it is effective as a lightening agent, slowing production of melanin. With continued use, Kojic acid may make your skin more susceptible to sun also so the importance of SPF on the skin is a must when using this acid.

Retinoids

Examples of retinoids include retinol, retinal aldehyde, and retinyl esters. They are used to improve acne and acne scarring, mottled pigmentation, skin aging, skin texture, tone and colour, the skin's hydration levels are also increased with the use of retinoids. Retinol is derived from vitamin A, tretinoin, which is the active ingredient in prescription Retin-A® and Renova® creams, are a stronger version of retinol. Here are why skin responds to skin care products with retinol: vitamin A has a molecular structure that is small enough to get into the lower layers of skin. Retinyl palmitate is another ingredient related to retinol but is less potent to the skin's cells. Retinol is larger than all the other AHA and BHAs and is more lipid soluble than the acids.

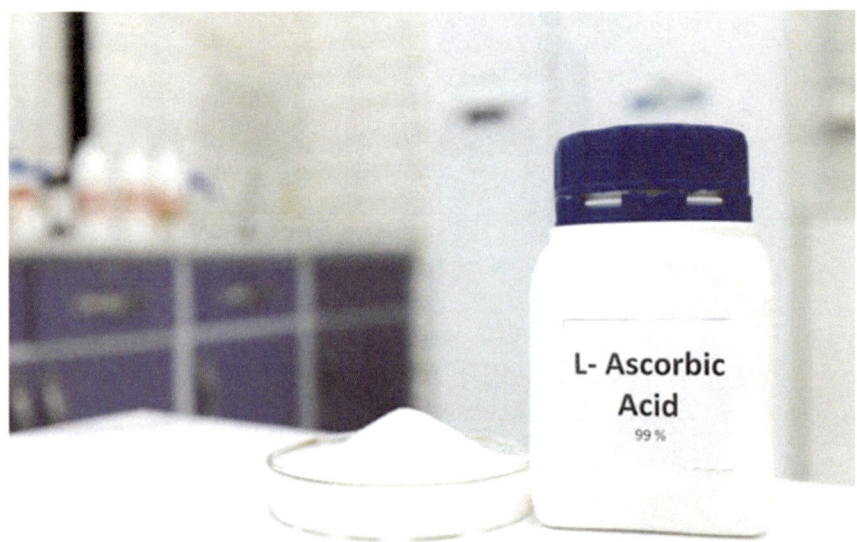

L-ascorbic acid

This is the only form of vitamin C that you should look for in your skin care products. There are many skin care products on the market today that boast vitamin C derivatives as an ingredient (magnesium ascorbic phosphate or ascorbyl palmitate, for example), but L-ascorbic acid is the only useful form of vitamin C in skin care products. With age and sun exposure, as collagen synthesis in the skin decreases, leading to wrinkles. Vitamin C is the only antioxidant proven to stimulate the synthesis of collagen, minimizing fine lines, scars, and wrinkles. Proven clinical studies suggests that L-ascorbic acid significantly improves the appearance of photodamaged skin. Initial use of vitamin C containing creams can cause slight stinging and/or redness, but these side effects generally subside with continued use.

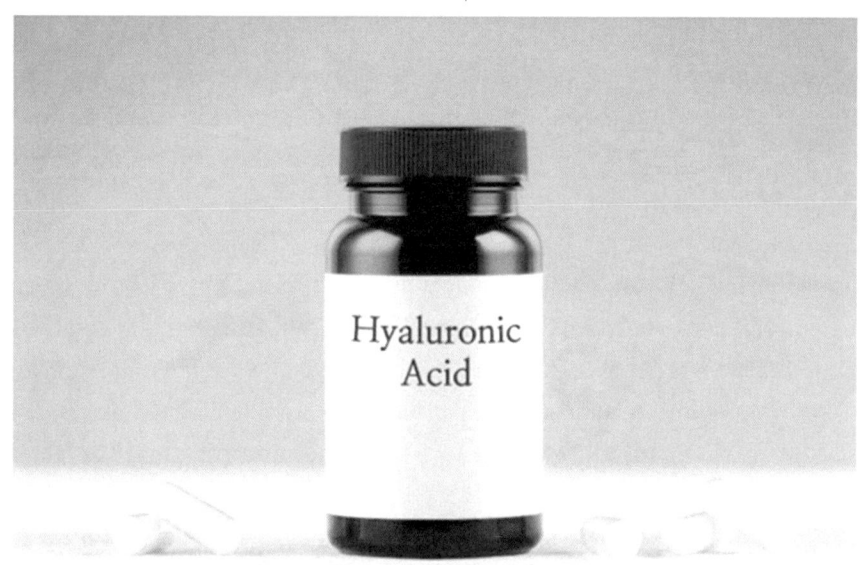

Hyaluronic acid

Skin care products containing this substance are often used with vitamin C products to assist in effective penetration. Hyaluronic acid (also known as a glycosaminoglycan) is best known for its ability to hydrate the skin resulting in fine lines and wrinkles being less pronounced. In news reports, you might have heard of hyaluronic acid as the "key to the fountain of youth." This is because the substance occurs naturally and quite abundantly in both humans and animals. Hyaluronic acid is a component of the body's connective tissues and is known to cushion and lubricate. As you age, however, the forces of nature diminish hyaluronic acid. Diet and smoking can also affect your body's level of hyaluronic acid over time. Skin care products with hyaluronic acid are most frequently used to treat dry, dehydrated, and ageing skin as it will improve the skins hydration and firmness.

Copper peptide

Copper peptide is often referred to as the most effective skin regeneration product, even though it has only been on the market since 1997. Here is why: Studies have shown that copper peptide promotes collagen and elastin production, acts as an antioxidant, and promotes production of glycosaminoglycans. Studies have also shown that copper-dependent enzymes increase the benefits of the body's natural tissue-building processes. The substance helps to firm, smooth, and soften skin, doing it in less time than most other anti-aging skin care products. Clinical studies have found that copper peptides also remove damaged collagen and elastin from the skin and scar tissue because they activate the skin's system responsible for those functions.

Alpha-lipoic acid

You may have heard of alpha-lipoic acid as "the miracle in a jar" for its anti-aging effects. It is a newer, ultra-potent antioxidant that helps fight future skin damage and helps repair past damage which is apparent when looking at top level skincare. Alpha-lipoic acid has been referred to as a "universal antioxidant" because it is soluble in both water and oil, which permits its entrance to all parts of the cell. Luc Rochette and Steliana Ghibu in a 2015 publication of *Can J Physiol Pharmacol* state alpha lipoic acid is a potent antioxidant with insulin-mimetic and anti-inflammatory activity. Due to this quality, it is believed that alpha-lipoic acid can provide the greatest protection against damaging free radicals when compared with otherantioxidants. Alpha-lipoic acid diminishes fine lines, it gives the skin a healthy glow, and boosts levels of other antioxidants, such as vitamin C. Nicholas V. Perricone, MD in the *Aesthetic Surgery Journal, 2000* stated topical alpha lipoic acid cream, at a concentration of 5%, resulted in the reduction of facial lines, and almost complete resolution of fine lines in the periorbital region and upper lip was noted in most patients.

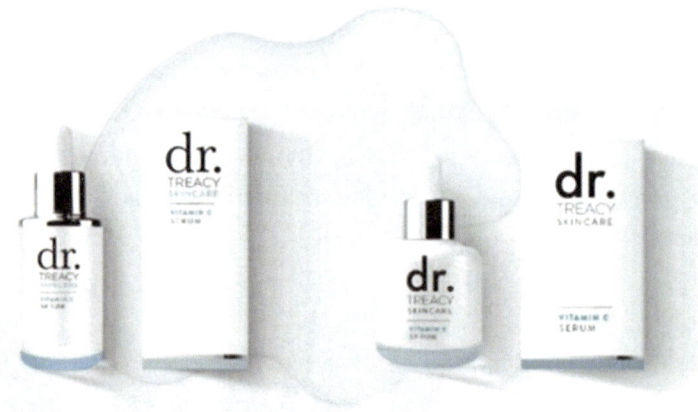

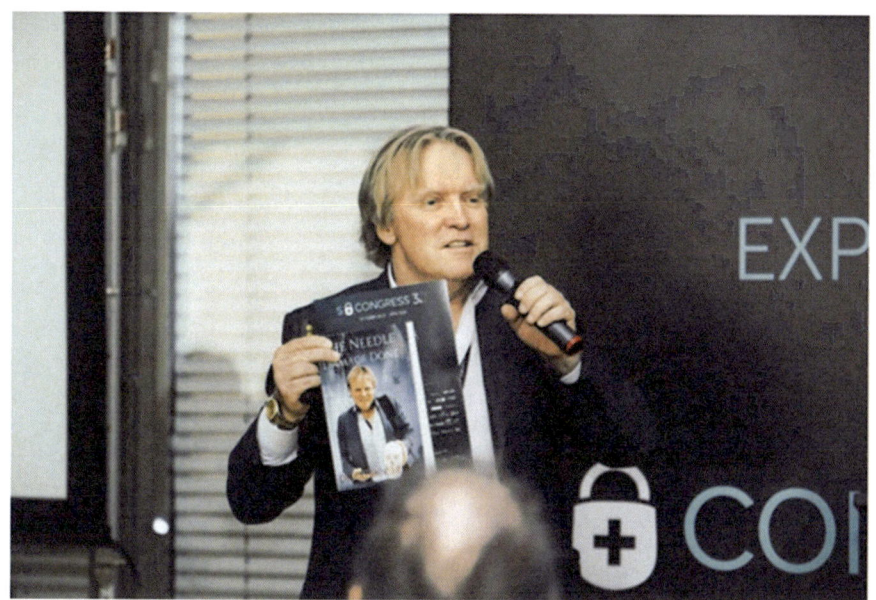

The author lecturing on cosmeceuticals

I am in the middle of launching new 'Dr Treacy' skin brand and thought it would be an interesting topic for one of the chapters of this book. I must give credit to my good friend, Dr Leslie Baumann's recent blog 'The interesting history of dermatologist-developed skin care' in Dermatology News. Leslie and I did a television show in Ireland at the start of aesthetic medicine and have lectured together in Miami since. Dr Baumann takes us on a journey over the years and recognises the criticism previously respected dermatologists endured from their colleagues whenever they promoted cosmeceutical products. This level of scrutiny deterred other doctors from entering the cosmeceutical business for many decades and left the skin care field wide open for imposters, charlatans, and non-dermatologists who had no real concern for either scientific efficacy or patient outcomes. Consequently, I will try and focus on some of the newer entrepreneurial dermatologists later in the chapter, but first want to start at the beginning. There is little doubt that ancient cultures were as preoccupied with the aesthetics of appearance as individuals are today.

I am also grateful to Dr Feliciano Blanco-Dávila and his colleague Prof. R. M. Chandler-Burns for their published discussions on the history of cosmetology and reference them when possible. Feliciano, in his well-researched article

Beauty and the Body: The Origins of Cosmetics published in Plastic and Reconstructive Surgery: March 2000 states that the practice of applying peels, ointments and tints to the body originated in prehistory.

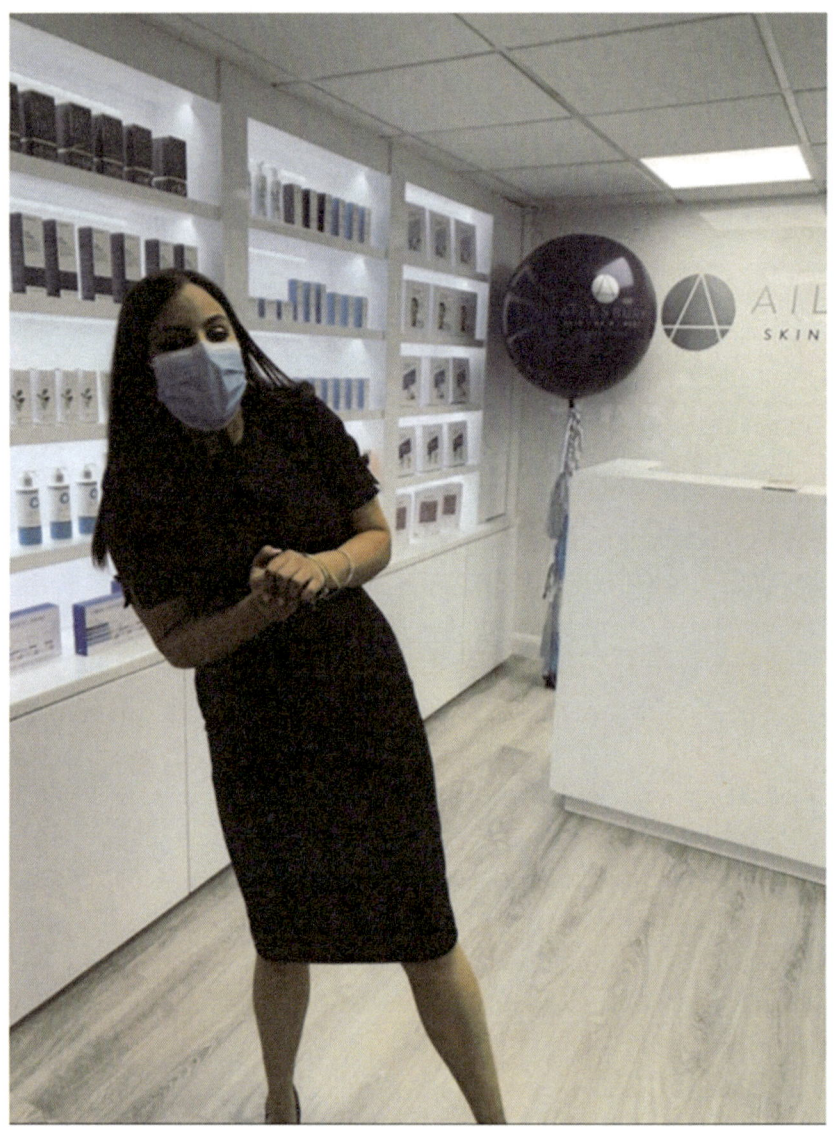

Dr Treacy skin brand at Ailesbury Dublin

Chapter 9: The Story of Cosmeceuticals

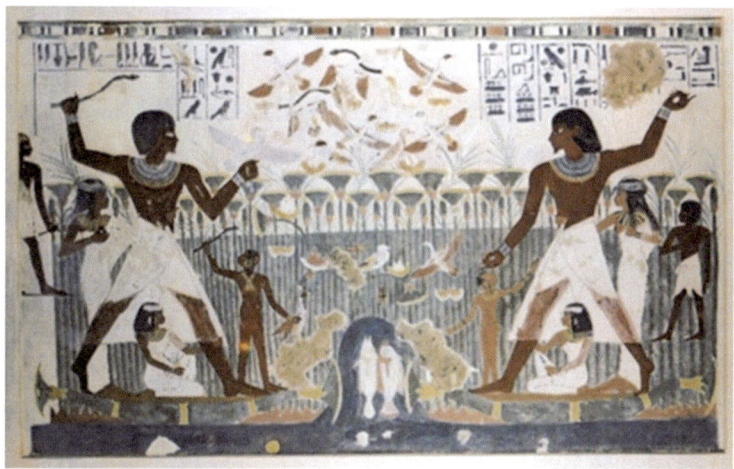

Egyptian Dress and Facial Dyes

Dr Feliciano Blanco-Dávila states the first cosmetic procedures were tattoos, which made tints permanent by placing them under the skin, and beauty marks were tattooed on the face or other parts of the body. Dermabrasion by pumice stone was also an early cosmetic practice. It is also of interest to note that the practice of peeling to which I devote a chapter of this book was also widely practiced in ancient times. Although many believe this is a recent phenomenon, peeling of the face was obtained by applying acids (acetic acid in vinegar and sulfuric acid in oil of vitriol) has been in existence for many millennia. E.J. Van Scott, and R. J. Yu, in their book Alpha hydroxy acids, state that hydroxy acids (malic acid from apple pomades, tartaric acid from aged wine, lactic acid from sour milk, and glycolic acid from sugar cane), have been used for facial chemical exfoliation since historical records began.

The Roman Influence

H.W. Johnston, in his book *The Private Life of the Romans* tells us that the modern term "cosmetic" originated in the ancient Roman public baths, which were used for an elaborate system of physical hygiene. He details the men's bath contained an unctuarium in which ointments for skin and facial care were applied to bathers by aliptes (masseuses). In the women's bath, the ornatrix managed female slaves who styled and dyed hair, applied facial makeup, performed manicures, and applied ointments to the skin. The term for these slaves, *cosmetae* from the Greek *cosmetikos,* evolved into our modern word "cosmetic, "meaning to "beautify the body."

C.P Bryan, in his book *Papyrus Ebers* states Egyptians were particularly concerned with physical appearance; their two greatest fears in life were of losing their hair and it appears that they used ointments made from the fat or blood of a variety of animals and reptiles. They also used incense, wax, cypress bark ground and fresh olive oil rubbed on the face to try and remove wrinkles. It is also apparent that they used ostrich eggs mixed with bullock's bile and milk to treat acne. L. Cottrell, in his novel, *Life Under the Pharaohs* states Egyptians used many facial dyes and henna, which gave a golden red hue to the nails and the soles of the feet. The same apothecaries who prepared medicines for physicians prepared substances and treatments to be used in perfumes and cosmetics. In the next periods, the Persians, Babylonians, Greeks, Hebrews, and Arabs all maintained the practice of cosmetology and practiced medicine to the best of their abilities.

In 332 B.C.E., Alexander the Great conquered Egypt. Ptolemy became ruler of Egypt when Alexander died and promoted the learning centre of Alexandria in honour of his cousin. Alexandria became the intellectual nucleus of the Mediterranean world. During the reign of Ptolemy, medical schools flourished, and many cultures, Egyptians, Greeks, Jews, and Arabs—showed an interest in learning medicine. Research carried out in Alexandria on anatomy, physiology, diet, and body care spread to the rest of the world. The physicians of the period promoted exercises and diets for good health and advocated the Oriental practice of bathing, but cosmetology and cosmetic procedures were excluded from the work of the doctor and these lay practitioners were often branded as charlatans.

Some minor cosmetic surgery procedures were practiced but are they were not deemed necessary to health; this was done mostly by lay practitioners. Those echoes of what is considered medical still echo today during the businesses allowed to open during the Covid lockdowns.

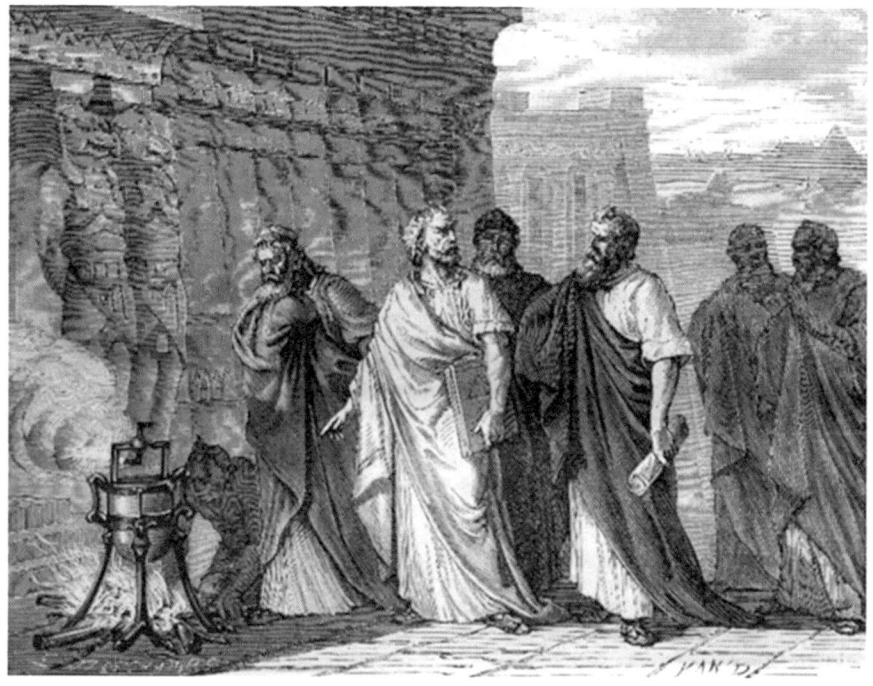

Hero demonstrating his aeolipile in front of the scholars of the school of Alexandria

The Greek and Egyptian Influence

Although the school of Alexandria gained an international reputation for training physicians of diverse cultures, the ruling monarch in Egypt was Cleopatra VII, the popular epitome of beauty. Cleopatra is said to have written a book on cosmetology, but it has been lost to antiquity. She is alleged to have bathed in goat's milk to maintain her beauty, unknowingly using lactic acid to produce smooth skin. In this early period, many thousands of years before the coming of Christ, dermabrasion or face resurfacing was regularly performed by lay practitioners using ground materials such as alabaster, seashell, limestone, pumice, ground grains, bone, and horn. It is also of interest to note that although medicine, was included in the school of Alexandria, along with astronomy and philosophy, the practice of cosmetology was not as it was considered by these physicians to be minor, without healing purpose, and left to lay practitioners.

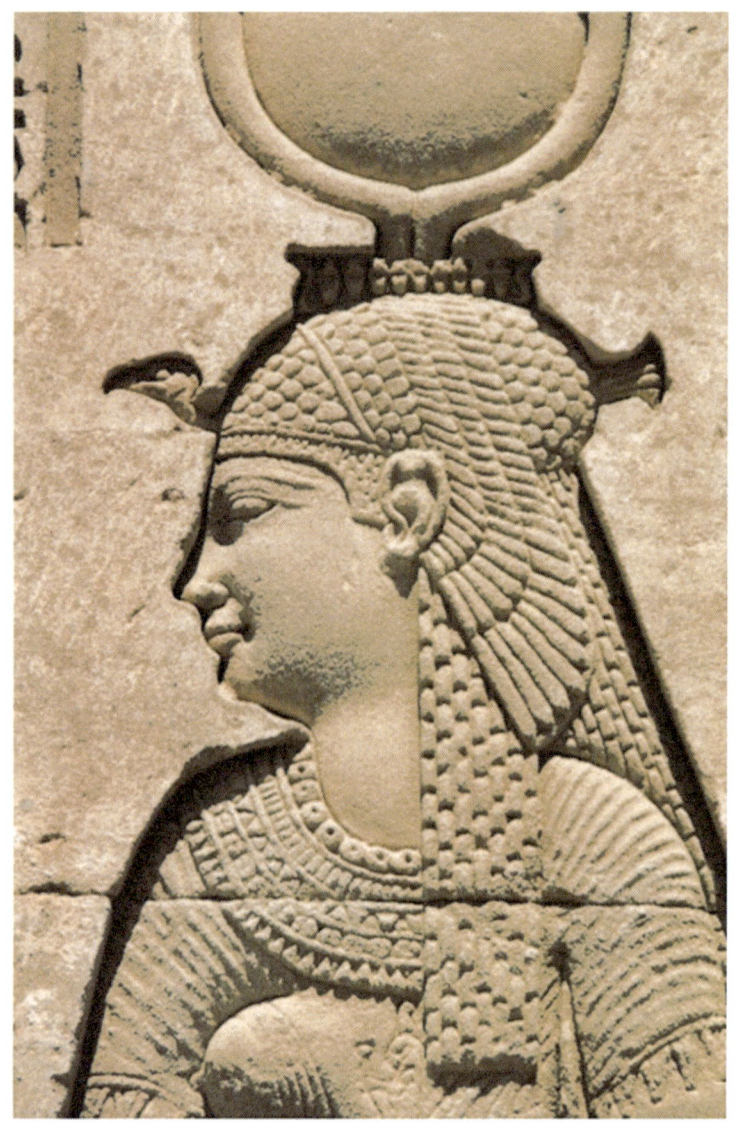

Cleopatra 69 - 30 BC was the last was the last pharaoh of Ancient Egypt

In his *Natural History*, Pliny the Elder describes the composition of some ointments to smooth facial wrinkles and beautify the face. The Greek physician Galen was a follower of Hippocratic ideas, and had the opportunity to learn, teach, and practice in the school of Alexandria. One of his contributions to cosmeceuticals was the *unctum refrigerans*, or cold cream, prepared with essence of rose water and used as a hair tonic and face lotion.

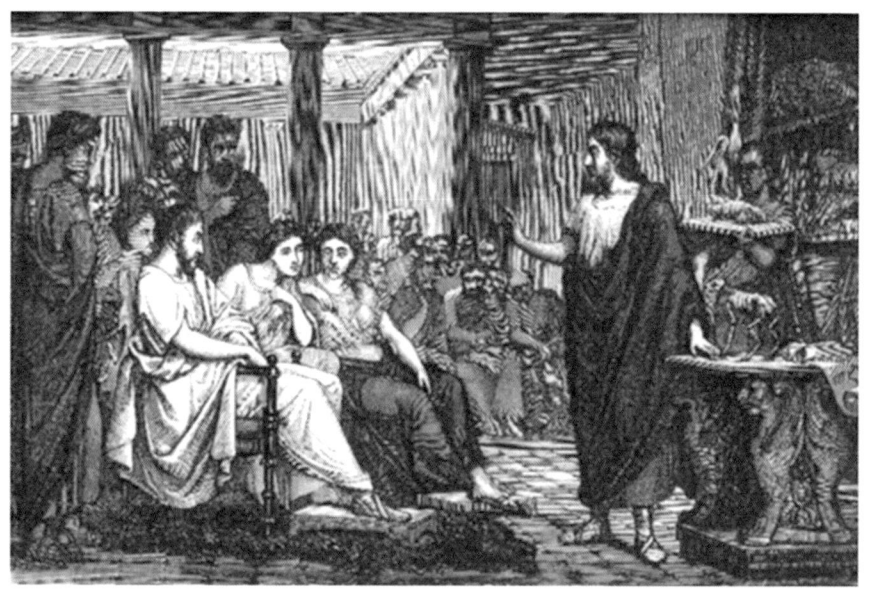

Galen the Greek physician, 129-216 B.C., teaching Anatomy in Rome

The Influence of the Catholic Church

We must look closer at the rise of Christianity, and the influence of its anti-scientific stance. For at least the next five centuries, healing became a matter of faith, and the sick being cared for by monks in monasteries. Medicine became dominated by the Church, and practices like exorcism, amulets, holy engravings, sacred oil, relics of saints, and other supernatural paraphernalia became valued over the kind of science practiced at Alexandria.

In fact, St. Benedict even forbade the study of medicine and dissections. There is no doubt that medicine suffered in this period, because of a complete breakdown in the relationship between religion and science. This was a period reflecting the decline of Greco-Roman polytheism and the Christianization of the Roman Empire. Joshua J. Mark, a freelance writer and director of Ancient History Encyclopaedia states that the anti-intellectual stance of the early church is attested to by early Christian writers themselves. St. Justin Martyr (c. 100-165 CE) was openly hostile to classical learning and the early Christian apologist Tertullian (c. 160-230 CE) also rejected classical learning. Plato's Academy in Athens, the first university in the world was closed by the Christian emperor Justinian later in 529 CE. The Christian writer St. Gregory of Nazianos (329-390

CE), rejected the precepts of learning and stated classical Greek and Roman literature was considered part of the 'old way'.

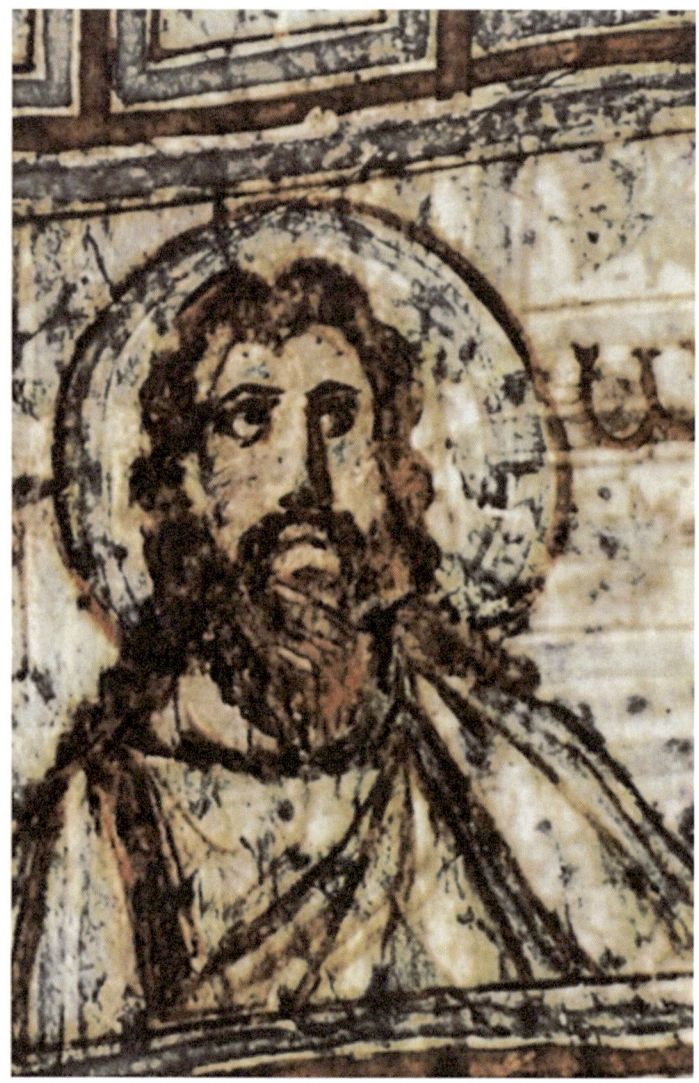

Early Christianity /Head of Christ, from the catacomb of St. Priscilla, Rome, Italy.

2nd or 3rd century A.D

Whether one believes in the Christian destruction of the library at Alexandria or not, there is no arguing that early Christianity destroyed an enormous amount of ancient knowledge and crushed intellectual thought. The ancient works we have today (such as Plato, Aristotle, and Plotinus) were preserved by the Islamic church because they supported the idea of an ultimate, objective truth.

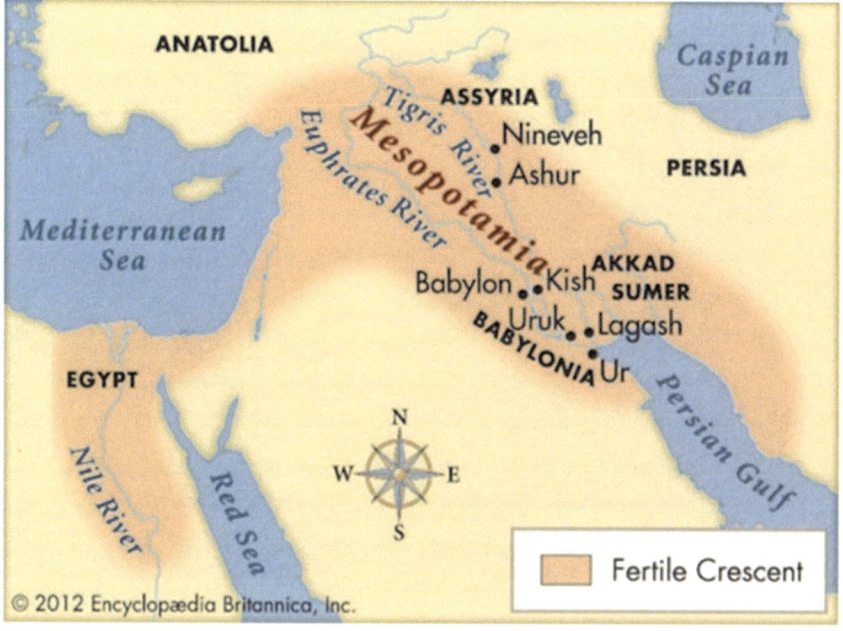

The rise of medicine in Mesopotamia

The Islamic Influence

The fall of the Roman Empire marked the end of Greco-Roman medicine and the rise of Islamic medicine. From the 9th to the 12th centuries, the Arabs consolidated a civilization. Arab physicians had learned alchemy and medicine in Alexandria. These physicians had deep knowledge of cosmetics, and they elaborated a facial mask, *batikha*, made of crushed rice grains, seashells, marble, crystal, limes, eggs, beans, and ground lentils. It was rubbed onto the face to produce a superficial dermabrasion. A skin cleanser, *hemsia*, was made of almond oil. Another facial ointment, *shnouda*, was scented with jasmine and benzoin. The Koran prohibited tattoos, and this technique died in the Islamic world. Avicenna (Ibn Sina), who was of Persian origin but whose works were widely known throughout the Arabic and Spanish worlds, is credited with the invention of the alembic and the first distillation of rose oil. Ibn Sina originated the idea of the use of oral anaesthetics, and he recognised opium as the most powerful *mukhadir* (an intoxicant or drug). He also used less powerful

179

anaesthetics such as mandragora, poppy, hemlock, hyoscyamus, deadly nightshade (belladonna), lettuce seed, and snow or ice-cold water.

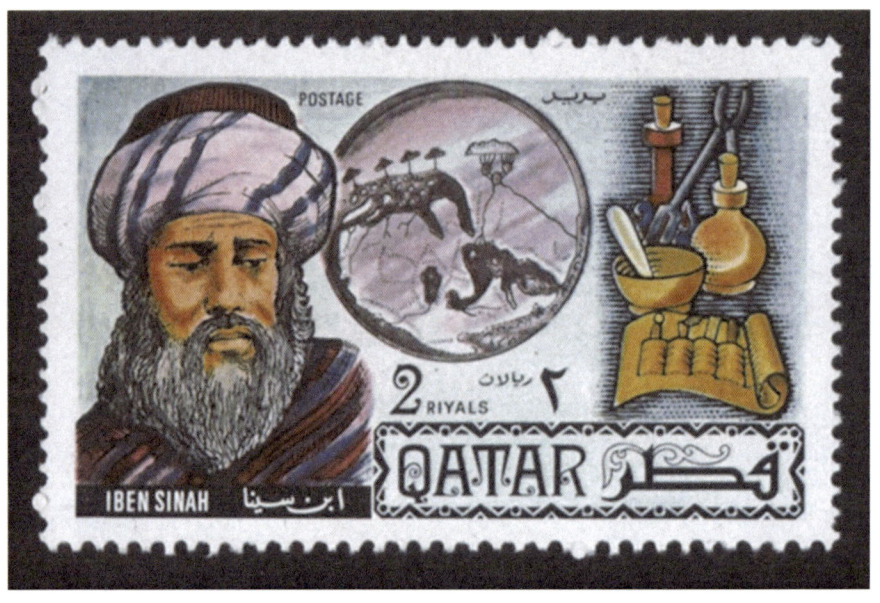

Avicenna (Ibn Sina)

Avicenna (Ibn Sina) described hay fever or allergic rhinitis. He wrote "The Diseases of Children," likely the first text to distinguish paediatrics as a separate field of medicine and pioneered ophthalmology. Records show, he was the first doctor to write about immunology and allergy. The new Al-Adudi hospital in Baghdad was built in 981 A.D. and had interns, residents, and 24 consultants.

Abu Bakr Muhammad ibn Zakariyya al-Razi, (854 CE – 925 CE), was a Persian polymath, physician, alchemist, philosopher, and important figure in the history of medicine. He became the chief physician of the Baghdad and Rayy hospitals. Razi was the first to recognize the reaction of the pupil to light and introduced mercury as a therapeutic drug for the first time in history, which was later adopted in Europe. Al-Razi is attributed to be the first to use animal gut for sutures. He is credited with many contributions, which include being the first to describe true distillation, corrosive sublimate, arsenic, copper sulphate, iron sulphate, saltpetre, and borax in the treatment of disease. As mentioned, he introduced mercury compounds as purgatives (after testing them on monkeys); mercurial ointments and lead ointments."

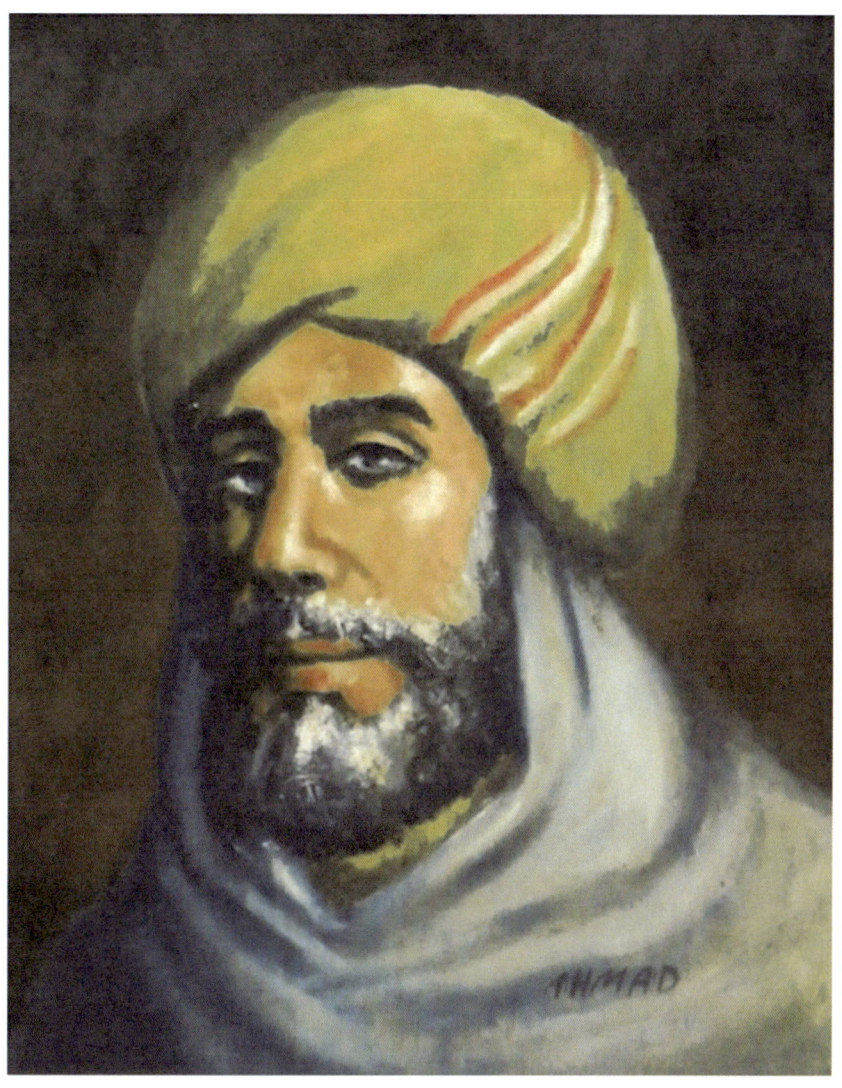

Abu Bakr Muhammad ibn Zakariyya al-Razi

Al-Razi moved to Baghdad where he became the Chief Physician of the Baghdad Hospital and the Court-Physician of the Caliph. He was the first to distinguish measles from smallpox, and he discovered the chemical kerosene and several other compounds. He suggested the communicable nature of tuberculosis long before the infectious nature of the pathogen was discovered.

An Abbasid minister, Ali ibn Isa, requested the court physician, Sinan ibn Thabit, to organise regular visiting of prisons by medical officers. Abu al-Qasim

Khalaf ibn al-Abbas al-Zahrawi al-Ansari, popularly known as Al-Zahrawi was an Arab Muslim physician, surgeon and chemist who lived in Al-Andalus. Considered the greatest surgeon of the Middle Ages, he has been described as the father of surgery.

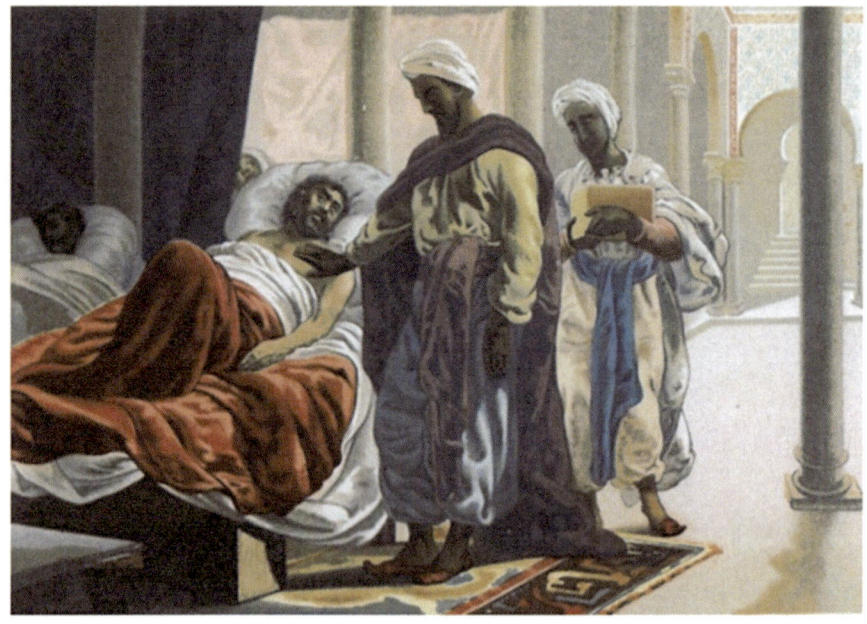

Al-Zahrawi in his hospital in Cordoba

Al-Zahrawi introduced what is called today Kocher's method of reduction of shoulder dislocation and patellectomy to orthopaedic surgery, 1,000 years before Brooke reintroduced it in 1937. He described tracheotomy, orthodontia and described the different types of fracture before the introduction of X Rays. He completed his medical encyclopaedia, *al-Tasfif liman 'Ajiza 'an al-Talif*, toward the end of the 10th century. It contains a treatise, entirely devoted to cosmetology, the art of beautification. Al-Zahrawi considered cosmetics a definite branch of medication (*adwiyat al-zinah*), "used generally by women and many men." In this treatise, Albucasis provides a detailed description of many drug formulae, their therapeutic virtues, their use as beautifying agents, the techniques of their preparation, and the methods of dispersing and storing them. Just when it seemed that medicine and cosmetology had again united under the one discipline, the great age of Islam's contribution to aesthetic medicine came to an end when a confederation of nomadic tribes led by Genghis Khan, first conquered China and spread out to attack the rest of the Muslim Empire.

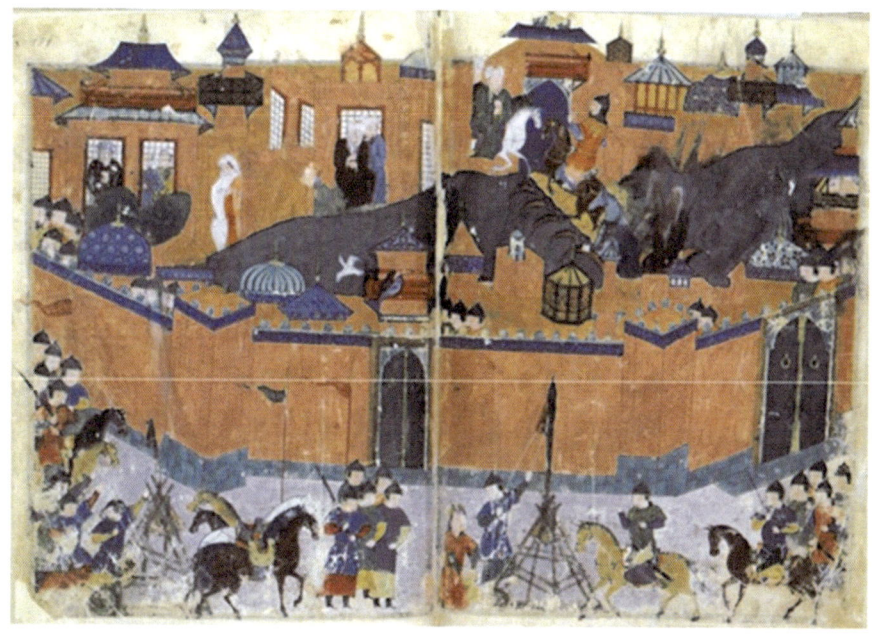

Siege of Bagdad (1258)

The Mongol Invasion

In 1258, Hulagu Khan invaded Baghdad and destroyed the ancient systems of irrigation with such extensive devastation that even today agricultural recovery in this nation is still incomplete. While in Baghdad, Hulagu made a pyramid of the skulls of Baghdad's scholars, religious leaders, and poets, and he deliberately destroyed what remained of Iraq's canal headworks. The medical knowledge of centuries was swept away, and Mesopotamia became a neglected frontier province ruled from the Mongol capital of Tabriz in Iran. In 1380, another Turko-Mongol confederation was organised by Tamerlane the Great, who claimed descent from Genghis Khan. They swept down on Baghdad again destroyed the hospitals and burnt the libraries with their irreplaceable works. It is said that the waters of the Tigris ran blue with the ink of the medical and scientific works destroyed by these barbarians. The result was to wipe out much of the priceless cultural, scientific, and medical legacy that Muslim scholars had been preserving and enlarging for some five hundred years. In 1401, he sacked Baghdad and massacred many thousands of its inhabitants.

His rule virtually extinguished Islamic dominance of medicine and Baghdad, long a centre of trade suffered severe economic depression. The medico-social innovations of the Baghdad scholars totally disintegrated. By the end of the Mongol period, the medical knowledge of the people of Mesopotamia had shifted from the urban-based Abbasid culture to the tribes of the river valleys, where it has remained well into the twentieth century.

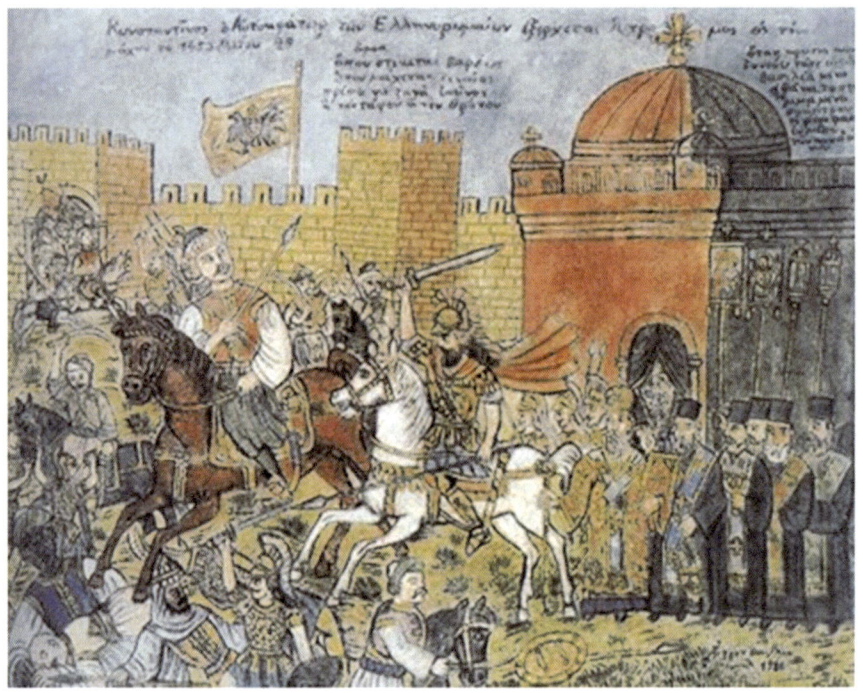

Constantinople, the capital of the Byzantine Empire fell to the Ottoman Turks in 1453

The Italian Renaissance

The Renaissance was a period in European history marking the transition from the Middle Ages to modernity and covering the 15th and 16th centuries. It occurred after the Crisis of the Late Middle Ages and was associated with great social change. The intellectual basis of the Renaissance was the rediscovery of science and classical Greek philosophy. I often wondered whether it was knowledge brought to Europe after the fall of Constantinople. In Renaissance Europe, magic and medicine based on miracles began to lose their power.

Barber-surgeons, who had not always practiced with scruples, were harshly criticized by Renaissance society, which did not discriminate between these conjurers and the physicians of that time. Paracelsus was a Swiss physician, alchemist, and philosopher of the German Renaissance who recommended using artichokes and aloe to prevent baldness and wine vinegar for the treatment of facial wrinkles. The rediscovery of ancient texts and the invention of the printing press allowed a faster propagation of more widely distributed ideas. In the first period of the Italian Renaissance, we saw a reverence for Aristotelian and Ptolemaic views of the universe. Despite scientific advances and the downfall of the barber-surgeon, this period of cosmeceuticals could only be explained as dangerous. Because fashion from the Elizabethan through the Georgian era (about 150 years) called for a white complexion, women began in their early teens to paint their faces with ceruse, a mixture of white lead and vinegar that could cause trembling.

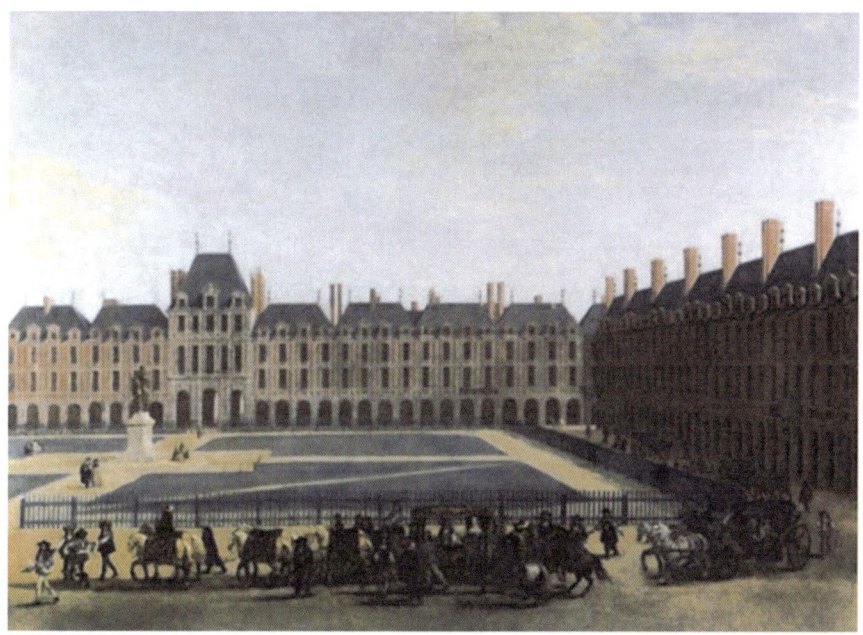

Place Royale, Paris, c1655. The King (Louis XIV) riding in royal coach pulled by six white horses

The influence of Louis XIV

George IV is said to have used leeches to achieve fashionable pallor. France in the Seventeenth Century was dominated by its kings; Henry IV, Louis XIII and Louis XIV. Each expanded royal absolutism at the expense of the nobility. Perfumes became popular and Louis XIV is said to have had perfumer-cosmetologists in the courts. The first stores to prepare perfumes appeared in Paris and they also made ointments to treat facial wrinkles. These original pomades, treated as secret formulae, were made from apples (in French, *pommes*), which contain malic acid, an alpha-hydroxy acid. The formulae of these products were kept secret and because their manufacturers had no chemical knowledge, references to the contents are very scarce. The tradition crossed the English Channel and soon perfumeries sprung up in London.

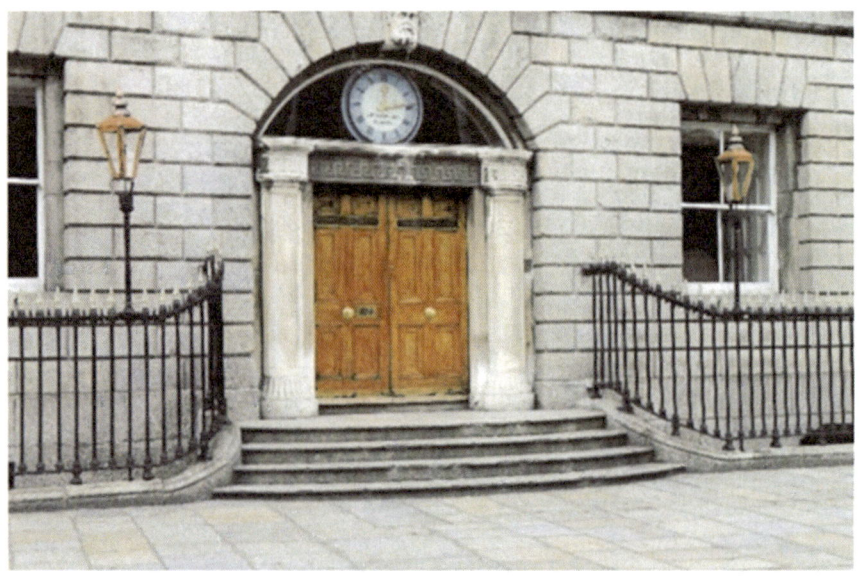

The Royal College of Surgeons in Dublin

The Georgian Period

It was in this period that pharmacies began selling cosmeceuticals and perfumes with that of medicine. Barber-surgeons flourished again, offering teeth extraction, and bloodletting. In 1745 George II created a legal separation between physicians and barber-surgeons. Afterward, barber-surgeons regrouped to form what would become, some decades later, the Royal College of Surgeons.

The Royal College of Surgeons in Dublin still portray a barber's pole in their coats of arms. The traditional barbershop red and white pole symbolised blood and bandages. Susan Leyden, archivist of the Royal College of Surgeons of Ireland (RCSI) says that the bloody land battles and naval battles in the late 1700s gave rise to increased demand for surgeons. The establishment of the Royal College of Surgeons of Ireland in 1784resulted in hundreds of students joining the Dublin school to learn how to perform battlefield surgery. The traditional barbershop red and white pole symbolized blood and bandages. Patients would grip the pole tightly to bring up the veins on their arms, if needed. To this day, a barber's pole is still used at ceremonial occasions at the Dublin college. In an interview with the Irish Independent, she continued "Surgeons' reputations were based on how fast they could amputate a limb," said Ms. Leyden. "Surgery was a skill like that of a carpenter. It was a very manual profession."

The 18th to 20th Century

By the middle of the 18th century, cosmetic disease was well recognized. When the Countess of Coventry, one of the famous Gunning sisters, died on October 1, 1760, she was identified in the press as "a victim to cosmetics. The dreaded leaded white face staged a comeback in the post-Civil War salons of the United States. Land's Bloom of Youth, a lead oleate preparation, was a favourite at the time, and lead palsy increased alarmingly in frequency. Typical of the tragedy was a 19-year-old Ohio woman who, after prolonged use, became so incapacitated from the metal that she could no longer apply the whitening to her face herself.

The modern use of cosmetics was facilitated by several practical yet powerful inventions: the toothpaste container, the compact makeup, the safety razor, the aerosol can, and lately the retractable lipstick container springing from the nimble mind of one Maurice Levy. [56] But the assault on bourgeoise reluctance that altered the cosmetic zeitgeist in the 20th century can be attributed to the verve and the daring business ventures of a Polish immigrant to the United States, the remarkable Helena Rubinstein. By 1908, when Ms. Rubenstein began to work her magic, actresses were the only women in America who dared to be seen in public with, as she put it, "anything but the lightest glim of rice powder."

Doctors and Cosmeceuticals in the twentieth century As Dr Leslie Baumann mentioned in her Dermatology News blog, the first doctor to market his own cosmetic product, was Erasmus Wilson. She states that many doctors who were involved with marketing dermatological skin products faced the ire of their medical colleagues, either through professional jealousy or because it was not seen to be appropriate to make profit from this source. This separation of what is deemed to be in accordance with treating sickness, has its origins in the school of Alexandria and possibly even long before. She states Dr Wilson faced a medical backlash because he promoted a turtle soap and a hair wash. Erasmus makes an interesting subject as he wrote and lectured about dermatology when it was not fashionable. Erasmus Wilson was born in London in 1809 and studied at Dartford Grammar School. He qualified in medicine at the University of Aberdeen and in 1840 began practicing as a doctor at St Bartholomew's Hospital in London. He began working as a surgeon but developed a sympathy with the poor of London and the treatment of their skin disease, and it was his overt humanitarianism that earned him a knighthood. As well as being a subeditor for The Lancet, he wrote several books on dermatology including in 1854 "Diseases of the Skin – A Practical and Theoretical Treatise," and the "Student's Book on Diseases of the Skin". I have reviewed some of the ones noted below and his attention to detail is quite phenomenal.

In 1869 he founded the chair and museum of dermatology in the Royal College of Surgeons and became the first professor of dermatology there. In 1878 he earned the thanks of the people of London, by bringing the Egyptian obelisk inaccurately called Cleopatra's Needle from Alexandria to London, where it was erected on the Thames Embankment. At this time, he was thought to be the leading English-speaking dermatologist in the world. In 1881, he was chosen president of the dermatology society, and was awarded with its s honorary gold medal just before his death in 1881. He contributed much to dermatology, including his pioneering work on rosacea, lichen planus, exfoliative dermatitis, and roseola. He visited the East to study leprosy, Switzerland to investigate the causes of goitre, and Italy with the purpose of adding to his knowledge of the skin diseases affecting an ill-nourished peasantry. He was knighted by Queen Victoria in 1881,and he devoted a great deal of the fortune made from his cosmetic products to charitable and educational purposes.

It was the same year Sioux chief Sitting Bull led the last of his people in surrender to United States troops at Fort Buford in Montana. Wilson died a few years later but his contributions to dermatology will be remembered. He was a prolific writer and his contributions to dermatology include the following.

- Wilson, Erasmus (1852). Fifteen Plates for the third edition of Wilson on the Skin
- Wilson, Erasmus (1854). Healthy Skin: A Popular Treatise on the Skin
- and Hair, their Preservation and Management

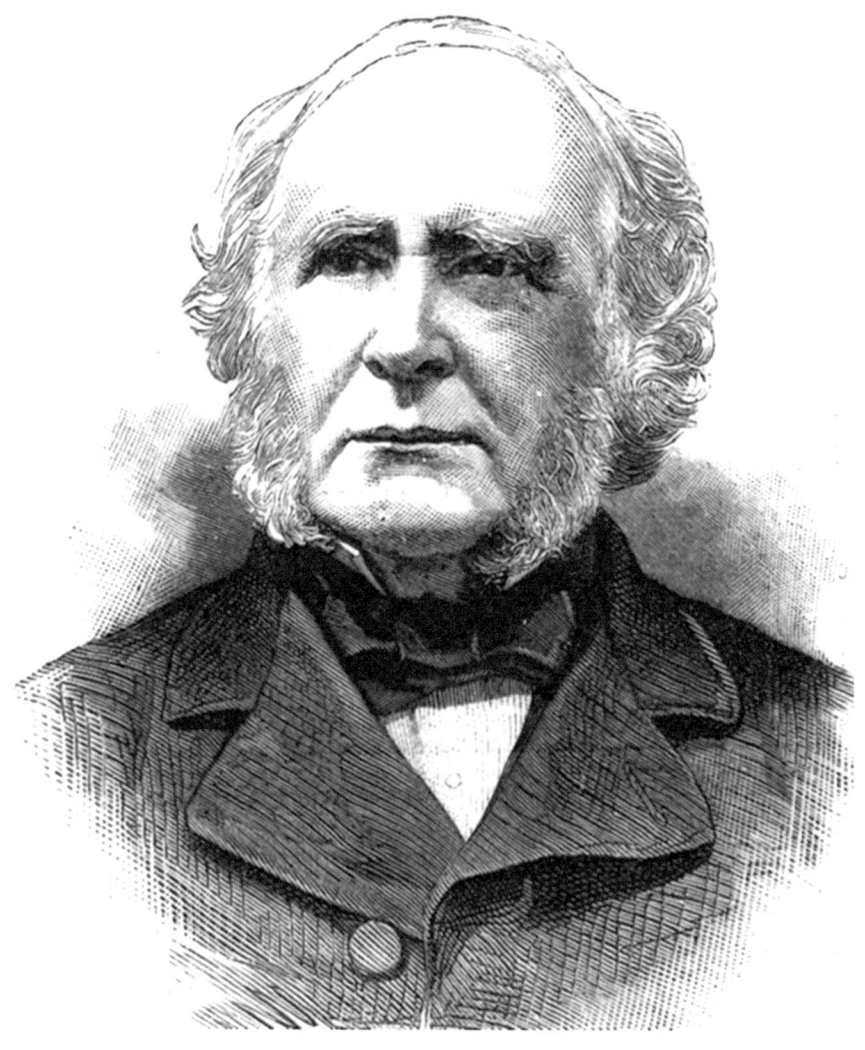

Erasmus Wilson

- Wilson, Erasmus (1865). The Student's Book of Cutaneous Medicine and Diseases of the Skin
- Wilson, Erasmus (1868). On Diseases of the Skin; A System of Cutaneous Medicine
- Wilson, Erasmus (1870). Lectures on Ekzema and Ekzematous Affections. With an Introduction on the General Pathology of the Skin
- Wilson, Erasmus (1875). Lectures on Dermatology; delivered in The Royal College of Surgeons of England in 1874–1875

The next doctor in Dr Baumann's story, is Dr William Pusey, who was a past president of the American Medical Association and head of the new dermatology department at the College of Physicians and Surgeons of Chicago. During his term as AMA president, Pusey complained that the costs associated with medical education meant that medical schools remained out of reach for those from poor rural backgrounds, which he said resulted in physician shortages in many rural areas. He wrote the first English language history of Dermatology as well as "The Principles and Practices of Dermatology," and "History of Dermatology" among others. In 1907, he became the first doctor to use solid carbon dioxide to treat skin lesions. During his term as AMA president, Pusey decried the costs associated with medical education. He criticized the fact that medical schools remained out of reach for those from poor rural backgrounds, which he said resulted in physician shortages in many rural areas. He created a backlash from his dermatological colleagues for allowing his name to endorse a Proctor and Gamble 'Cany' soap advertisement, which ran from 1926-1929. It was the same year that Henry Ford announced the forty-hour working week. This criticism concerned many dermatologists who refrained from getting involved with commercial cosmeceutical products for many decades after that.

Pusey regretted his actions, but before the negative reactions of his dermatologycolleagues, he had become an expert in the treatment of syphilis and criticized the widespread use of arsenic in the management of the condition. One wondersthen, what he would have thought about another of his pioneering American dermatology colleagues, LeGrand N. Denslow (1852-1918) whose controversial career brought him around the cities of New York; St. Paul; Minnesota; and London, England. In 1885, he became professor of skin diseases at St. Paul Medical College, thus making him one of the earliest dermatologists to practice in the state of Minnesota.

In 1908, he presented a paper before the New York Academy of Medicine claiming that he had cured, through urologic procedures on male patients, one of syphilis's most dreaded neurologic manifestations: *tabes dorsalis*. This created a media sensation, and his colleagues denounced his treatments as being totally worthless and hastened the end of his medical career. Denslow was a pioneer of American dermatology in St. Paul, Minnesota, serving as professor and secretary of the St. Paul Medical College during the late 1880s. He contributed to prestigious medical journals such as the *Boston Medical and Surgical Journal,* now known as the *New England Journal of Medicine.*

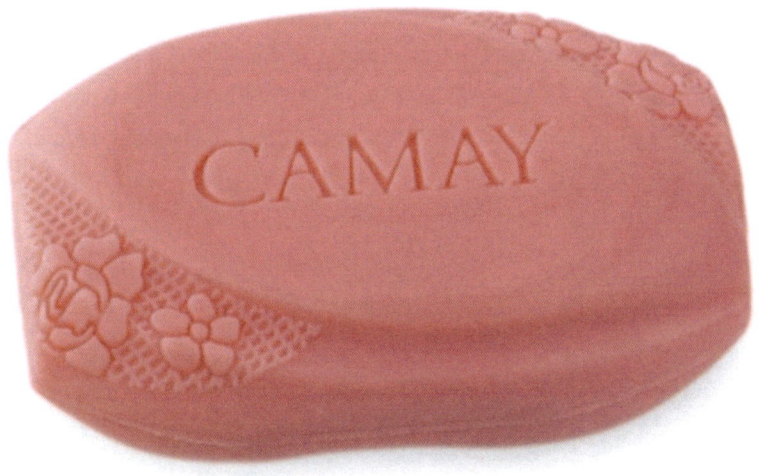

He is of special interest to me, as I worked with the dermatology department at the Mayo Clinic in Minnesota in 1984 and published a paper on malignant melanoma in the Rochester population, along with Neil Popescu and Leonard Kurland. During the period Denslow was dermatology professor at St. Paul's many American physicians travelled to Europe for more advanced medical education. His neurology colleagues went to Hopital Salpêtrière in Paris to learn from Dr Jean Martin Charcot who was first to describe Charcot Marie Tooth disease (CMT) and multiple sclerosis.

Neurology was in its infancy in the United States the multitude of battle injuries to the central nervous system and peripheral nerves of soldiers fighting the Civil War was a stimulus to the study of the neurological consequences of trauma. Fifty years later, the American neurosurgeon, Harvey Cushing became a pioneer of brain surgery, and the world's the first exclusive neurosurgeon.

In 1862, both the Sioux uprising and the civil war between states severely hindered progress of medical education in Minnesota. Many physicians served during the civil war and were eager to improve upon the medical training after the war ended. In 1879, St. Paul Medical College became affiliated with Hamline University. In 1908, as Denslow was in New York making ridiculous claims about syphilis, the medical colleges and faculties of Hamline University merged with the University of Minnesota and the era of the private medical schools largely ended. When the medical faculties of Hamline University merged with the University of Minnesota, this led to a conflict of interest between the medical school faculty, and former faculty with the Mayo Clinic. Many suspected that Dr Mayo was using his position as University Regent to retard the development of the clinical departments of the medical school and of the University hospital. Following the death of Dr Charles Horace and William Worrell Mayo in 1939, it was proposed that a memorial devoted to education and research be created on the campus of the medical school.

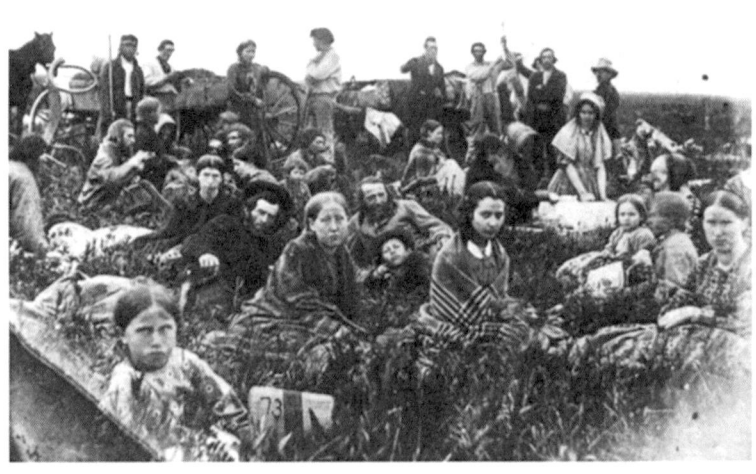

SIOUX UPRISING, 1862. /Settlers in flight from Sioux Native American massacres at rest on the prairie in Minnesota. Photographed in 1862

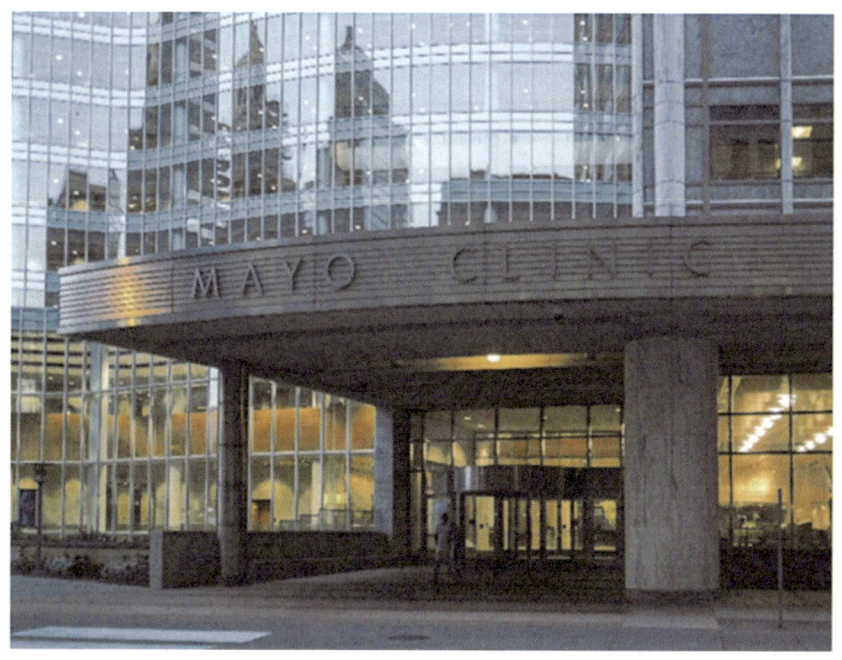

Mayo Clinic Connection

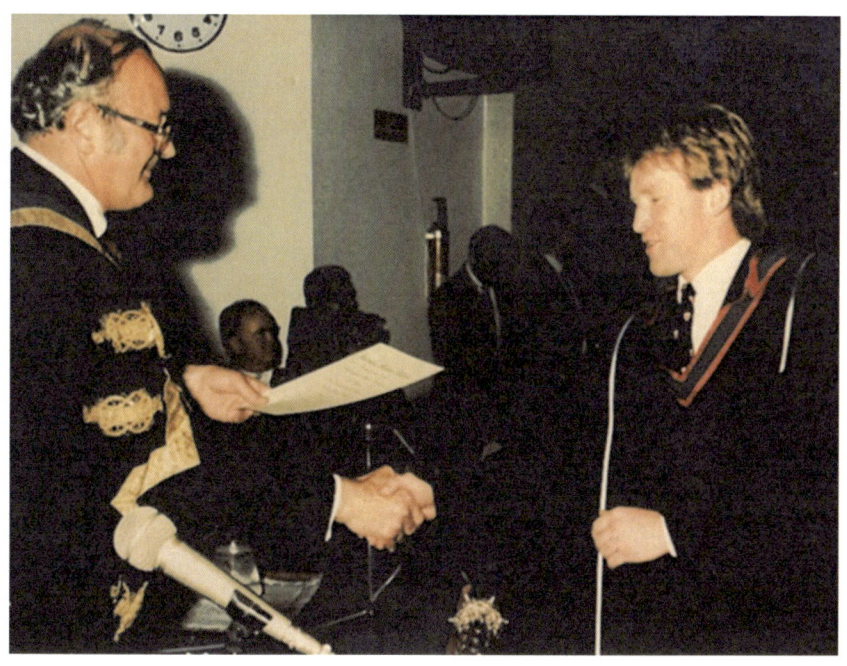

Author graduating from RCSI Dublin 1986

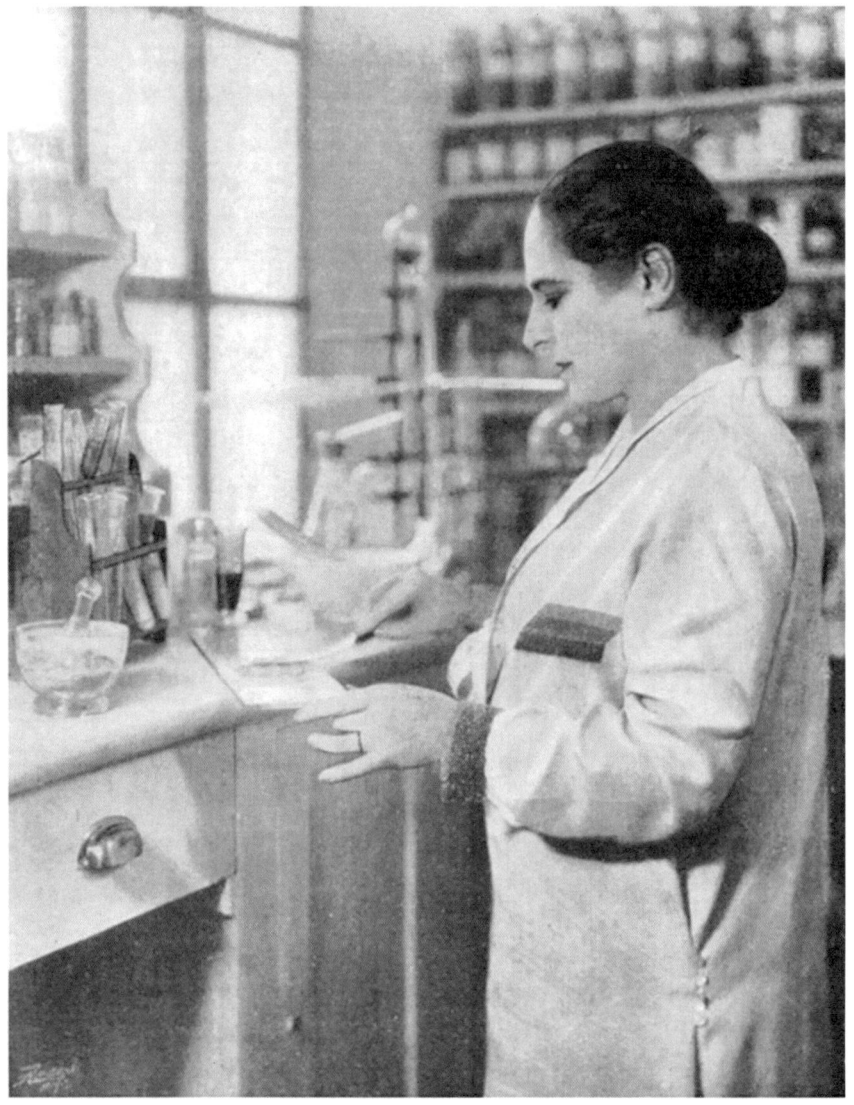

HELENA RUBINSTEIN (1872-1965) Polish American cosmetics entrepreneur

It is only with the emergence of medical specialties that some of these procedures such as peelings, face resurfacing, skin cosmetics, micropigmentation, and lately massages by means of endermotherapy have been incorporated into mainstream medicine.

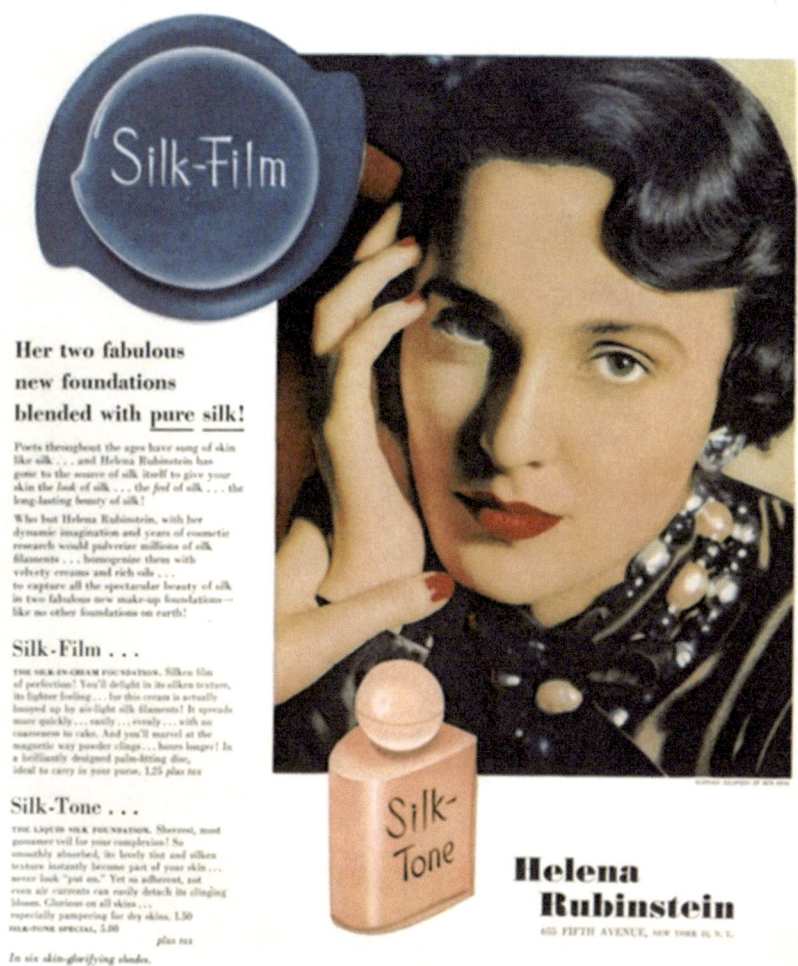

Helena Rubinstein was a Polish American businesswoman, art collector, and philanthropist. A cosmetics entrepreneur, she was the founder and eponym of Helena Rubinstein Incorporated cosmetics company, which made her one of the world's richest women.

In the 21st century we reached an age where dermatologists researched cosmetic products and even patented formulations. Despite the long two-thousand-year history of using Alpha Hydroxy Acids as a method of exfoliation, dermatologist Dr van Scott filed a method patent in the early 1970s on the effectiveness of using these chemicals to treat ichthyosis. He also invented the abbreviation "AHA" and continues work on organic acids to this day. Nicholas Perricone is a board-certified dermatologist, a businessman, and his company, N.V. Perricone, M.D. Ltd., sells branded skin products, which he markets on shows like Dr Oz, and as of 2008 had $50M in revenue. Dr Zein Obagi, is another Board-Certified Dermatologist, who has pioneered advanced skincare solutions based on his philosophy of creating healthy skin as opposed to merely treating disease and damage revenue.

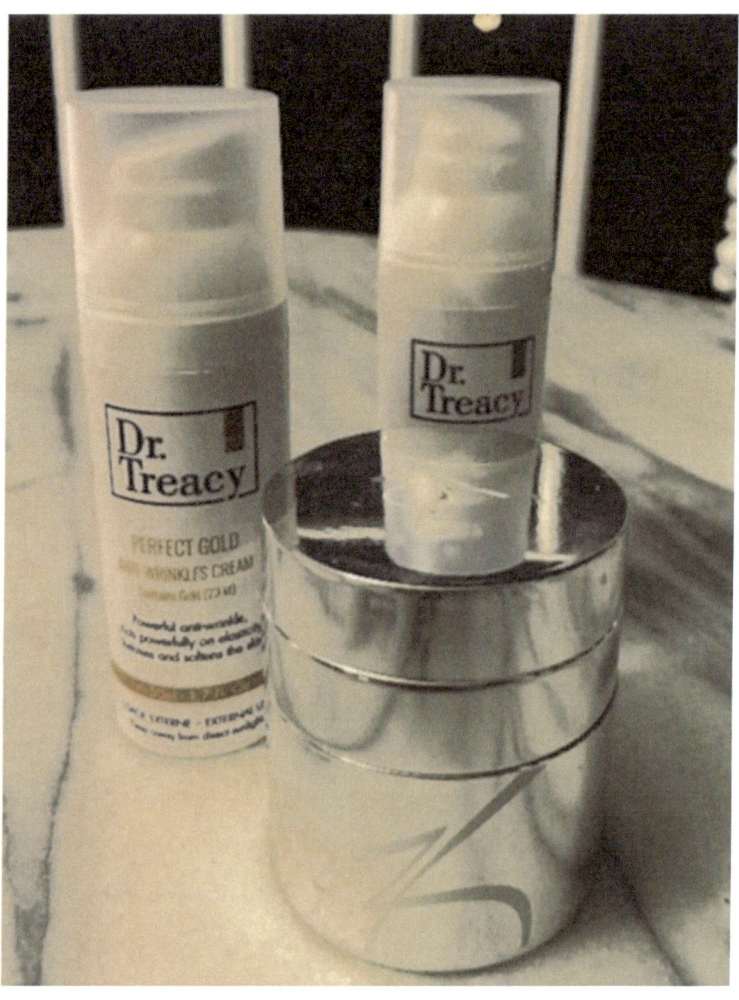

Zein Obagi product range and samples from the author

Dr Zein Obagi, is another Board-Certified Dermatologist, who has pioneered advanced skincare solutions based on his philosophy of creating healthy skin as opposed to merely treating disease and damage.

Cosmetology in the 21st Century

Cosmetology has grown, and modern plastic surgery must come to grips with this phenomenon. We are consulted now throughout the day on the safety and efficacy of cosmetic preparations, and if we are to discharge our responsibilities properly along these lines, it behooves us to become better informed. Restless innovators have originated many cosmetologic practices and cosmetic substances. Sometimes the medical community ignores them, but the procedures are still performed.

Chapter 10: Beauty

Beauty and ageing are intrinsically linked, neither dependent on each other. While beauty is a concept that is ethnically, racially, and culturally determined, the ageing process is slow, relentless, and irreversible.

So, what is beauty? Many say it is a subjective experience and that "beauty is in the eye of the beholder." Others say that beauty scientifically can be defined numerically: - 1.6180339887. So how do we assess beauty? Does it change with time? Does it change with culture? Can we use this type of information to our benefit? Is beauty just a visual experience; representing features of the human face that excite aesthetic admiration, attraction, desire, or love or does it provide a perceptual experience to all the other senses: the ear, the intellect, the aesthetic faculty, or even the moral sense. Can we say that beauty is the characteristic of a person that provides a perceptual experience of pleasure or are we being naive, failing to realise that it is just a principle of evolutionary biology representing fertility, health, and vitality, which ultimately is programmed to improve an individual's chance of survival and reproduction.

The golden ratio
This figure 1.6180339887 is called the golden ratio, first described by Euclid and the Pythagorean mathematicians, and is present in many shapes that we find pleasing, be it in nature, people's faces, or architecture. The golden ration shows that the distance between the navel and the foot to the height and the ratio of the distance from the top of the head to the fingers to the height are exact. Hence, this ratio represents balance and symmetry and the logical conclusion that within our species it most probably provides a perceptual experience of how to maximise reproductive fitness, hence improving the individual's chance of survival and reproduction.

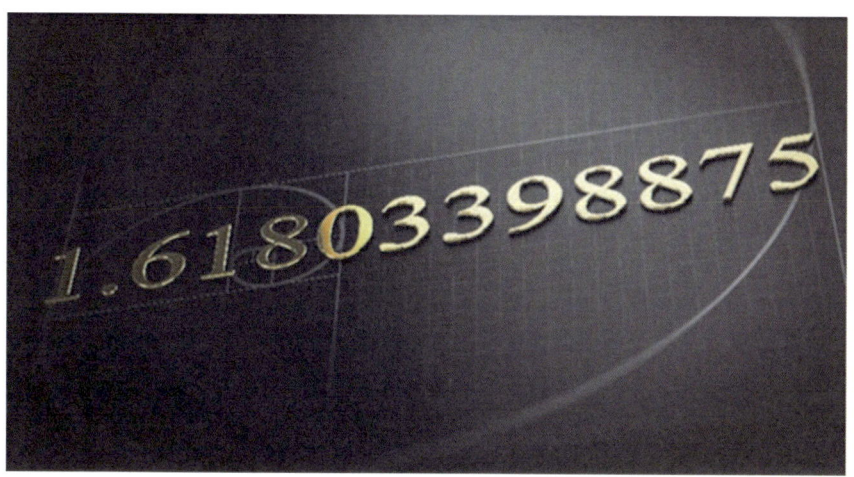

The Golden Ratio 1.61803398875

Aldous Huxley stated, 'beauty is worse than wine, it intoxicates both the holder and beholder', whereas Aristotle said, "Personal beauty is a greater recommendation than any letter of reference." Interestingly, he continued, "The chief forms of beauty are order and symmetry and definiteness" and further claimed that science proved this wherever you looked. He found great beauty in 'the golden ratio' mentioned above that mathematical formula found all over nature, such as the growing of shells and the human body. George B. Mere possibly came closer to beauty's relevance to Aesthetic Medicine when he said, 'Beauty is the first present nature gives to women and the first it takes away'. Men and women have developed different strategies to appear attractive and have different interests in identifying beauty in people. For every historical period and human culture, people have had their own ideal of beauty. It has resulted in social and economic benefits to those who possess it, and that ideal has never been constant and is still subject to changes. Though we opened this chapter with the maxim "beauty is in the eye of the beholder", some qualities, features and proportions are universally esteemed. For instance, Pierre Fournier once told me 'cuteness' is a feature that is universally esteemed throughout the animal kingdom and in his mind, it was related to having 'babylike' features.

Fibonacci Golden Ratio

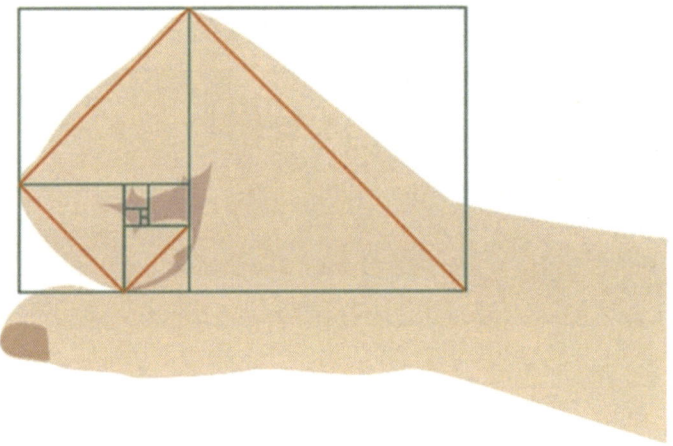

The head forms a golden rectangle, and the mouth and nose are placed at golden sections of the distance between the eyes and the chin, and there are many others present and when we look at the human body. I gave a lecture on the concept of beauty to three hundred doctors at an aesthetic conference in the Royal Society of Medicine in 2017. Later that year, I won the 1st AIDA Award in Abu Dhabi for showing that the concept of beauty and symmetry remains constant across all cultures throughout the world. In this sense, symmetry is universally regarded as a reflection of health, vitality, sexual allure and social appeal, and we use it as a primordial means of mate selection.

****

Each succeeding finger bone is 1.618 times the length of the preceding one. The distance from elbow to wrist is 1.618 times the length of the wrist to the fingertip. When analysing an ECG, the distance between the last two peaks is 1.618 times that of the first two. This ratio remains the same across all cultural groups.

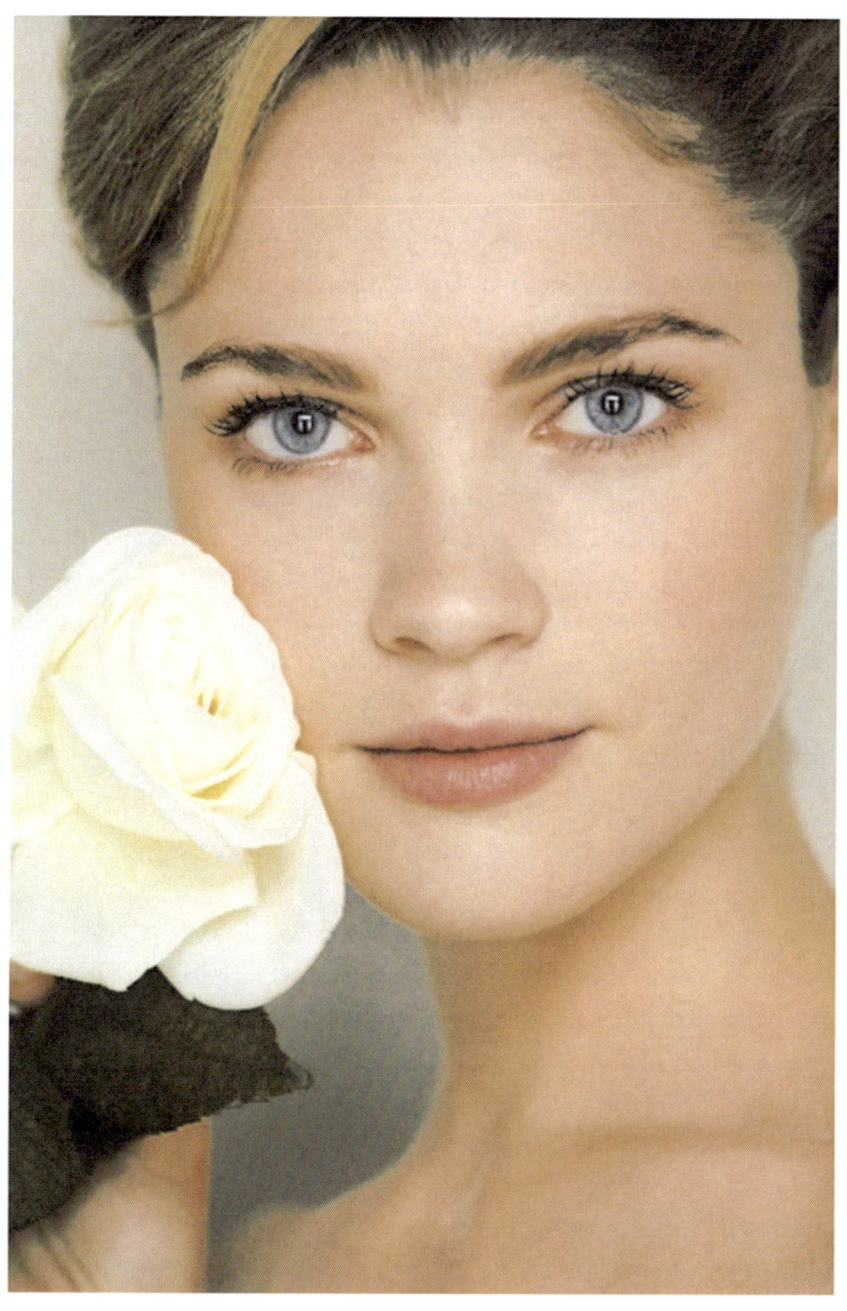

Attractive youthful features

A set of youthful features and proportions (e.g., large forehead, wide set eyes, round cheeks, small, short nose, full lips, and smooth unblemished skin) appears to be attractive to in both males and female faces. Hence, women have used facial cosmetics for millennia. There is evidence that women used green malachite on their faces in Ancient Egypt in 4000 BC and lead was used on female skin in the Mycenean period 1944 BC. As late as 1300 BC, European women were using male urine as an exfoliant, and covered their faces in bat's blood in the belief that is made their skin look healthier.

This existence of *infantile schema* was first identified mammals (including homo sapiens) by Konrad Lorenz in 1939. Research shows that most people will infer positive characteristics when viewing a bilateral symmetrical face. In 1994, Watson and Thornhill in a review of symmetry in mate selection, researchers found that animals from scorpion flies to zebra finches showed a preference for symmetrical patterns and shapes and concluded that asymmetry is seen as a sign of weakness or disease. The same year, Perret, May, and Yoshikawa published a paper showing a study of American and Japanese observers of female attractiveness rated high cheekbones, large eyes, a short distance between the mouth and the chin (and the nose and mouth) and a thin lower jaw are preferred qualities in men's and women's faces alike.

Infantile Schemata

In 1995, Cunningham noted in a study utilizing Asian, Hispanic, and Caucasian judges, the most attractive had larger, wider-set eyes, smaller noses, larger lower lips, larger smiles, dilated pupils, and well-groomed fuller hair. Research by Dan Ariely (MIT School of Management) and Hans Brieter (Massachusetts General Hospital) published in the 2001 issue of the journal *Nature,* indicates that female beauty stimulates the same pleasure centres in the brain as cocaine. Characteristic features of an unsexy face include, *wide* facial shape, fat, bigger distance of eyes, low cheek bones, wide nose, eye bags, sunken nasolabial lines, thin lips and wrinkles. These are all the features that Aesthetic Medicine serves to change. Darker skin apparently looks more 'unsexy' on a male than a female, as is a weak lower jaw and lighter eyebrows. Jaw size is also important as vertically excessive or deficient prognathic (protruding), or retrusion of the upper and lower jaws affect our perceptions of facial beauty.

This existence of infantile schema was first identified mammals (including homo sapiens) by Konrad Lorenz in 1939. Research shows that most people will infer positive characteristics when viewing a bilateral symmetrical face.

They include larger, wider-set eyes, smaller noses, larger lower lips, larger smiles, dilated pupils, and rounded cheekbones.

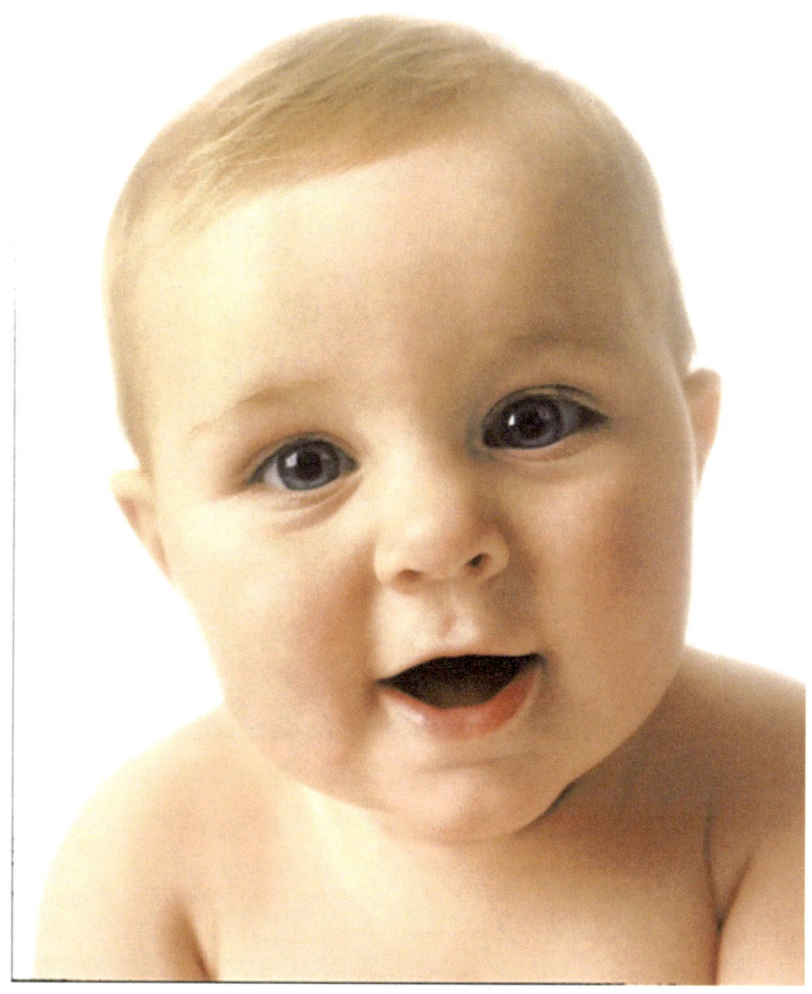

Infantile schema

Facial Disfigurement

Facial disfigurement is the state of having one's facial appearance harmed medically, either from a disease, birth defect or trauma. Although this perceived defect does not usually affect a patient's health, the condition leads to social stigmatisation, isolation and incurs limitations of privileges and opportunities otherwise afforded to those without the problem. It is estimated that presently, there are about 40,000 adults and children in the UK (1 in 150 people) with significant facial disfigurements and 1 in 500 children is seriously affected by facial disfigurement to result in severe psychosocial problems, poor self-esteem, and depression. Studies have shown that the general population respond to people with a facial disfigurement with prejudice, intolerance, less trust, and respect and often try to avoid making contact or having to look at them.

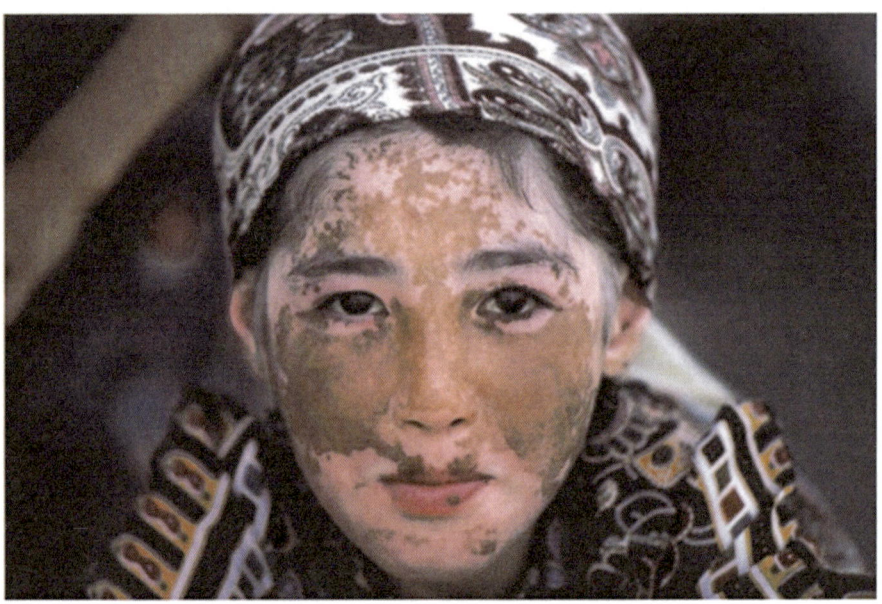

Young Uzbek child in traditional costume, Samarkand, Uzbekistan, Central Asia

Although modern reconstructive surgery and medical treatments help in making some of the unusual features less noticeable, usually it does not remove them completely and the patients must employ coping strategies that include avoidance of social contact, alcohol misuse and aggression. For those affected, it can turn a simple social event into a major ordeal.

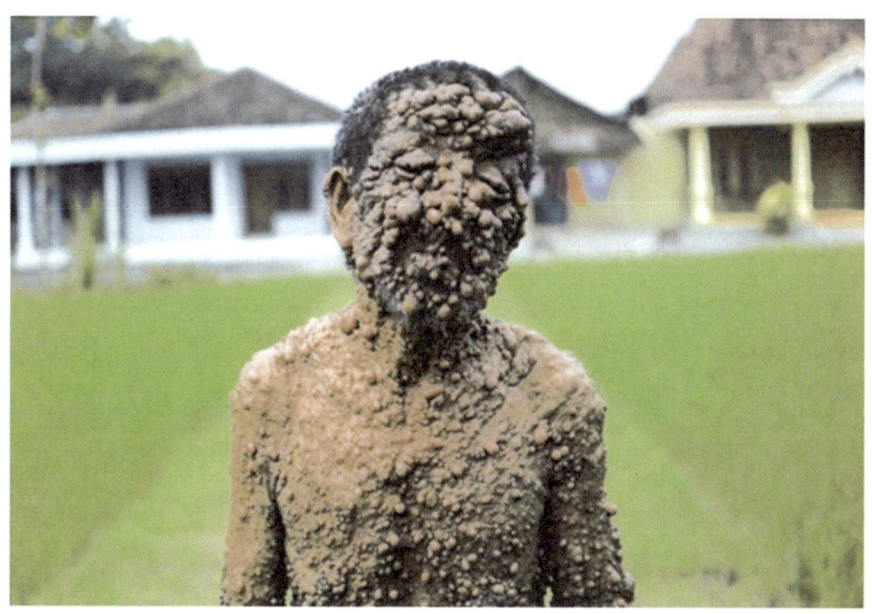

Patient with neurofibromatosis

The causes of facial disfigurements are highly variable. At one end of the scale are patients who are born with significant craniofacial abnormalities such as Apert syndrome, while at the other, we have less aesthetically challenging problems secondary to skin conditions such as cystic acne, birthmarks or possibly vitiligo. In between, we have a myriad of cases secondary to diseases such as elephantiasis or leprosy or because of congenital disfigurements caused by conditions like neurofibromatosis.

Weaved into this myriad of pathologies are those who have already suffered great emotional trauma because of benign or malignant facial cancers, scarring secondary to road traffic accidents or burns, etc. While skin conditions like acne into this myriad of pathologies are those who have already suffered great emotional trauma because of benign or malignant facial cancers, scarring secondary to road traffic accidents or burns, etc. While skin conditions like acne scarring or vitiligo may not immediately appear to be of major psychological concern, these patients often disguise their facial disfigurements through camouflage techniques and live a life behind a mask of coloured creams.

I personally witnessed this phenomenon treating one of the most famous faces in the world for vitiligo a few years ago. Whatever the cause, society presently dictates that people with a facial disfigurement are perceived to be less physically attractive, less socially desirable, and less likely to find an acceptable spouse. In this article, I will try and analyse what drives such a bias in every cultural society on earth, especially as it is guided towards people who already have been the victim of gross trauma or unfairness.

Prejudice and belief

Before we start this exploratory journey, let us define two underlying words: prejudice and belief. The word *prejudice* comes from the word prejudgment, deciding before becoming aware of the relevant facts of a case. In recent times, this word has gained prominence when used to refer to legal judgments toward people or a person because of a bias against their gender, religion, race/ethnicity, sexuality, or possibly social class. Prejudice is a baseless and usually negative attitude towards the members of a group. Common features of prejudice include negative feelings, stereotyped beliefs, and a tendency to discriminate against members of the group. While specific definitions of prejudice given by social scientists often differ, most agree that it involves prejudgments (usually negative) about members of a group.

Belief, on the other hand, is the psychological state in which an individual holds a conjecture or premise to be true. Because our beliefs are the primary determinant of what we do and feel, and even what we perceive, all prejudice can usually be traced to belief systems. Both beliefs and prejudices themselves change with time. Twentieth-century Britain has seen many prejudices enacted against differing races and religions.

A few years ago, facial lipodystrophy syndrome (HLS) was a major problem for many HIV patients undergoing long-term use of highly active antiretroviral therapy (HAART). The psychological facial wasting effects of the condition were extremely distressing, and these patients had high levels of depression, suicide as well as social withdrawal and isolation. In fact, a UK study showed that 47% of patients with HLS had HRSD scores for severe depression.

It was for this reason and the lack of proper aesthetic therapy to manage this complex condition that I pioneered a facial endoprosthesis technique to replace the malar fat pad in the Ailesbury Clinic some years. It restored dignity to these otherwise socially isolated patients. Thankfully, the new anti-AIDS drugs thankfully do not give rise to these types of problems. Just as we look back at cultural practices of ancient Rome with repulsion, future generations will probably look back at these prejudices with similar reactions.

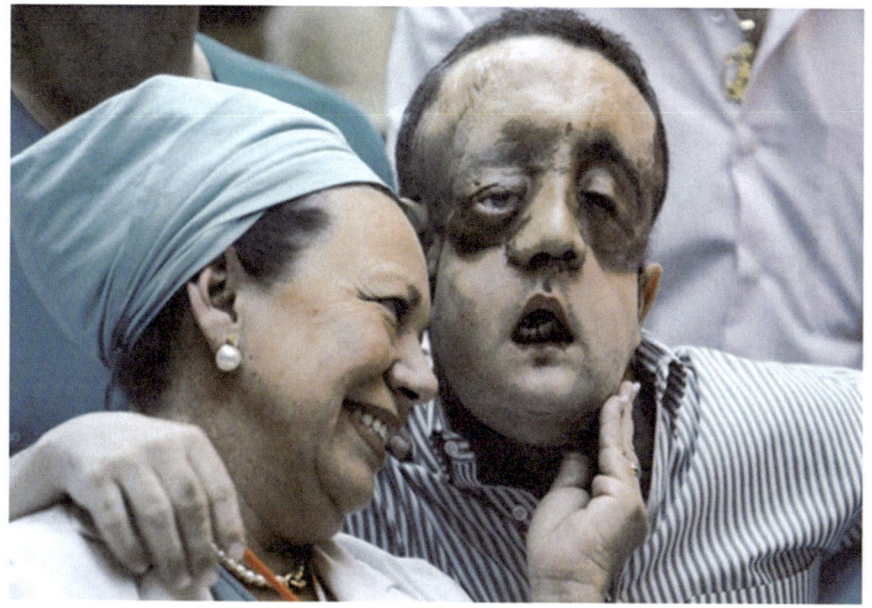

Rafael with neurofibromatosis

The image above shows face transplant recipient Rafael embracing a nurse during a news conference at Virgen del Rocio hospital in Seville May 4, 2010. Rafael, who received the lower face transplant at the hospital in January, suffered from neurofibromatosis, a genetically inherited disorder which caused facial tumours.

It is impossible for us to try and understand the Roman thinking that feeding Christians to lions was acceptable as a spectator sport. These beliefs were accepted two thousand years ago as these people were a threat to the society that existed then. And they were probably right. History has decided that Christian religion would displace the Roman deities and their ministers would give rise to their own prejudices in turn, especially in the period after the reformation. So, a belief is just a statement about a perceived reality that we individually experience as the truth at that time. But, in fact, no belief describes the truth about reality. Without exception,beliefs are arbitrary interpretations of events by individuals.

Physical objects and events certainly occur in the world, but the meaning that we give the events exists only in our minds, not in the material world. If this is so, why is the prejudice against facial disfigurement so strong and why has it survived the ages?

At the outset, it would be easy to blame the stigmatisation of people with facial disfigurement on the emphasis that our modern image-conscious society places on physical appearance. There is continual pressure, through media and other marketing tools, for people of every age to conform to what is a perceived normal appearance. However, throughout the centuries, facial beauty has been perceived by many cultures as a human quality that provides a sensory experience of pleasure or goodness.

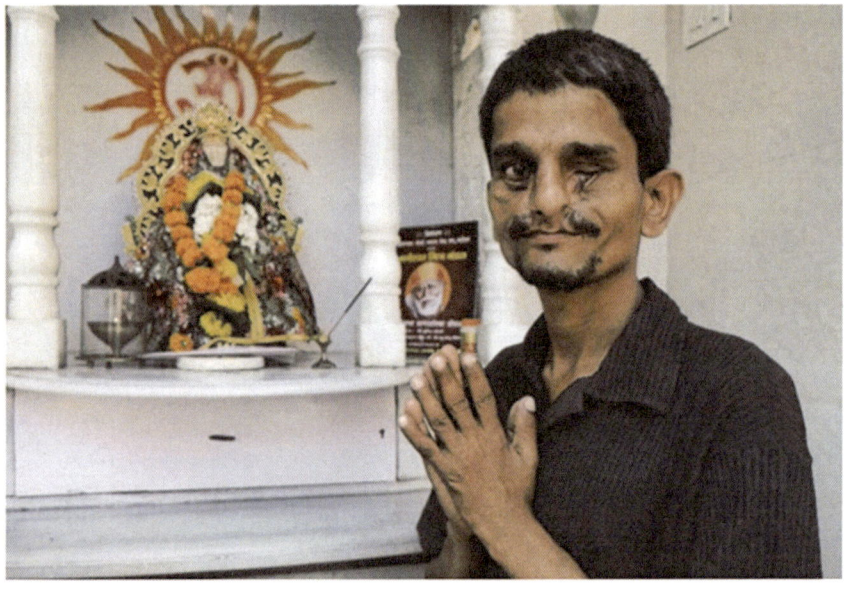

A victim of an acid attack praying at a shrine to Hindu saint Sai Baba, Mumbai, India

Beauty has generally been associated with that which is good, and ugliness has been associated with evil. The Byzantine Emperor was considered God's Vice-Regent on Earth and his beauty was taken as an essential complement to the perfection of heaven. For this reason, many deposed emperors were facially disfigured by being blinded or having their noses cut off to disqualify them from ever reclaiming the throne. During this period of history, society believed that facial 'disfigurement' involved the entity being out of balance and harmony with nature and ugliness engendered a deeply negative perception of a person. This simplistic approach to ugliness and by association to facial disfigurements is still reinforced today at every stage by the media and by our education system.

Consider our current classic children's fairy tales, where the Ugly Sisters equate ugliness with evil and Cinderella with all things wonderful, or indeed the tale of Sleeping Beauty or the evil old witch in Hansel and Gretel.

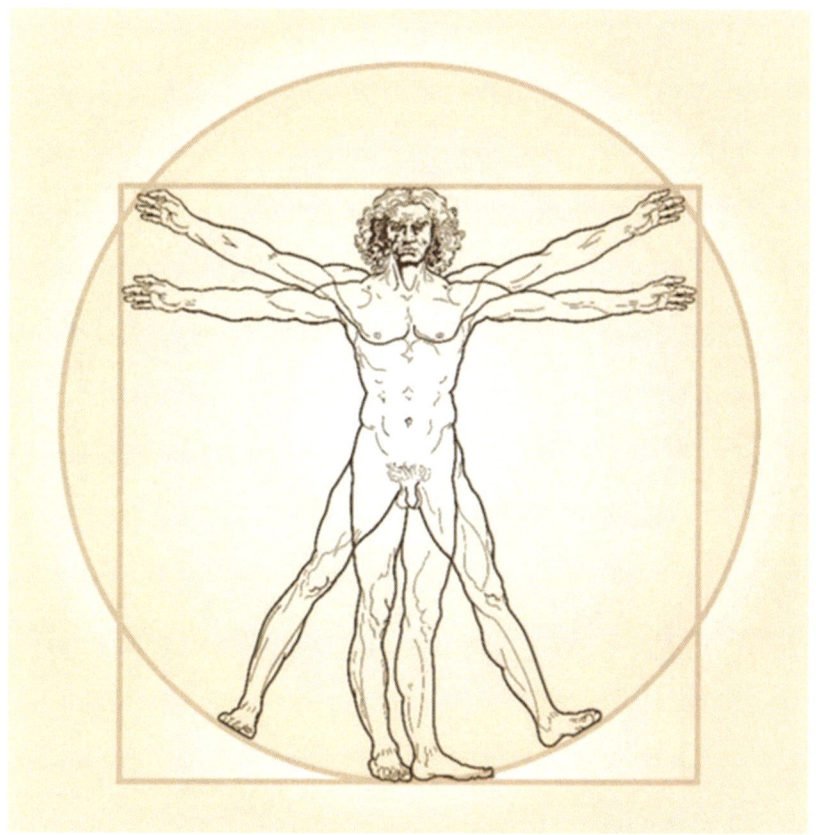

The Golden Ratio

It is also reinforced on our TV screens (*Ugly Betty*) and with film and video villains such as Freddy (*Nightmare on Elm Street*) and John Merrick (*Elephant Man*). If filmmakers or novelists were to treat race or sex in the way that they presently portray beauty or ugliness, they would probably be subject to society's revulsion and possible legal prosecution. Then why is society still disrespectful and uncompassionate to people who are usually not contributory in any way to their condition? What causes us to turn away in revulsion from a person with a congenital, traumatic, or malignant facial condition rather than being compassionate and comforting them?

Let us for a moment reflect on these two celebrities, both of whom sustained recent excessive facial disfigurement.

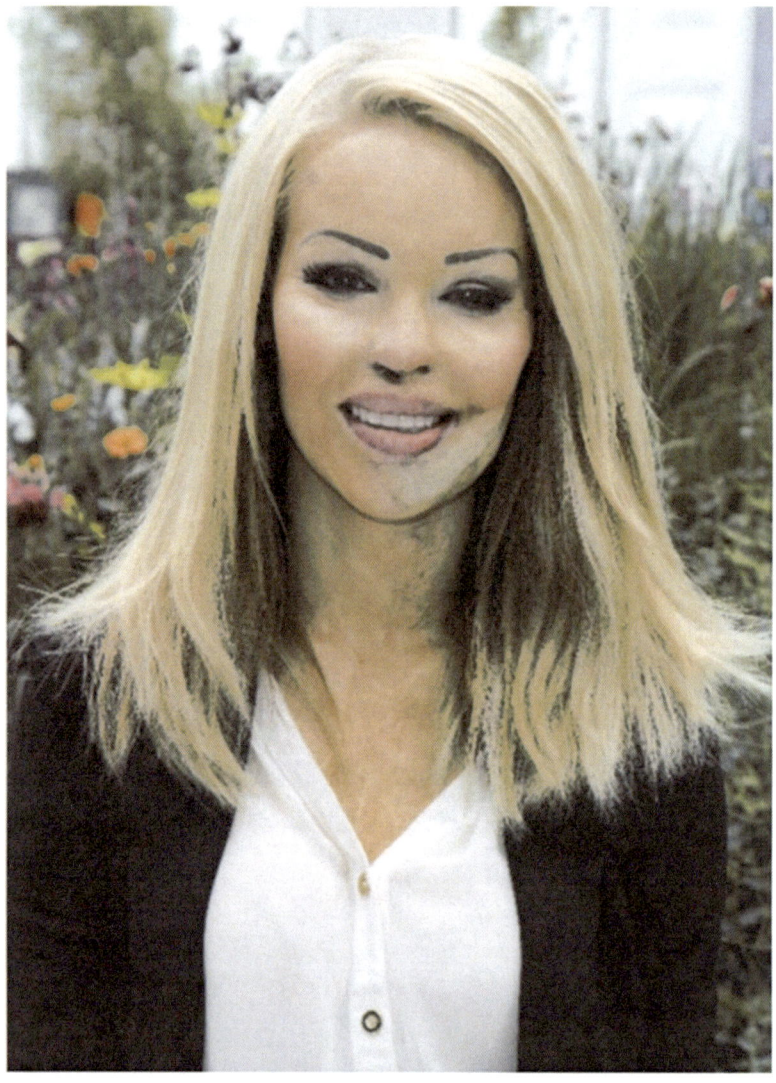

Katie Piper at the RHS Chelsea Flower Show

(1) Kate Piper is an English writer, activist, television presenter and model from Andover, Hampshire. In March 2008, she was attacked with acid by her ex-boyfriend and an accomplice, causing major damage to her

face and blindness in one eye. Piper underwent pioneering surgery to restore her face and vision. Both attackers were convicted and given life sentences. In 2018, one of the attackers was released after serving nine years in prison. In 2009, Piper gave up her right to anonymity to increase awareness about burn victims.

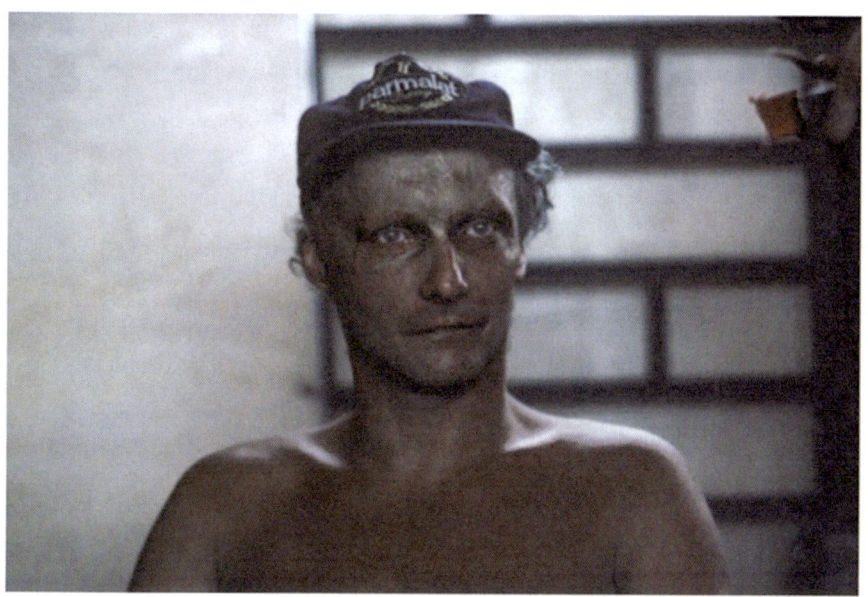

Niki Lauda after receiving severe facial burns – 1980s

(2) The late Niki Lauda was a three-time F1 World Drivers' Champion, (1975, 1977 and 1984). He is widely considered to be one of the greatest F1 drivers of all time. He was severely burned, when his car went on fire at the 1976 German Grand Prix at the Nürburgring, even though he had urged his fellow drivers to boycott the race, largely because of circuit's safety arrangements, including lack of fire marshals, fire and safety equipment and safety vehicles. He was trapped in his car and suffered severe burns to his head, especially his face as well as damage to his lungs. However, he overcame his disfigurement and became a consultant for Scuderia Ferrari and team manager of the Jaguar Formula One racing team for two years and founded and ran three airlines: Lauda Air, Niki, and Lauda.

An experiment by the BBC *Inside Out* team demonstrated presenter Julia Hankin made up with tattoo ink by a make-up artist to give the appearance of a prominent port-wine stain. During the programme, she took a seat on a busy bus route. It took 65 minutes before someone would sit next to her. Later, on the same journey, with the make-up off, it was a quite different story, and someone took the seat next to Julia after about 30 seconds. Professor Nichola Rumsey, from the Centre for Appearance Research at the University of West England, performed similar research on the London tube and found that people chose not to sit next to someone when they had a disfigurement on their face.

Psychologists like Valerie Curtis, a behavioural scientist at the London School of Hygiene and Tropical Medicine, believe that the emotion of disgust is like fear. "Fear evolved to keep you away from large animals that want to eat you from the outside" but "disgust evolved to keep you away from smaller animals that kill you from the inside". Our subconscious minds constantly scan the environment for signs of potential diseases, she says. If we see one, disgust kicks in and we avoid that object or person like the plague. It appears that even if we know that these people are perfectly healthy, our minds are responding to them as if they are not.

Why is facial symmetry so important?

Symmetry of facial form leads to a person having more sexual partners and more satisfactory relationships and this is similar across every culture. In fact, if facial symmetry as a means for determining beauty has indeed an evolutionary basis, then this would explain why it is present in every human culture and even suggests that our stigmatisation of facial disfigurement may be innate. This would happen if there was an evolutionary benefit to society to allow it to remain in every culture across so many millenniums.

Many scientists now believe that this revulsion may be an innate defence mechanism designed to protect society against disease and bad genes. It is well known that a three-month-old baby will smile and develop a bonding relationship quicker with a symmetrical face than they will with their own mother. This is probable evidence that this is not learned behaviour. More recently, some British papers carried a story that nobody wanted to bring home a cat that had developed an unusual face after being infected with the fungus *cryptosporidium*. It seems our prejudice does not only relate to humans.

So, is there anything we can do to change our behaviour?

Education is probably a good start. We should strive to make atypical appearance more familiar and mundane, possibly following the lead set by Channel 4 and showing people with these types of appearances on television more often. As doctors, we must respect and give supportive care to patients with facial disfigurements.

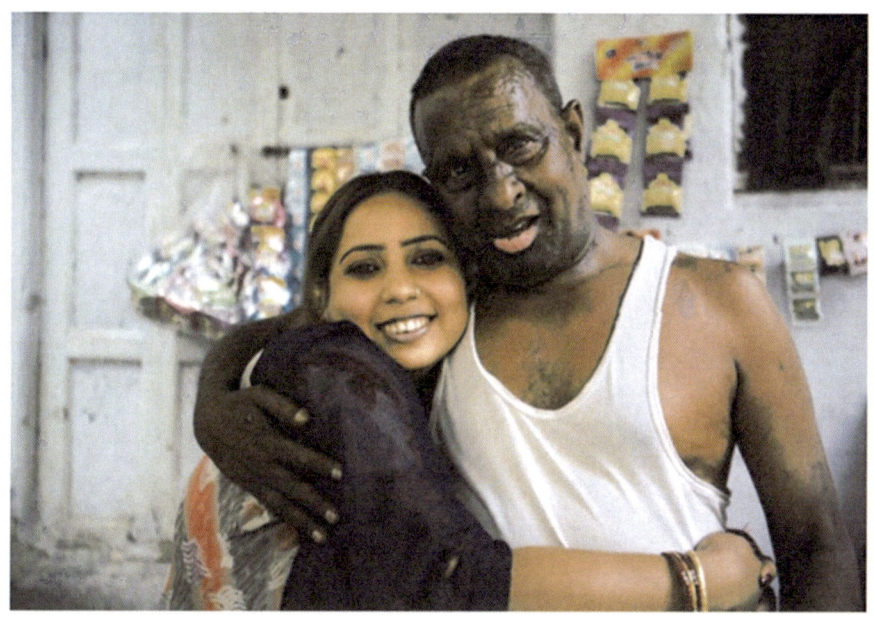

An Indian man with a facial disfigurement

For this reason, I have provided an extensive list of specialist organisations such as Changing Faces or the Disfigurement Guidance Centre in the UK, who provide support to people living with facial disfigurement and offer advice on all types of treatment.

It is important for parents to learn about their child's condition and not be afraid to ask their consultant as many questions as possible. Being better informed about your child's condition will help them learn how to cope with it. There are also easy-to-learn, practical skills to help parents overcome some of the common challenges and uncertainties they may face. Children start becoming curious about their appearance from an early age and learn from watching their parents deal with challenging situations.

UK and Irish disfigurement support groups offering support, information, and advice on specific conditions:

Bell's Palsy Association
The only UK-registered charity dedicated solely to providing help and information to people with Bell's palsy.

Facial Palsy, UK
Charity supporting people who are affected by facial paralysis.

The Birthmark Support Group
A UK-based support group for anyone with a birthmark.

The Children's Burns Trust
The Children's Burns Trust is committed to providing support for burn- and scald-injured children and their families.

Cleft Lip and Palate Association (CLAPA)
CLAPA is the only UK-wide voluntary organisation specifically helping those with, and affected by, cleft lip and palate.

Headlines
Support for those affected by craniosynostosis and associated conditions.

The Craniofacial Society
A society for the study of cleft lip and palate and other craniofacial anomalies.

Changing Faces
Support for people who have disfigurements of the face or body from any cause.

DEBRA
A UK charity for people with the genetic skin blistering condition, epidermolysis bullosa (EB).

The Neuro Association

Help, support and advice for those affected by either form of neurofibromatosis, or their families.

Proteus Family Network

A UK support group for families and individuals affected by Proteus syndrome.

Childhood Eye Cancer Trust (CHECT)

A UK-wide charity for families and individuals affected by retinoblastoma.

The Scar Information Service

Providing information on scarring, scar therapies and support organisations.

Sturge-Weber Foundation

Support and information on different aspects of Sturge-Weber syndrome, a rare neurological disorder.

Treacher Collins Family Support Group

Support, advice, and friendship for people with Treacher Collins syndrome, and their families.

The Vitiligo Society

Support for people with vitiligo and their families in the UK and the Republic of Ireland.

XP Support Group

Support for people with xeroderma pigmentosum and other related conditions, and their families.

Chapter 11: Facial Ageing

Facial aging is a consequence of many interacting intrinsic and extrinsic factors. The most important of these include sun exposure, or photoageing and the intrinsic changes associated with chronological aging. Many skin functions deteriorate with time as the cellular activity of the skin begins to slow down, which is why we require active ingredients within a cosmeceutical regimen. This is mainly seen in reduced keratinocyte and fibroblast production, leading to decreased barrier function and stem cell activity, as well as slow wound healing.

The face is the area for which most patients seek cosmetic rejuvenation as the convex lines of a youthful appearance tend to flatten and droop as one grows older. Facial aging is a consequence of many interacting intrinsic and extrinsic factors. The most important of these include sun exposure, or photoageing and the intrinsic changes associated with chronological aging. Over a period, the muscles of facial expression produce dynamic and static facial lines and folds. The younger face is characterized by a balance captured in the classic shape of the inverted triangle.

The reversal of this "triangle of beauty" as aging proceeds is considered generally less aesthetically appealing. At present, a variety of differing dermatologic and volumising treatments are available for facial rejuvenation. These include chemical peels, dermal fillers, IPL and RF lasers, plasma rich platelets, micro-needling, microdermabrasion, botulinum injections and laser resurfacing. Each has their own relative benefits as well as their own risks. In recent years, facial rejuvenation has been revolutionized with the development of CO_2 fractionalised laser skin resurfacing (FLSR).

Laser resurfacing has long been recognised as a skin rejuvenation procedure for tissue that has lost its elasticity and become less able to resist stretching. However, despite the advent of newer fractionalised lasers, it has adverse risks and does not adequately address the problems associated with chronological aging as gravity exerts its toll on the facial structures. This procedure has benefits of faster recovery time, more precise control of ablation depth and reduced risk of post procedural problems. However, there have been cases of hypopigmentation, hypertrophic scars and skin mottling most often seen on the face, neck, and chest when the laser parameters are used more aggressively. The technique does not also attend to chronological aging problemssuch as volume deficits resulting from the loss and repositioning of facial fat. We need to apply adjunct methods such as dermal fillers or plasma rich platelets to address nasolabial or marionette lines and volume deficits resulting from the loss and repositioning of facial fat.

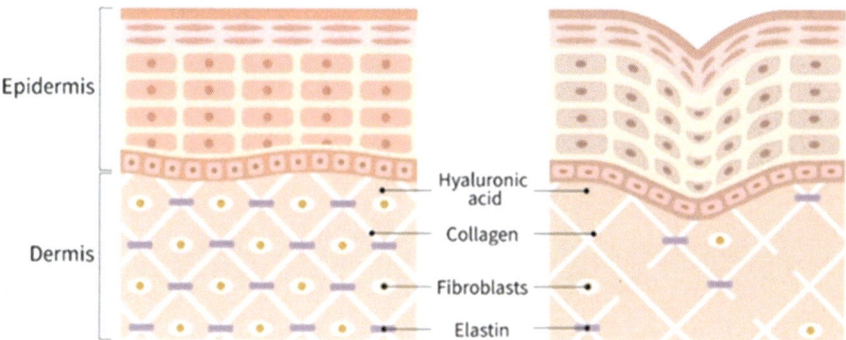

The Science of Facial Ageing

The aetiology of age-related facial changes has been related to many theories over the past 100 years related to skin, soft tissue, muscle, and bone. Gonzalez-Ulloa and Flores described facial ageing in relation to descent of the soft tissues, while the more recent discovery of anatomical facial fat compartments has made us consider adding volume to specific deflated soft- tissue compartments to create a youthful restoration to the face. Environmental factors such as body mass index, hormones, alcohol consumption, cigarette smoking, and unprotected sun exposure have all been associated with contributing to an accelerated appearance of facial ageing. General changes that occur with facial ageing include the following.

Collagen Loss

Loss of collagen and elastin from the skin of the face. Skin elasticity decreases and the skin becomes thinner. Lifestyle choices such as diet and sun exposure have an impact on the rate these factors come into play. Areas with thin epidermis (eyes and lips) receive wrinkles first.

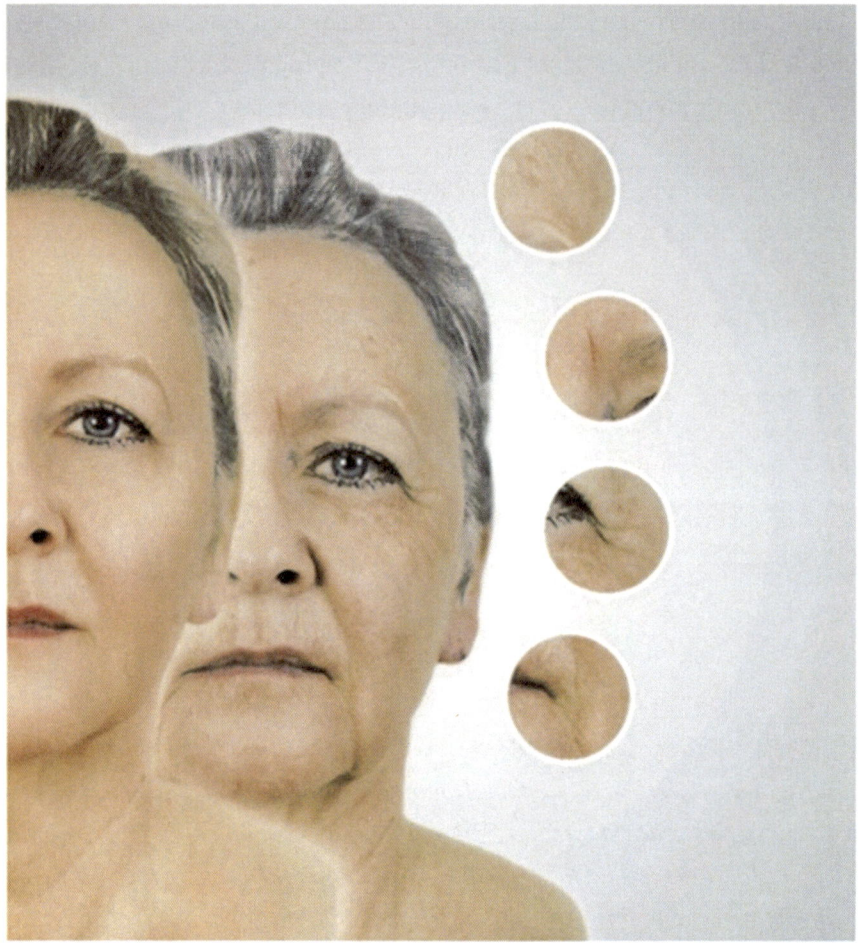

Collagen loss

- 20-30 years: Collagen levels start to fall resulting in crow's feet and frown lines.

- 30-40 years: Collagen and elastin levels continue to fall resulting in edge of brow drooping. Extension of nasolabial folds. Lips begin to thin.

- *Correction: Botox® to frown lines and eye area. Retinol or Vit-C.*

Glabellar (between the eyebrows) and forehead wrinkles. appear. With advanced filling techniques, we tend to look at changes that are occurring inthe mid face and lower face.

- *Correction: Botox® to most of upper face and to elevate eyebrows. Hyaluronic acid such as Restylane, Juvederm or Teosyl to enhance lips and nasolabial lines to hold malar fat pad in place. Sculptra and resurfacing lasers.*

- 40-50 years: Collagen and elastin levels continue to fall resulting in eyelid bags and lines start to appear in upper and lower lips. Forehead wrinkles deepen. Gravity and the pull of muscles cause drooping or sagging of the skin and deeper structures from areas of deeper attachment.

- *Correction: Hyaluronic acid fillers to upper lip. Botox® to upper face. Radiofrequency skin tightening treatments such as Polaris, ReFirme and Thermage. Infrared skin tightening such as Titian and LuxIR. Resurfacing skin lasers such as ActiveFx.*

- 50-60 years: Menopausal effects. Fat hangs in saggy skin. Nasolabial and marionette lines substantially deepen if not corrected. Neck wrinkles. More of the eyebrow droops. The nasal tip droops. The lips thin so there is less dry vermillion (pink area where lipstick is applied) showing. Perioral wrinkles deepen. Platysmal banding appears in the neck.

- *Correction: Hyaluronic acid fillers to upper lip. Botox® of diminishing effect.*
- *Face lift, brow lift, blepharoplasty or neck lift often required.*

Fat loss

For many years, we thought that the human face aged uniformly. We now know from the work of Dr Pessa that fat disappears from different fat compartments in the face at a differing rate. Most cosmetic doctors now agree that the rate of fat disappearance is related to how the face ages. The knowledge of the location of these facial fat compartments and the order in which they deflate allows a doctor to make a patient's face look younger. There are many different fat pads locations, including malar fat, nasolabial fat, superior medial fat, and the inferior infraorbital fat compartments. Precise volumisation with targeted dermal fillers by injection or cannula can restore a youthful appearance to the face.

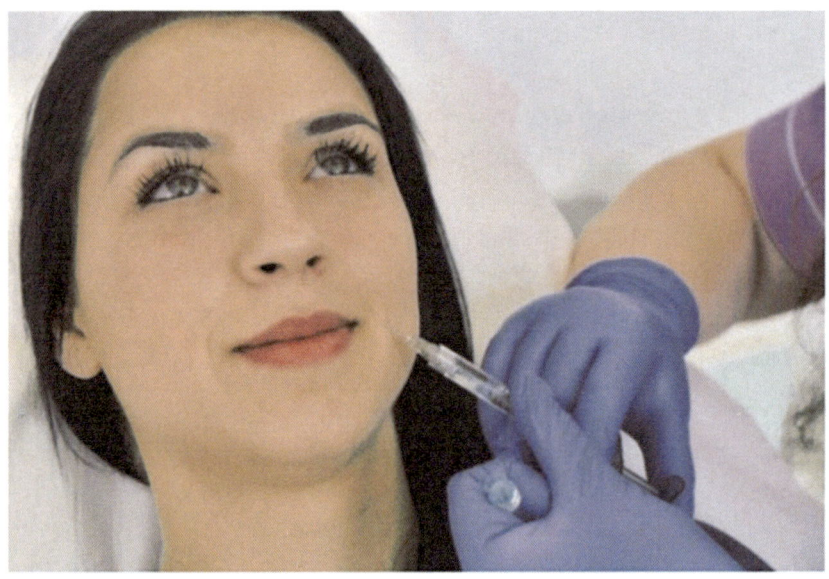

Hyaluronic acid to nasolabial line

- 20-30 years: Fat begins to disappear from under the eyes. Dark shadows cause us to look older and tired. Correction: Hyaluronic acid to lower eye area.

- 30-40 years: Malar fat pad descent begins. Nasolabial lines appear. The result is wrinkles and jowls in the face. Those due to muscle motion are referred to as dynamic wrinkles while those that are merely due to ageing of the skin are referred to as dynamic wrinkles.
- *Correction: Hyaluronic acid to nasolabial line to hold malar fat pad in place and lower eye area.*

- 40-50 years: Cheek begins to flatten. Malar fat pad descent becomes more obvious. Nasolabial lines deepen. Facial fat atrophy or wasting becomes evident with concavity of the surface contour in the temple area and cheeks appearing. In some individuals, the eyes become sunken because of fat atrophy rather than forming eyelid bags.

- *Correction:* Fortunately, multiple fillers are available to replace cheek volume lost with age. In the US, these include hyaluronic acid fillers such as Juavderm Voluma, Restylane Lyft, *Restylane Volume, or non-HA such as* Radiesse and Sculptra. Each of these dermal fillers has unique advantages and disadvantages if injecting *to central face to hold malar fat pad in place and achieve volumisation.*

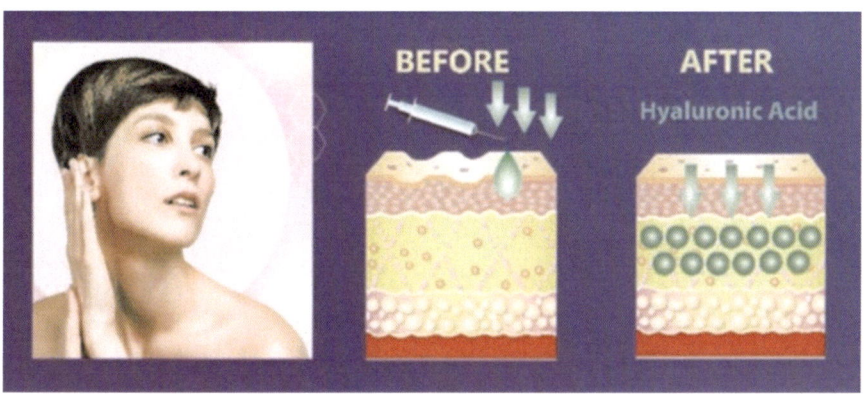

- 50-60 years: Menopausal effects. Fat hangs in saggy skin. Nasolabial and marionette lines substantially deepen if not corrected. Marionette lines and jowls become more obvious. Double chin and 'turkey neck' appear. *Correction: Short scar facelift. MACS facelift. Anterior neck lift.* Excess fat appears under eyes. *Correction: Blepharoplasty.*

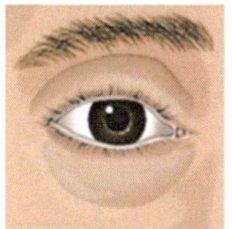 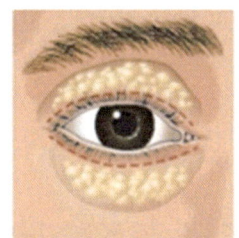 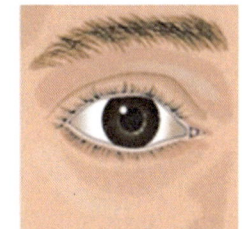

Bone loss

Facial bones lose density and thickness. This causes some minor changes in facial shape. Loss of bone along the bony rim under the eye and in the region of the nose-cheek junction. The remaining upper and lower jaw bones do not change if teeth remain intact.

- 20-30 years: Little effect of bone loss seen in this age group. *No correction required.*

- 30-40 years: Base of nose gets bigger. Some changes seen in chin area.

Correction: Enhance facial contours with hyaluronic acid to change nasolabial line to marionette ratio. Fat grafting such as autologous fat transfer.

Marionette lines and jowls now appear. Double chin appears.

Correction: Vaser LipoSelection, SmartLipo or Lipodissolve.

- 40-50 years: Chin area continues to enlarge. Eye sockets begin to widen. *Correction: Many cosmetic doctors feel the changes are too subtle to require correction.*

- 50-60 years: Menopausal effects. Bone density gets less as combination factors such as reduced growth hormone and oestrogen levels occur. *Correction: Many cosmetic doctors feel the changes are too subtle to require correction.*

- 60-70 years: Facial skin thins. Skin pigment cells increase in number and size in a blotchy pattern giving rise to brown spots of the back of hand and face (senile lentigo). *Correction: IPL lasers. Skin cancer screening.*

Ageing occurs at different rates from individual to individual as well as in each person at any given time. It is related to a combination of loss of bone, fat, collagen, and elastin, each of which is causally related to genetic composition and environment. During this ageing process, the general outline of the face

changes from a triangle with the apex pointing downward to a trapezoid or
rectangle due to sagging skin and downward descent of the cheek soft tissues.

The Effect of Glycation on Ageing

Ingrid Bergman once said, 'Getting old is like climbing a mountain; you get a little out of breath, but the view is much better!". No matter how you define ageing, it is at the end of the day (no pun intended!) a progressive loss of the efficacy of biochemical and physiological processes[1] that occur until one dies. There are many theories to explain what happens whenever we age. Many theories have been advanced to explain ageing. In this article, I want to focus on two main issues:

1) Exposure to sugars, and how it affects or modifies proteins and lipids
2) Advanced glycation end products (AGEs) and their harmful effects on the body and skin

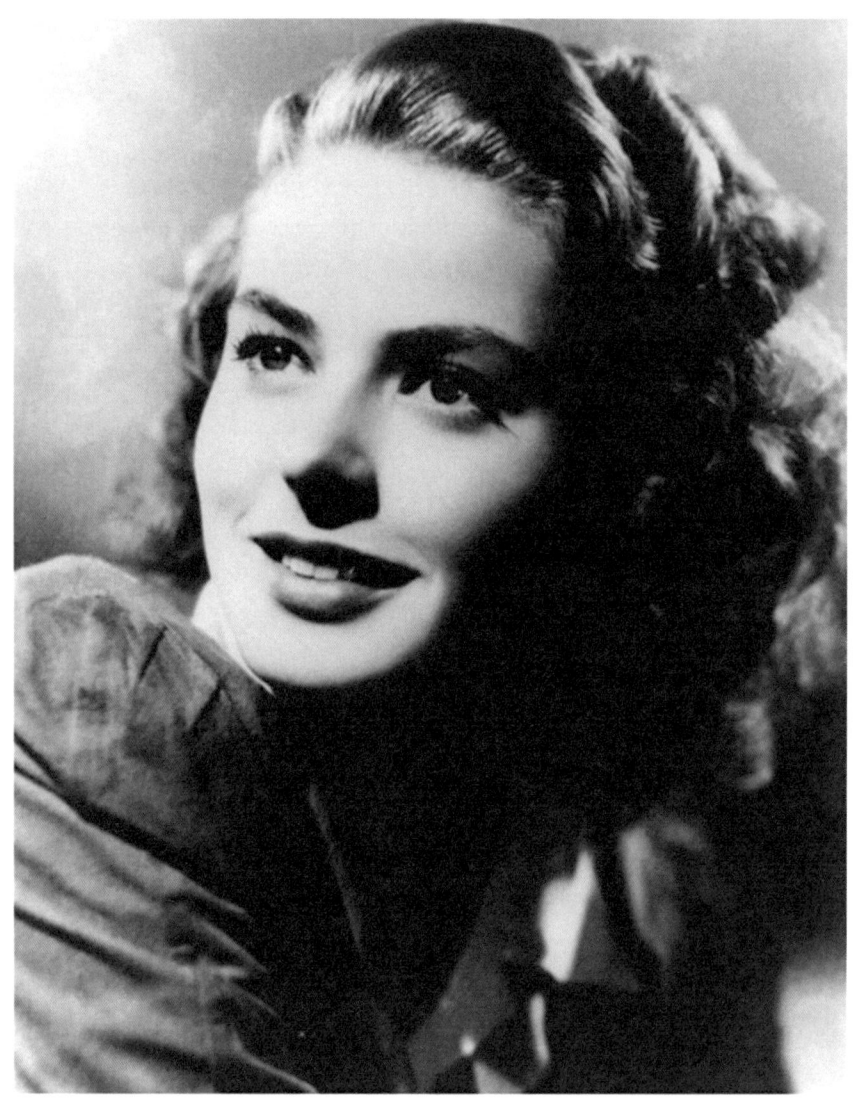

Ingrid Bergman

Glycation and Aging

Numerous publications have demonstrated advanced glycation end products (AGEs) being involved in the acceleration of the aging process. The progressive accumulation of these AGEs in the body is a hallmark of the aging process in humans, animals, and other organisms. Besides external stimuli, that would include sunlight, UV radiation, chemicals, pollutants, and smoking, exogenous

AGEs in dietary foods also trigger organ dysfunction and tissue aging. Endogenous processes that trigger the aging process include reduced cell proliferation, impaired immune functioning, excessive free radical production, shortening of the telomere, nuclear/mitochondrial gene mutation, and cellular senescence. Oxidative stress, more specifically oxidative damage to proteins, plays an important role in the mechanism by which AGEs form and accumulate, and has been implicated as a key factor in the progression of various diseases, including chronic diseases, especially Alzheimer's disease, and aging.

Glycation and the Skin

Although most research into the changes in skin with age focus on the unwelcome aesthetic aspects of the aging skin, skin deterioration with age is more than a merely cosmetic problem. The characteristic features of aging skin include wrinkles, dryness of the skin, reduced skin thickness, loss of elasticity, dermal and epidermal atrophy, reduced rate of epidermal cell proliferation and cellular senescence. In recent years, many scientific studies have revealed that Advanced Glycation End products (AGEs) are also among the crucial contributory factors of skin aging. Accumulation of AGEs in the skin has been observed both in diabetes and during chronological aging.

Proteins with a slow turnover rate, such as collagen I and IV, as well as long-lived proteins, such as fibronectin, are primary targets of glycation reaction in the skin. Moreover, excessive deposition of AGEs in sun-exposed skin areas suggests that solar radiation, especially UV radiation, may play an important role in the formation of AGEs. Receptors for AGEs are generally expressed in the epidermis and dermis, and it has been observed that the expression is higher in the sun-exposed areas of the skin as compared to sun-protected areas. Most commonly found AGEs in the skin include carboxymethyl-lysine, carboxyethyl-lysine, pentosidine, methylglyoxal and glyoxal, glucosepane and fructose-lysine. The degenerative changes that occur in the aging skin are increasingly understood at both the molecular and cellular level, facilitating a deeper understanding of the structural and functional deterioration that these changes produce.

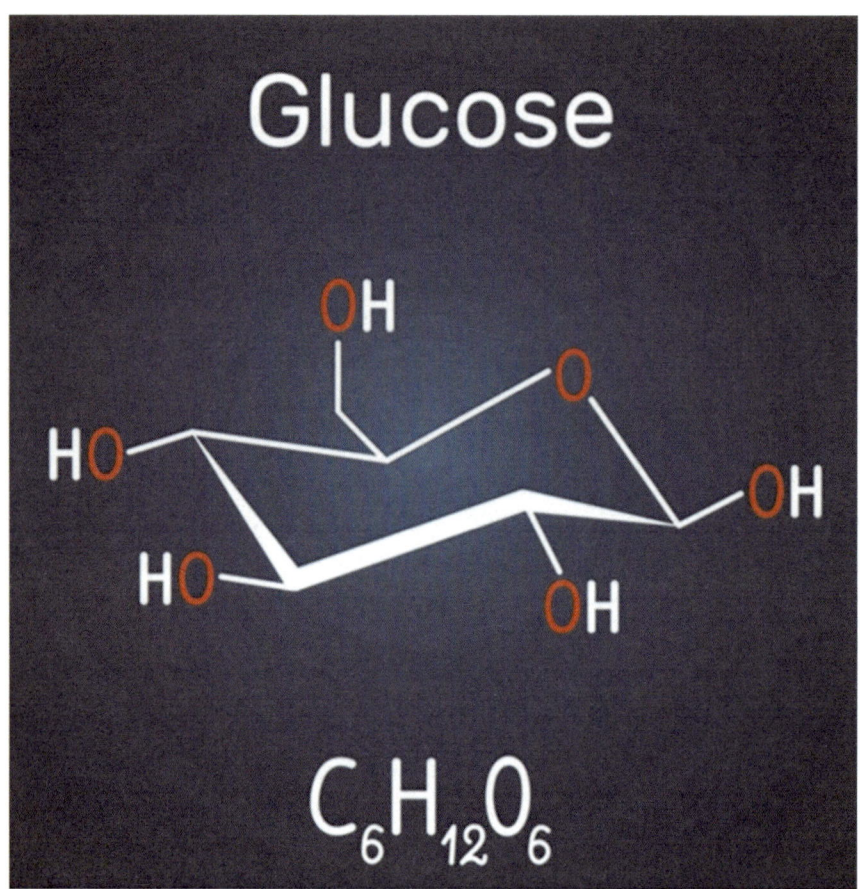

The Effect of Glucose on aging

The chemistry of Glycation

- Glycation is a general term describing the addition of a carbohydrate to another molecule, in this instance a protein, lipid, or DNA.
- Typical sugars that participate in glycation are glucose, fructose, and their derivatives.
- Glycation may occur either enzymatically or nonenzymatically.
- The common term for enzymatic glycation is glycosylation
- Nonenzymatic glycation, is commonly used in reference to reducing sugars with proteins or by the reaction of glucose with lysine residues in protein to form a ketoamine (Amadori) product (Figure 1).

- Glucation, fructation, ribation, etc. are used in reference to glycation by specific sugars.

O
$\|$
$\sim\!\!\sim$NH$-$CH$-$C$\sim$
$|$
$(CH_2)_4$
$|$
NH_2

Lysine

$+$

H $\ce{->[] }$ O
C
$|$
$H-C-OH$
$|$
$(CHOH)_3$
$|$
CH_2OH

Glucose

$\rightleftharpoons$

O
$\|$
$\sim\!\!\sim$NH$-$CH$-$C$\sim$
$|$
$(CH_2)_4$
$|$
NH
$|$
CH_2
$|$
$C=O$
$|$
$(CHOH)_3$
$|$
CH_2OH

Fructoselysine

Amadori
adduct

$[O_2]$

$[O_2]$
Arginine

O
$\|$
$\sim\!\!\sim$NH$-$CH$-$C$\sim$
$|$
$(CH_2)_4$
$|$
NH   CML
$|$
CH_2
$|$
COOH

Carboxymethllysine

$\sim\!\!\sim$Lysine$\sim$

HN$-$
HN$^{\displaystyle\frown}$N

$\sim\!\!\sim$Arginine$\sim\!\!\sim$

Pentosidine

Glycation $\dfrac{[O_2]}{\text{Glycoxidation}}$ $\longrightarrow$ AGEs

The Glycation Effect

Louis-Camille Maillard

The Amadori products above undergo a series of chemical reactions that lead to the formation of advanced glycation end products (AGEs). This process, which requires high temperatures or low water concentrations was first noticed by Louis-Camille Maillard in 1912. Maillard was a French physician and chemist, who made important contributions to the study of kidney disorders, but we remember him in this article for the "Maillard reaction", the chemical reaction by which amino acids and sugars react in foods via contact with fats, giving a browned, flavorful surface to everything from bread and seared steaks to toasted marshmallows. Technically, because we evolved as hunter gatherers used to eating raw meat there are no enzymes to remove glycated products from the human body. Some would say the glycation process causes the accumulation of metabolic waste and this promotes ageing. Glycation is responsible for many vascular complications in diabetes mellitus and is implicated in skin aging.

How do we prevent glycation?

The most obvious way is to search for an inhibitor of AGE formation, which could prevent the glycation process. This has led to several natural products being identified, including medical herbs, dietary plants, and phytocompounds inhibit protein glycation. These natural products have high antioxidant capacity and may hold the key to prevent glycation and AGE formation. Their anti-AGE activity may be one mechanism of their beneficial actions on human health. Since autofluorescence is an intrinsic property of AGEs, measurement of skin fluorescence is an effective method of detecting AGE deposition in the skin.

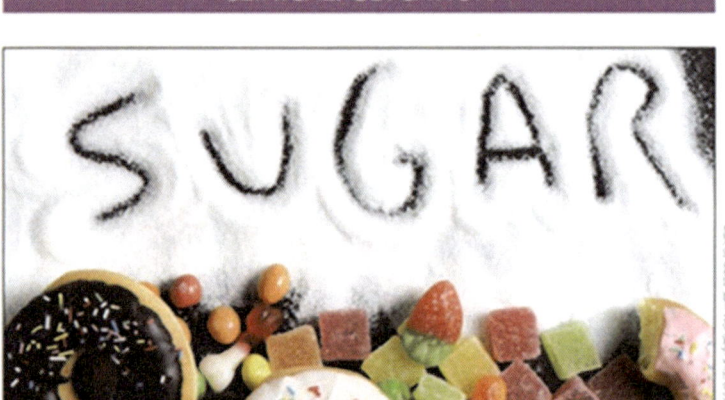

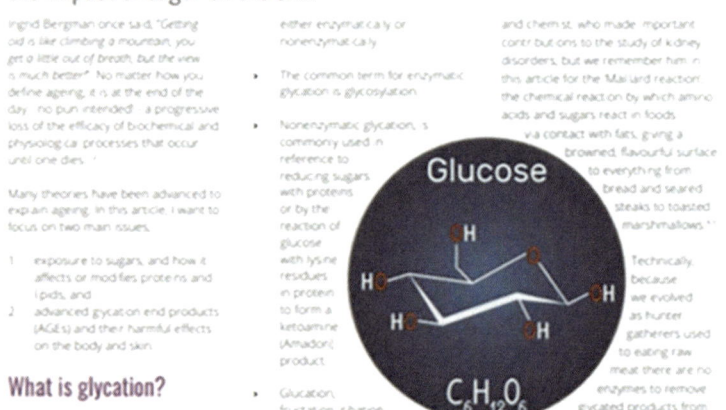

Article by the author and Rebecca McMahon in Consulting Room Magazine

Inhibition of AGE formation – Pimagedine, also known as *aminoguanidine*, is an investigational drug for the treatment of diabetic nephropathy that is no longer under development as a drug. It is known to prevent AGE formation by sequestering early glycation products, such as carbonyl intermediates. However, it has many side effects and apparently has no little effect on advanced glycation products. Another such compound is *pyridoxamine*, one form of Vit B6, which is used to prevent or treat low levels of vitamin B6 in people who do not get enough of the vitamin from their diets. It has been shown to have good results in phase II clinical trials involving patients with diabetic neuropathy. This compound is known to inhibit advanced glycation products.

Chapter 12: Rejuvenation

Platelet rich plasma (PRP)

Platelet-rich plasma (PRP) is a preparation of autologous human plasma with an increased platelet concentration produced by centrifuging a larger volume of a patient's own blood. Platelets contain a plethora of growth factors and mediators in their alpha granules (TGF-β1, PDGF, bFGF, VEGF, EGF, IGF-1), which are concentrated through the centrifugation process to release concentrated amounts of these growth factors and cytokines to an injury site and augment the natural healing process.

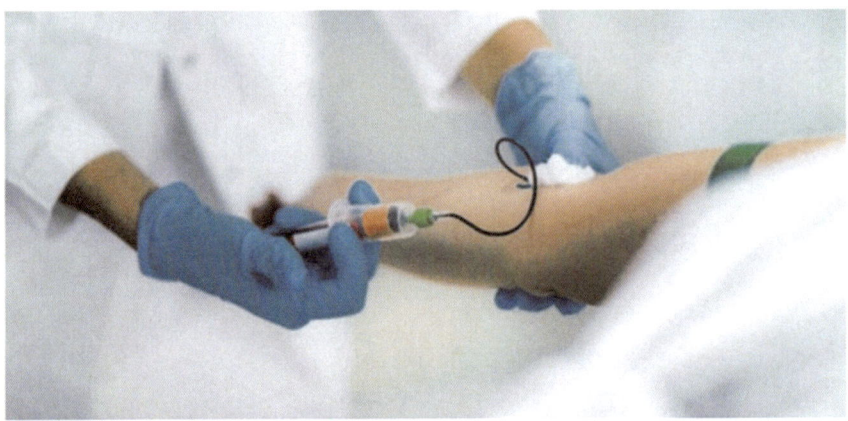

Removing blood for PRP

The normal human platelet count ranges anywhere from 150,000 to 350,000/μL. Improvements in bone and soft tissue healing have been demonstrated with concentrated platelets of up to 1,000,000/μL, representing a three- to fivefold increase in growth factor. PRP preparations are typically further categorized into platelet rich PRP (PR-PRP) preparations, and platelet poor PRP (PP-PRP) preparations, depending on the type of centrifuge used to complete the process. Castillo and Pouliot in their publication 'Comparison of growth factor and platelet concentration from commercial platelet-rich plasma separation systems' state that there is no consensus on the optimal PRP preparation with respect to concentration of blood components and there are currently many different commercial PRP systems that are available on the market.

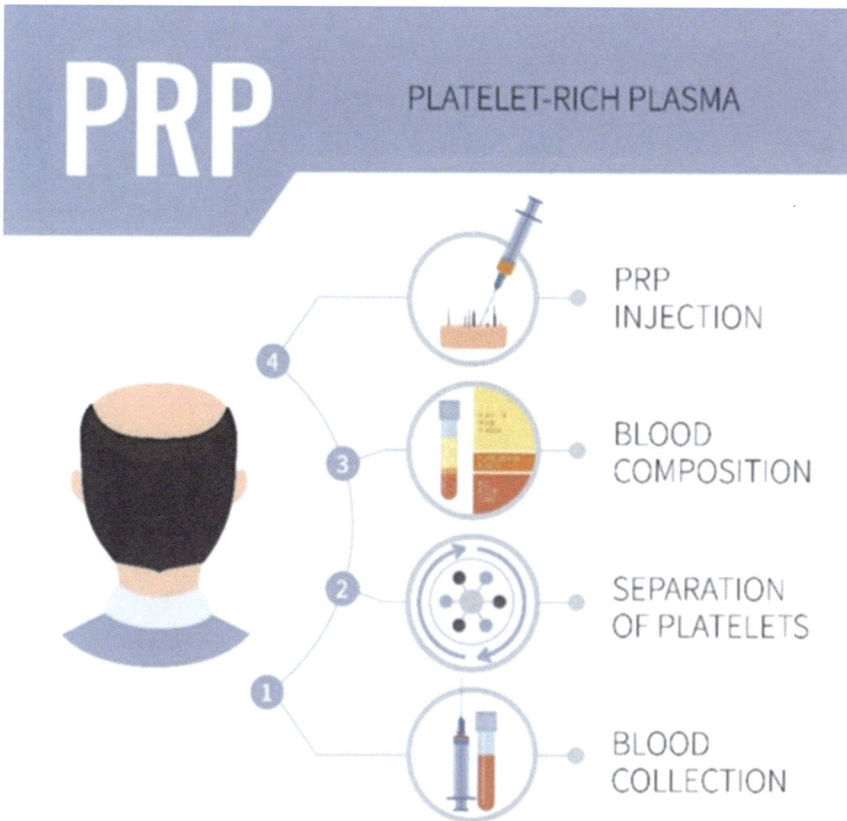

As such, variation exists in the PRP collection protocols and preparation characteristics depending on the commercial system. Controlled studies have suggested that the application of autogenous PRP can enhance wound healing in both animals and humans. Five major growth factors such as TGF, insulin-like growth factor (IGF), PDGF, EGF and VEGF are known to be related to the wound-healing processes. These growth factors are released from platelets and the production of collagen of fibroblasts is stimulated by IGF, EGF, interleukin-1 (IL-1) and tumour necrosis factor (TNF)-α. In vivo studies report TGFβ to be the most stimulative growth factor. PRP may be used for dermal augmentation and Sclafani observed aesthetic improvements of the nasolabial fold in less than 2 weeks and the results lasted for up to 3 months.

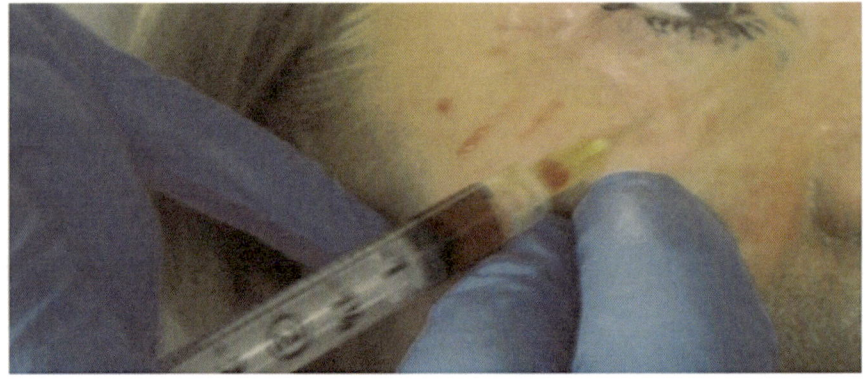

Using PRP in the periorbital area

****

The key growth factors in PRP are:

- Insulin-Like Growth Factor 1 (IGF-1).
- Fibroblast Growth Factor (FGF).
- Platelet-Derived Growth Factor (PDGF).
- Vascular Endothelial Growth Factor (VEGF).
- Epidermal Growth Factor (EGF).
- Transforming Growth Factor Beta (TGF-β).
- Nerve Growth Factor (NGF).

The author notes that evidence for benefit of PRP is mixed, with some evidence for use in certain conditions and against use in other conditions. In 2019, Health Canada stated that most autologous cell therapies have little evidence showing they work and can pose risks, such as cross-contamination between people if equipment is not sterilized properly or potentially dangerous immune reactions.

Red Light Therapy (RLT)

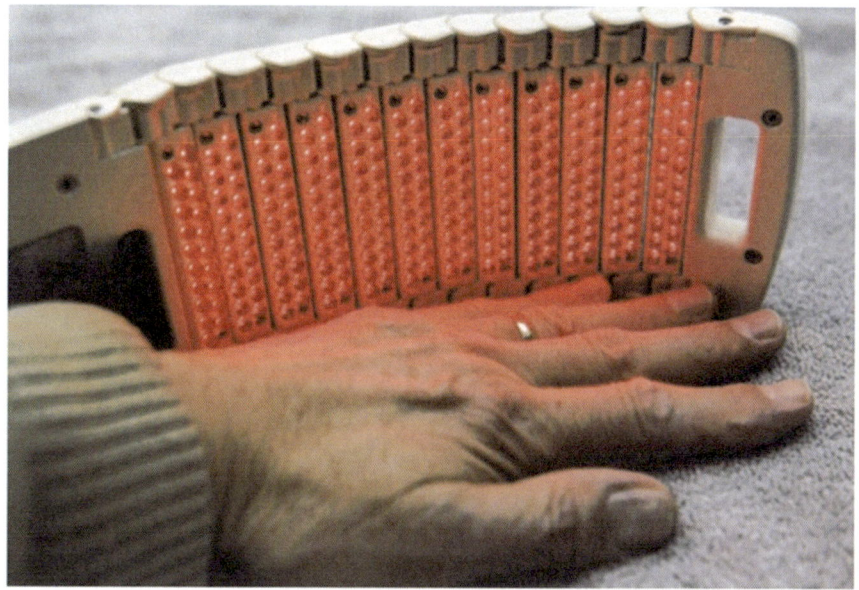

Omnilux ReviveTM (633nm) therapy stimulates fibroblast activity, leading to faster and more efficient collagen synthesis and ECM proteins. It also increases cell vitality by increasing the production of cellular ATP and stimulates the contractile phase of the remodeling process producing better lineated collagen.

Ever since the initial experiments in space, there have been hundreds of clinical studies and thousands of laboratory studies conducted to determine if RLT has medical benefits. It is generally accepted that red light accelerates cell renewal and repair by increasing collagen and elastin synthesis, hence reducing scars, and forming better skin. B A Russell and N Kellett in a study, *J Cosmet Laser Ther* 2005 showed Omnilux red and near infrared LED therapy represented an effective and acceptable method of photo rejuvenation. Exposure to red light at 633nm is supposed to increase the body's natural form of cellular energy (ATP). By increasing the function of the mitochondriausing RLT, a cell can make more ATP. Many studies have had promising results,but the benefits of red-light therapy can still be a source of controversy. Some say additional clinical research is needed to prove that RLT is effective. The author hypotheses that 633nm light can act in conjunction with PRP and stem cells to produce an overall reepithelisation effect and has won international awards for his research into this. Red light proposed benefits

- promotes wound healing and tissue repair
- improves hair growth in people with androgenic alopecia
- reduces psoriasis lesions
- improves skin complexion and builds collagen to diminish wrinkles
- helps to mend sun damage
- prevents recurring cold sores from herpes simplex virus infections
- helps diminish scars
- relieves pain and inflammation

****

Microneedling

Collagen induction therapy (CIT) is an aesthetic medical procedure that involves repeatedly puncturing the skin with tiny, sterile needles. Typically, this is done with a specialized device called a microneedling device.

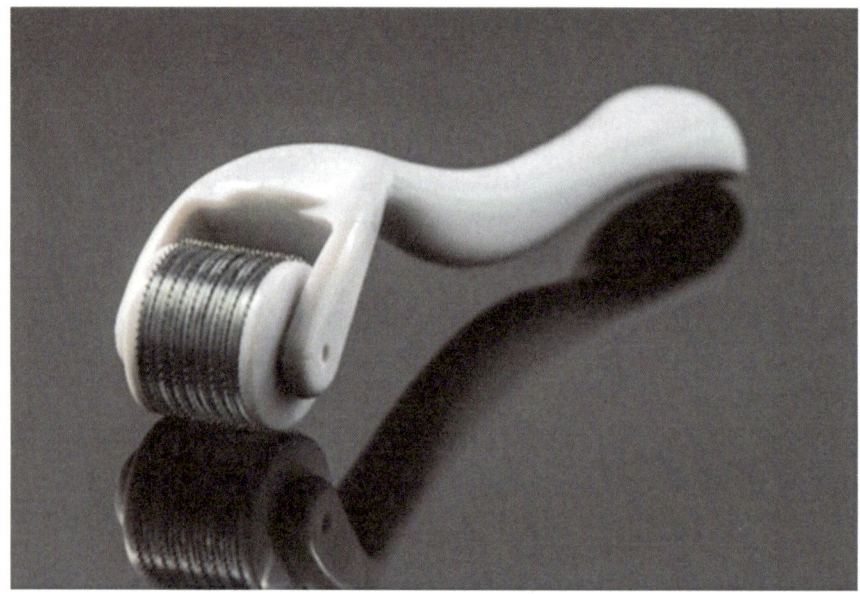

Dermaroller Device for stimulating new collagen

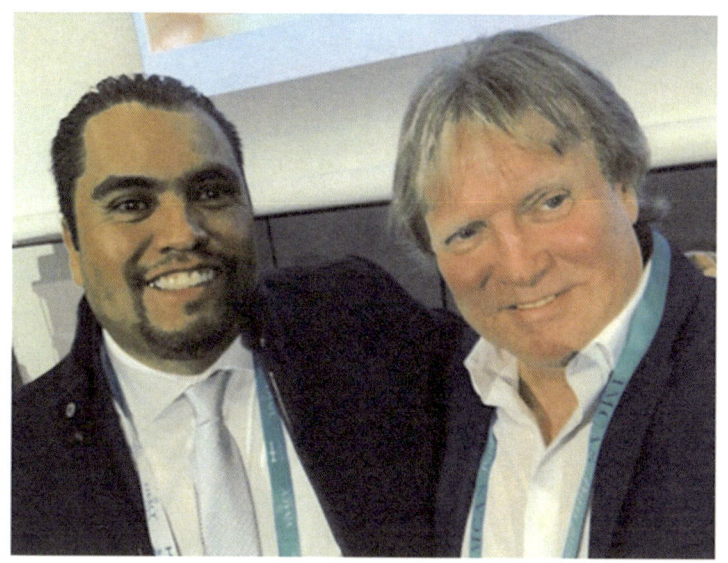

With Karim Dominguez speaking about DUBLiN Lift at CCME-Congress inMéxico 2018

The Dublin Lift

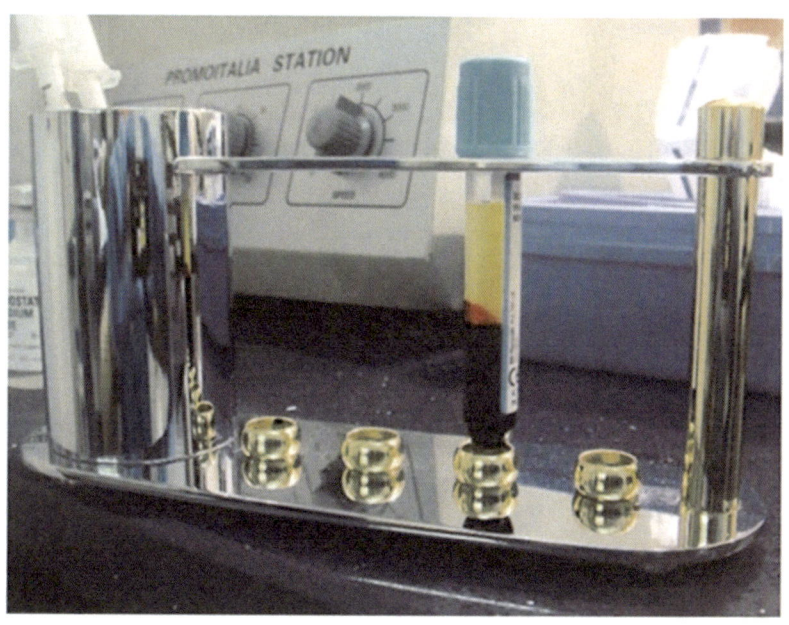

Platelet Rich Plasma used in facial rejuvenation

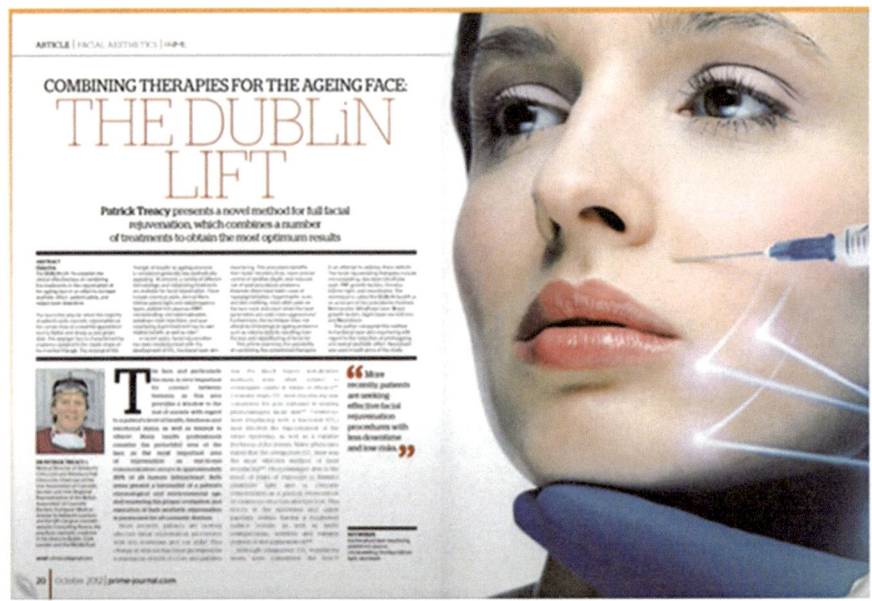

COMBINING THERAPIES FOR THE AGEING FACE:

THE DUBLIN LIFT

Patrick Treacy presents a novel method for full facial
rejuvenation, which combines a number
of treatments to obtain the most optimum results

The Dublin Lift combines five treatments in the rejuvenation of the aging face to increase aesthetic effect, patient safety. We need to apply adjunct methods such as dermal fillers to address nasolabial or marionette lines and volume deficits resulting from the loss and repositioning of facial fat. I developed this award-winning technique in 2007 by combining five established therapies to address these deficits. The facial rejuvenating therapies included microneedling, low dose Ultralase laser, (PRP) plasma rich protein growth factors, Omnilux 633 light and neurotoxins. The technique is called the Dublin facelift as an acronym of the procedures involved. D Dermaroller U Ultralase Laser B Blood growth factors Li Light (near red 633) N Neurotoxin.

Restoring the ageing face (periorbital area)

The face and more especially the eyes, is particularly important in contact between humans, as these areas provide a window to the rest of society regarding a patient's level of health, tiredness, emotional status as well as interest in others. Many doctors consider the periorbital area face is the most important area of rejuvenation as eye-to-eye communication occurs in approximately 80% of all human interactions. Both areas present a barometer of a patient's chronologic and environmental age and mastering the proper evaluation and execution of their aesthetic rejuvenation is critical to all cosmetic doctors.

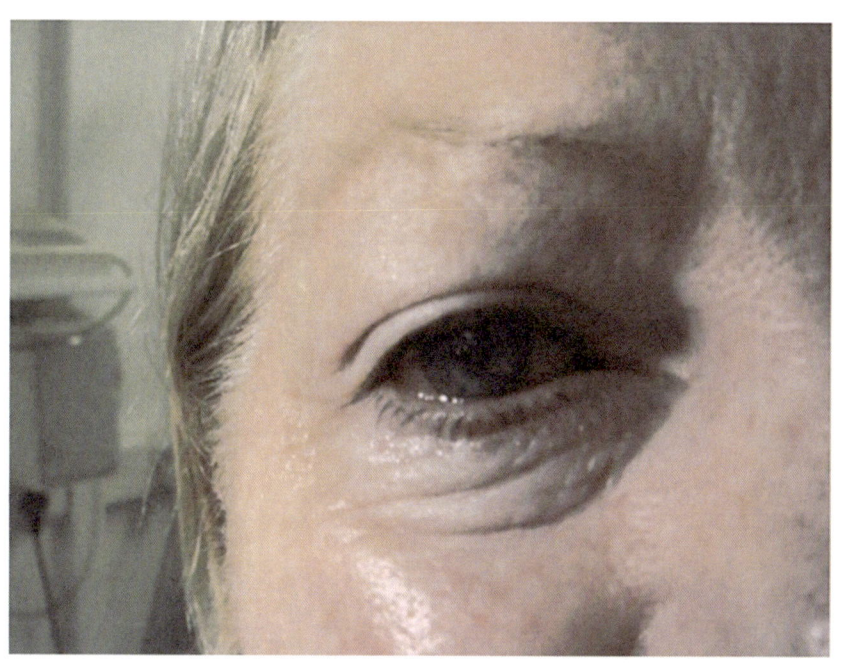

Periorbital area before DUBLIN Lift treatment

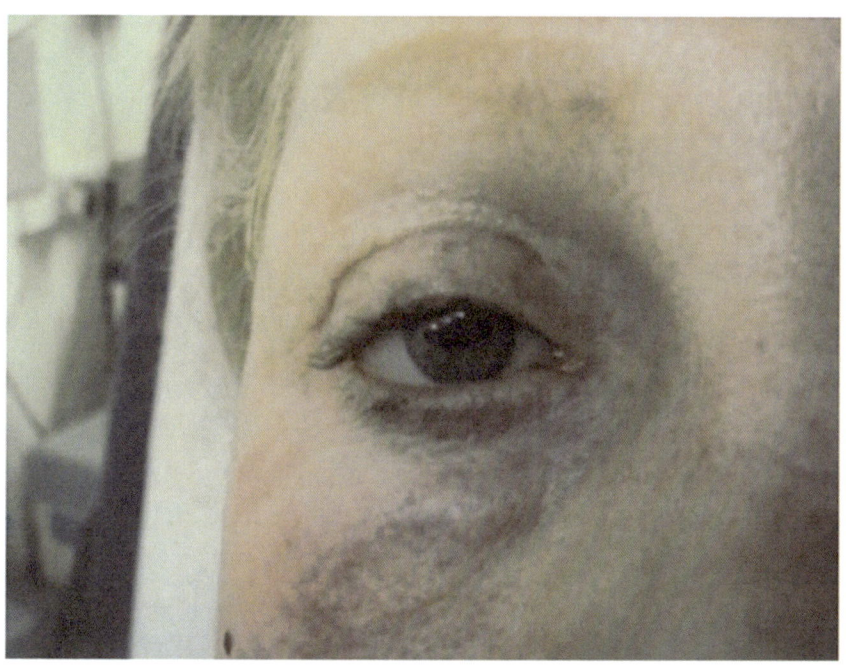

Periorbital area after DUBLIN Lift treatment

COMBINING THERAPIES FOR THE AGEING FACE:

THE DUBLiN LIFT

Patrick Treacy presents a novel method for full facial
rejuvenation, which combines a number
of treatments to obtain the most optimum results

ABSTRACT

Objective

The DUBLIN Lift. To establish the clinical effectiveness of combining five treatments in the rejuvenation of the ageing face in an effort to increase aesthetic effect, patient safety and reduce laser downtime.

The face is the area for which the majority of patients seek cosmetic rejuvenation as the common lines of a youthful appearance tend to flatten and droop as one grows older. The younger face is characterised by a balance captured in the classic shape of the inverted triangle. The reversal of this

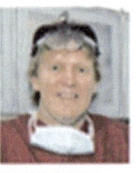

DR PATRICK TREACY is Medical Director of Ailesbury Clinics Ltd and Ailesbury Hair Clinics Ltd, Chairman of the Irish Association of Cosmetic Doctors and Irish Regional Representative of the British Association of Cosmetic Doctors, European Medical Advisor to Network Lipolysis and the UK's largest cosmetic website Consulting Rooms. He practices cosmetic medicine in his clinics in Dublin, Cork, London and the Middle East.

email: ptreacy@gmail.com

THE FACE AND particularly the eyes, is very important for contact between humans, as this area provides a window to the rest of society with regard to a patient's level of health, tiredness and emotional status, as well as interest in others. Many health professionals consider the periorbital area of the face as the most important area of rejuvenation as eye-to-eye communication occurs in approximately 80% of all human interactions. Both areas present a barometer of a patient's chronological and environmental age, and mastering the proper evaluation and execution of their aesthetic rejuvenation is paramount for all cosmetic doctors.

More recently, patients are seeking effective facial rejuvenation procedures with less downtime and low risks. This change in attitude has been prompted by a realisation of both doctors and patients

> **More recently, patients are seeking effective facial rejuvenation procedures with less downtime and low risks.**

KEYWORDS
fractionalised laser resurfacing, platelet-rich plasma, microneedling, Omnilux 633nm light, neurotoxin

More recently, patients are seeking effective facial rejuvenation procedures with less downtime and low risks. For many years CO_2 laser resurfacing was considered the 'gold standard' in treating photodamaged facial skin. Cutaneous laser resurfacing with fractionalised (CO_2) laser involves the vapourisation of the entire epidermis as well as a variable thickness of the dermis. Many physicians stated that the ultrapulsed CO_2 laser was the most effective method of laser resurfacing. Photodamaged skin occurs after years of exposure to harmful ultraviolet light and is demonstrated clinically as a gradual deterioration of cutaneous structure and function. This results in the epidermis and upper

238

papillary dermis having a roughened surface texture as well as laxity, telangiectasias, wrinkles and variable degrees of skin pigmentation. Care should be taken when treating sensitive areas such as the eyelids, upper neck, and especially the lower neck and chest by using lower energy and density. Scarring after fractional CO2 laser therapy is considered mainly due to overly aggressive treatments, lack of technical finesse. Physicians have also recorded postoperative infections leading to scarring although it is generally felt that these may be prevented by careful taking of history, vigilant postoperative monitoring and/or prophylactic antibiotic. However, in very deep rhytides, acne scarring and severe elastotic changes from sun damage, the fractional CO_2 sometimes requires multiple treatments to achieve the same results as the older lasers. Several studies have evaluated using different laser combinations in the same session to improve collagen deposition, with a wider zone of fibroplasia.

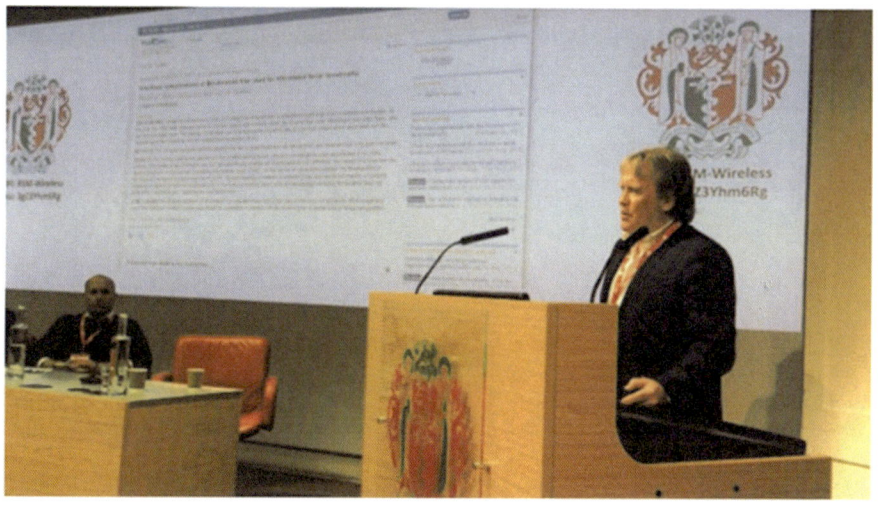

The author lecturing in the Royal Society of Medicine (London) about the DUBLiNLift

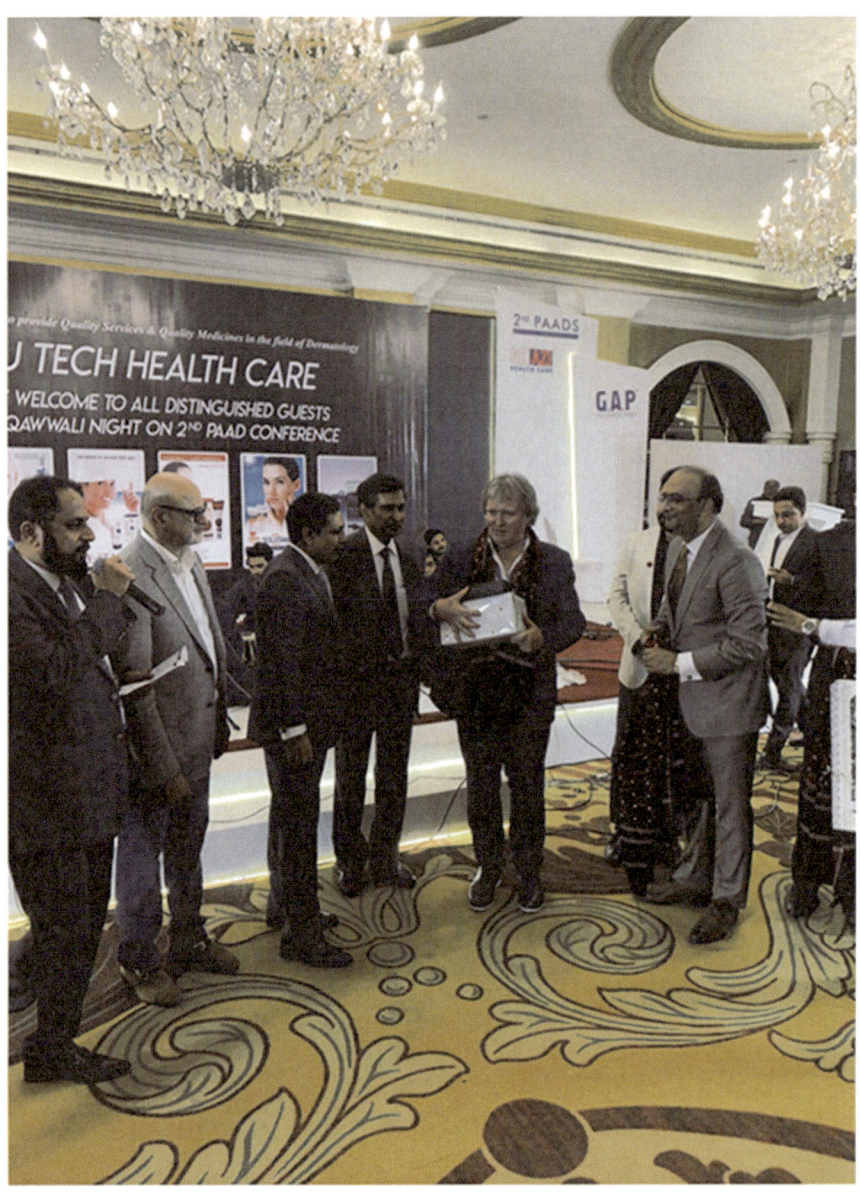

Receiving Award for lecturing about the DUBLiN Lift Karachi (Pakistan) 2019

Chapter 13: Medication

Are anti-ageing therapies effective?

There has been a lot of talk recently about anti-ageing. We must first look at what exactly is ageing and how can we control it? I suppose as a molecular biologist and doctor, I must say that ageing is really an accumulation of damage to molecules, cells, tissue and eventually organs. The maximum lifespan known for humans is 122 years, whereas the maximum lifespan of a mouse is about 3 years. There are many reasons this happens; genetic differences between humans and mice, fertility rate, efficiency of DNA repair and the old 'buzzword': different rates of free radical production, etc.

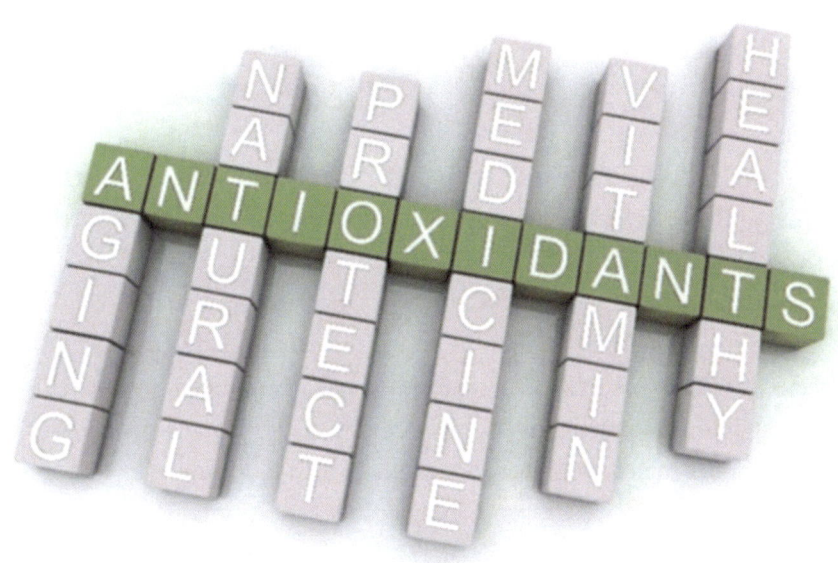

Antioxidants, including vitamins A, B-6, B-12, C and E, are believed to counteract free radicals and, in some way, prevent chronic disease such as heart disease and diabetes. There are many studies that point towards the benefits of beta-carotene, folic acid, and selenium. These antioxidants are found in a variety of fruits and vegetables. I suppose as a scientist, I am cynical about the advantage of these adjuncts in pill form.

Regarding hormone use, I am going to stand out on a limb and look at the evidence supporting their use. When people talk about hormones, they usually mean taking DHEA, testosterone, oestrogen, and probably human growth hormone.

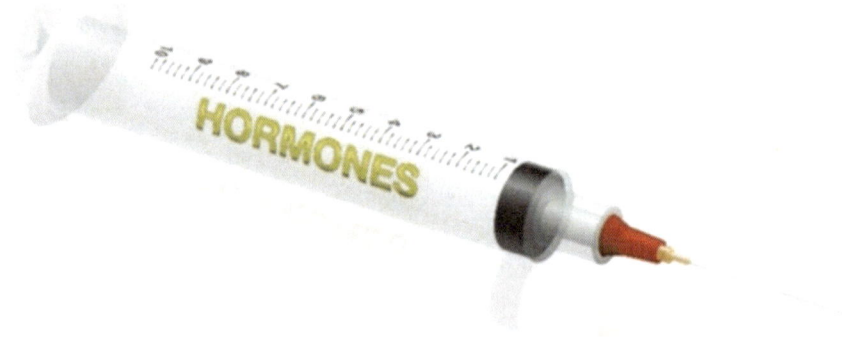

Hormones

Hormones are chemicals needed to help keep your vital organs working properly, which decline naturally as we age. It is easy to see why people would believe restoring their level to lead to previous levels. Unfortunately, life is never that simple. We all know that HRT can restore a woman's skin, vaginal secretions, energy, etc. but it has its risks in older age groups also. Look at the precursor hormone DHEA, which is converted in the body to oestrogen and testosterone. DHEA has long been touted as an anti-ageing therapy, used to ward off chronic illness and maintain energy and vigour. Proponents say it also slows ageing, increases muscle and bone strength, burns fat, improves cognition, and bolsters immunity. However, an October 2006 study published in the *New England Journal of Medicine* by Sreekumaran Nair, MD, an endocrinologist at Mayo Clinic, Rochester, found no evidence that taking DHEA reverses the effects of ageing.

DHEA is the most abundant naturally occurring hormone circulating in the human body. It is secreted by the adrenal glands and reaches its peak by the early twenties and then declines with age. The decline with age of DHEA levels correlates with many age-related changes, including peaking at games, of muscle

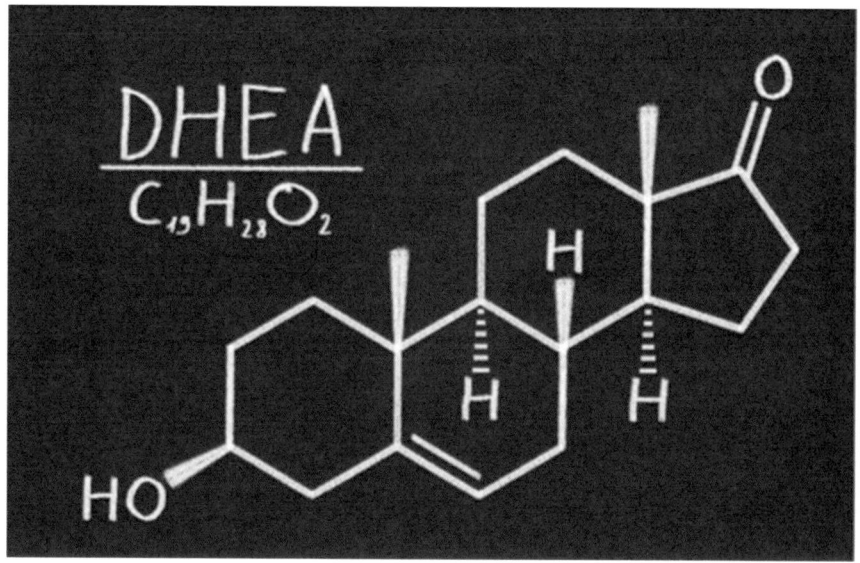

Dehydroepiandrosterone (DHEA) or androstenolone

muscle mass, of bone density, physical endurance, and ability to fight disease. The study tells of significant beneficial effects on any of those factors in men and women in their 60s and 70s. I do not mind standing out on a limb on some issues but not this one as I do not really know. I expect not, as its use is regulated by the FDA in the US. This hormone is extensively promoted and used as an anti-ageing nutrient supplement by people, hoping it will restore the pleasure of youth or increase longevity.

I expect science does not support its use, although I am sure there are many people who would disagree with me on this one. The increasing use of testosterone is also one to watch. The male menopause – does it really exist? We do know for many years that declining levels of testosterone have been linked with decreased energy and sex drive, decreased muscle mass, decreased mental ability and even osteoporosis. We also know that more and more men are taking testosterone but not enough is known about the long-term effects of testosterone therapy for this purpose.

Testosterone

Doctors feel uncomfortable about prescribing this hormone because of the lack of scientific evidence to balance whether the declining levels are unhealthy, especially as there is suspicion towards possible risks, including prostate problems. We do know that about 20% of men of age 60 and older have testosterone levels below the normal range (testosterone deficiency). The question is should not these men be treated?

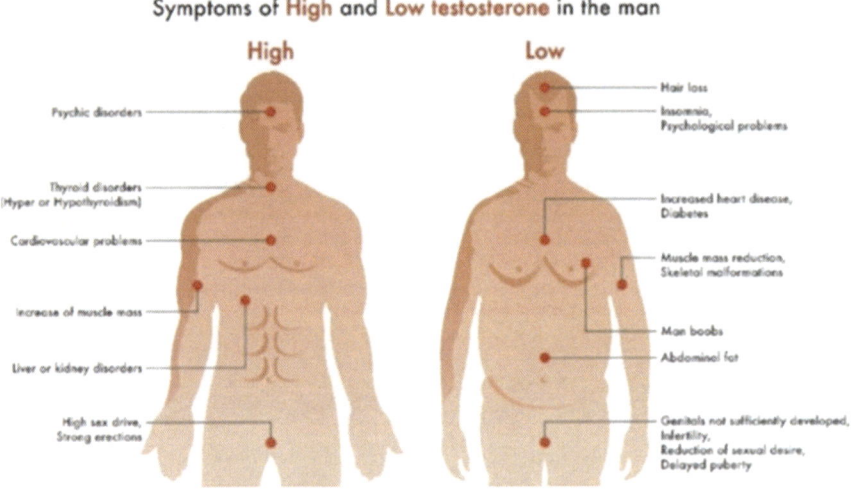

Symptoms of High and Low testosterone in the man

If a patient feels decreased energy, reduced strength or cognitive ability, less sexual interest, or potency, I will certainly check his testosterone levels as well as his thyroid levels, mood, and medication. If his testosterone proved to be low, I would treat him. In men with testosterone deficiency, testosterone therapy can restore sexual function and protect against heart disease (atherosclerosis). Also, some men taking testosterone therapy report an increase in energy, sex drive and well-being. In effect, I would not deprive a patient of testosterone if he were aware of the potential benefits and risks of the medication. Though potentially beneficial, high doses of testosterone may result in sleep apnoea, infertility and it may also pose problems for prostate and breast cancer in men. Probably, patients with a family history of prostate or breast cancer should be cautioned. It can be taken in tablet form, but many doctors say that testosterone taken by this method may cause an unfavourable cholesterol profile, thereby increasing the risk of blood clots and heart and liver problems.

Several other types of testosterone therapy exist. Intramuscular testosterone injections (Delatestryl, Depo-Testosterone) are safe and effective. Injections are given approximately every two weeks. A patch containing testosterone (Androderm) is applied each night to your back, abdomen, upper arm, or thigh.

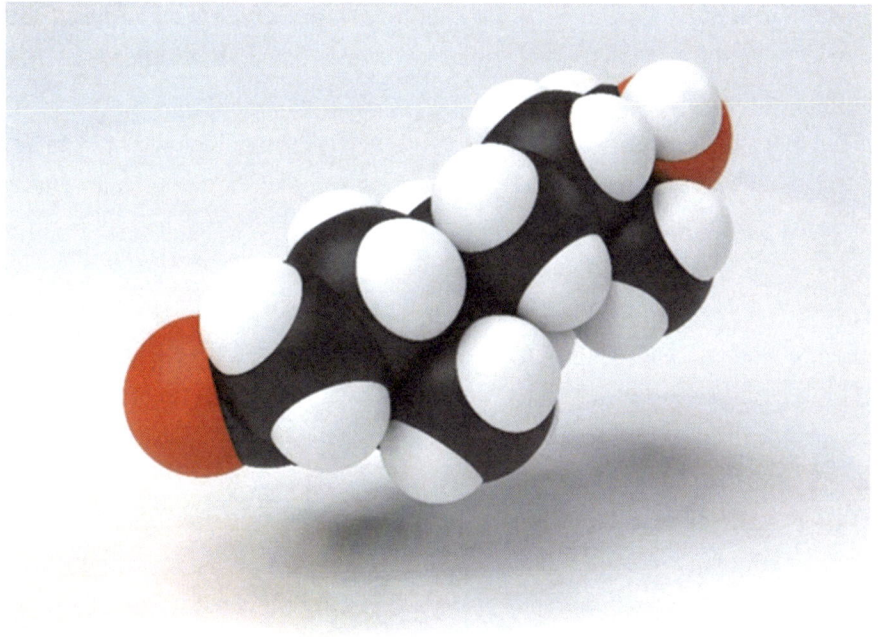

Testosterone

The site of the application is rotated to maintain seven-day intervals between applications to the same site to lessen skin reactions. In Ireland, your GP can prescribe a testosterone gel (TestoGel) to put on the skin of the lower abdomen, upper arm, or shoulder. I think it also comes in a chewing gum form.

Many patients ask me about my attitudes regarding the increasing use of growth hormone. I suppose, my early tempered memories are prejudiced because of my time working as a young doctor in Our Lady's Children's Hospital in Dublin in the late eighties when the news surfaced that the cadaver growth hormone, they had been using was implicated in multiple cases of Creutzfeldt-Jakob disease (CJD). This spurned an interest in limb-lengthening procedures in our orthopaedic department. The medicine was also used for children with kidney disease, Turner's syndrome, Prader-Willi syndrome, and muscle wasting associated with AIDS and HIV.

We know that growth hormone caused growth in childhood and helped maintain tissue throughout our life. We also know the level of growth hormone in our bodies begins to drop during midlife, in our 40s. Studies of adults with growth hormone deficiencies show that injections of growth hormone can: increase bone density, increase muscle mass, decrease body fat, improve mood and motivation, and increase exercise capacity. It is not hard to see why people believe that synthetic growth hormone could help healthy older adults, who have naturally low levels of growth hormone, regain some of their youth and vitality. We do not have a lot of clinical data, but most studies show that growth hormone injections can increase muscle mass and reduce the amount of body fat in healthy older adults. It was not exactly clear whether they became stronger or had increased moods. The studies pointed towards several side effects, including swelling in the arms and legs, arthritis-like symptoms, carpal tunnel symptoms, headaches, muscle pain and, worse still, unfortunately diabetes, hardening of the arteries and high blood pressure.

Many patients also ask me whether hormones will restore the vitality of youth. I really hate to sound like a killjoy, especially as I am continually asked to speak at anti-ageing conferences, and I realise that this part of medicine is in its infancy. I am also aware that the new science of nutrigenomics will become more important. In essence, I would really love to see a hormonal answer to stop the process of ageing but none of these supplements has sufficient medical evidence to back up the claims made by anti-ageing enthusiasts in view of the risks they carry. We all know that post-menopausal hormone replacement therapy also carries significant risks, including breast cancer and an increased risk of blood clots leading to heart disease and heart attack. However, unlike the other hormones, it has been the subject of extensive research and I have prescribed it for many years and valued its benefit in treating mental alertness, hot flushes, vaginal dryness, and poor skin. The real fifty-dollar question is whether calorie restriction theory really applies to humans. I believe that the theory is based on studies in animals, including rats, mice, fish, flies, and worms. These studies found that the lifespan of each species could be extended by reducing the number of calories consumed.

Clinical trials in humans tend to show that underweight people are more susceptible to disease and death. We would have to make sure that calorie-restricted diets were still rich in fruits and vegetables so that dieters still get the nutrients they need.

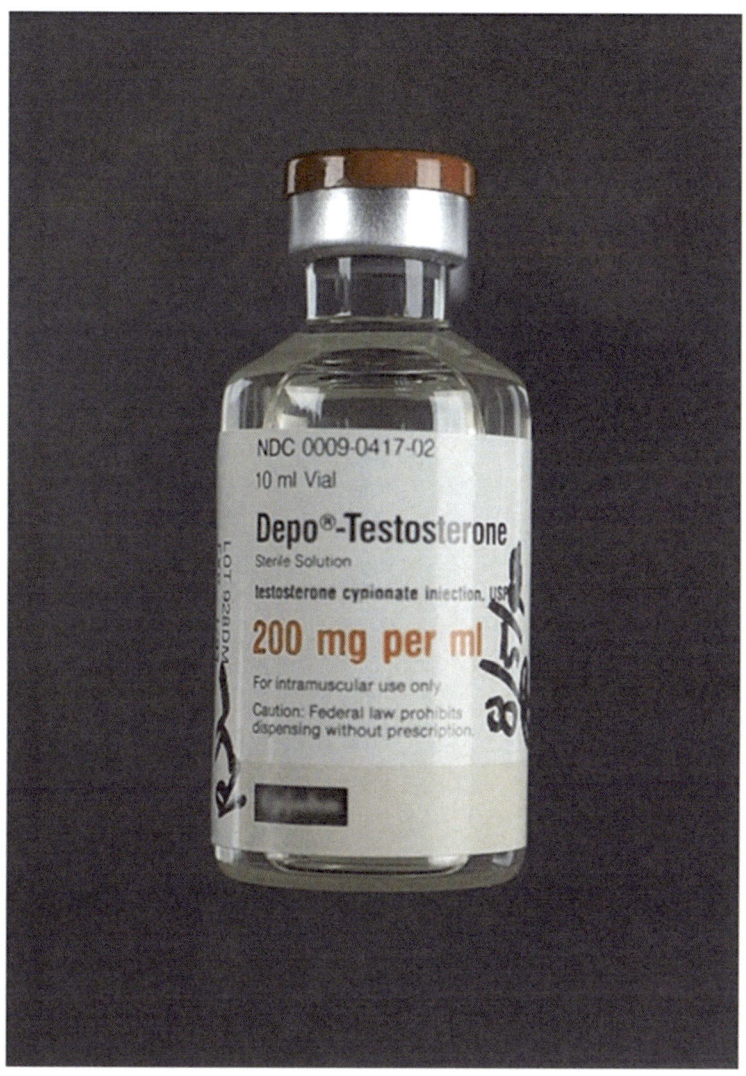

Depot Testosterone

To finish, I really think that ageing is a more complex process than presently perceived. It involves many aspects of tissue function, most importantly genetic makeup, and it's as yet unlikely that a pharmaceutical product can cure many of the ills age can bring. That is not to say that we should not continue to chase the elixir of youth. I suspect things such as heavy exercise in later years may increase free oxide radicals and shorten life. Any A&E officer will tell you about the number of myocardial infarctions brought in from badminton games, tennis games or even golf courses. Others say that is just what people do in retirement. Controlled exercise is, of course, beneficial for cardiac disease.

The influence of Testosterone

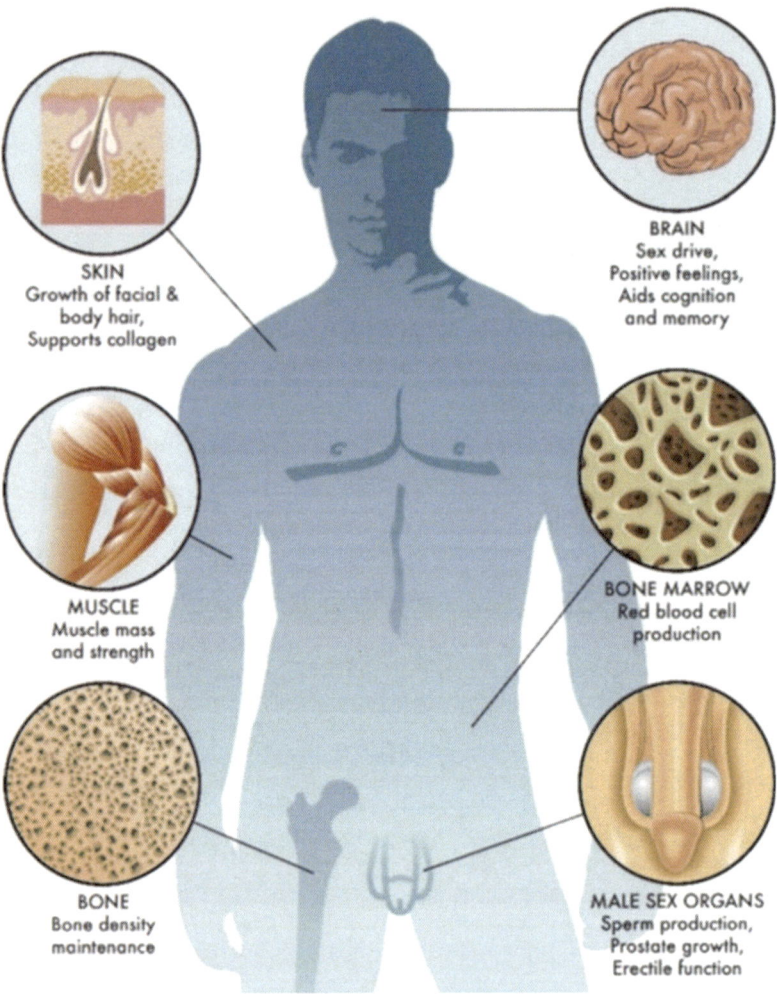

SKIN
Growth of facial & body hair, Supports collagen

BRAIN
Sex drive, Positive feelings, Aids cognition and memory

MUSCLE
Muscle mass and strength

BONE MARROW
Red blood cell production

BONE
Bone density maintenance

MALE SEX ORGANS
Sperm production, Prostate growth, Erectile function

Your best bet for a long and healthy life is to have the right parents, eating plenty of fruits and vegetables, maintain a healthy weight, exercise a little every day, do not smoke, use sunscreen, and laugh a lot… I suppose all the things that I do not do!

Chapter 14: Vitamin D

An estimated one billion people worldwide are either vitamin D insufficient or deficient. As vitamin D cannot be synthesised in adequate amounts by most mammals above 52 degrees of latitude there are insufficient photons falling per centimeter of skin to synthesis, it is essential, so technically a vitamin. After studying global data from the novel coronavirus (COVID-19) pandemic, researchers have discovered a strong correlation between severe vitamin D deficiency and mortality rates.

Sorano of Ephesus, a Greek physician, is often credited as being the first to mention some of the features of rickets. He was born in Ephesus but practiced in Alexandria and subsequently in Rome and was one of the chief representatives of the Methodic school of medicine. This medical school arose in reaction to both the Empiric and Dogmatic schools and its doctrines are well documented. Several of Sorano's writings still survive, most notably his four-volume treatise on gynaecology and a Latin translation ofhis on acute and chronic diseases.

The Methodic school asserted that the knowledge of the cause of the disease bears no relation to the method of cure and in some ways reminded me of the theories of Peter H. Duesberg, the professor of molecular and cell biology at the University of California, Berkeley, who played a major part in the AIDS denialism controversy as a proponent of the belief that HIV does not cause AIDS. Duesberg's views are cited as major influences on South African HIV/AIDS policy under the administration of Thabo Mbeki, which embraced AIDS denialism. Duesberg served on an advisory panel to Mbeki convened in 2000. The Duesberg hypothesis claimed that recreational and pharmaceutical drug use was the cause of AIDS, and that HIV (human immunodeficiency virus) was merely a harmless passenger virus. I wrote many articles against his theories and almost got banned from South Africa under the leadership of Thabo Mbeki.

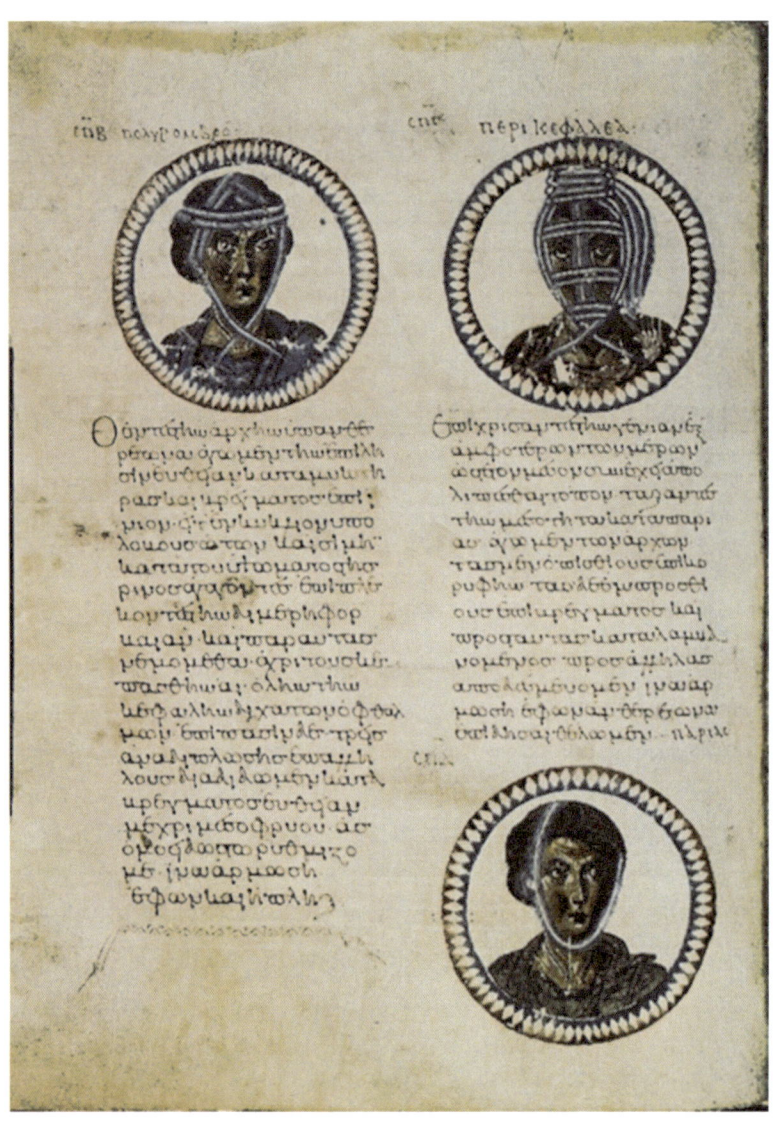

Works of Sorano of Ephesus

The History of Rickets: In 1582, it is said that Bartholomeus Reusner described a disease common among the inhabitants of Holland and Switzerland, characterised by 'the bending'. In 1614, Saint Willibrod is thought to have been referring to rickets when he described children with deformed legs. The word 'rickets appeared in 1632 with some remedies that were being considered and appeared a few years later in the records of the numbers and causes of death in the area around the Tower of London and St Paul's Cathedral, for that year.

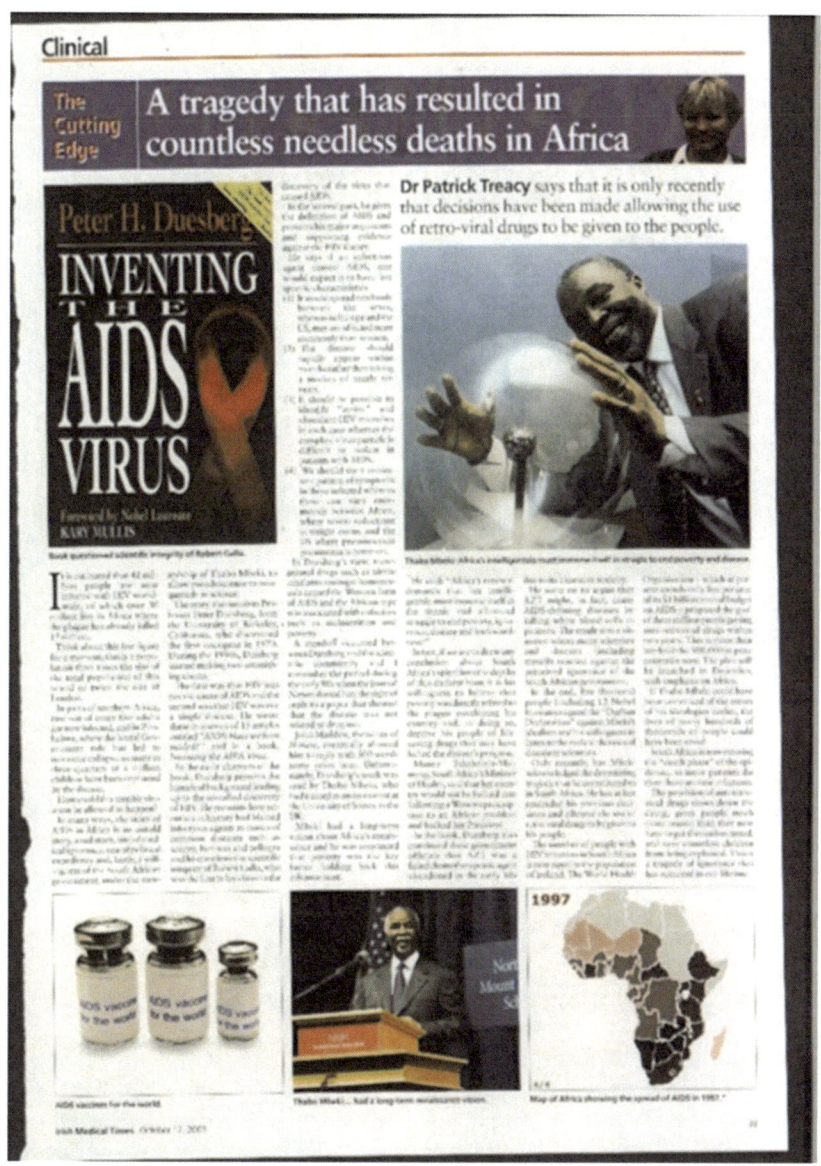

Theories of Peter H. Duesberg

In 1640, the apothecary and King Charles I's herbalist, John Parkinson, published a book with a chapter devoted to thistles, in which he claimed that Galen gave extracts of thistle to children suffering from rickets. Charles I, the second son of James VI of Scotland, was born in Fife in 1600, and became heir to the throne on the death of his brother, Prince Henry, in 1612.

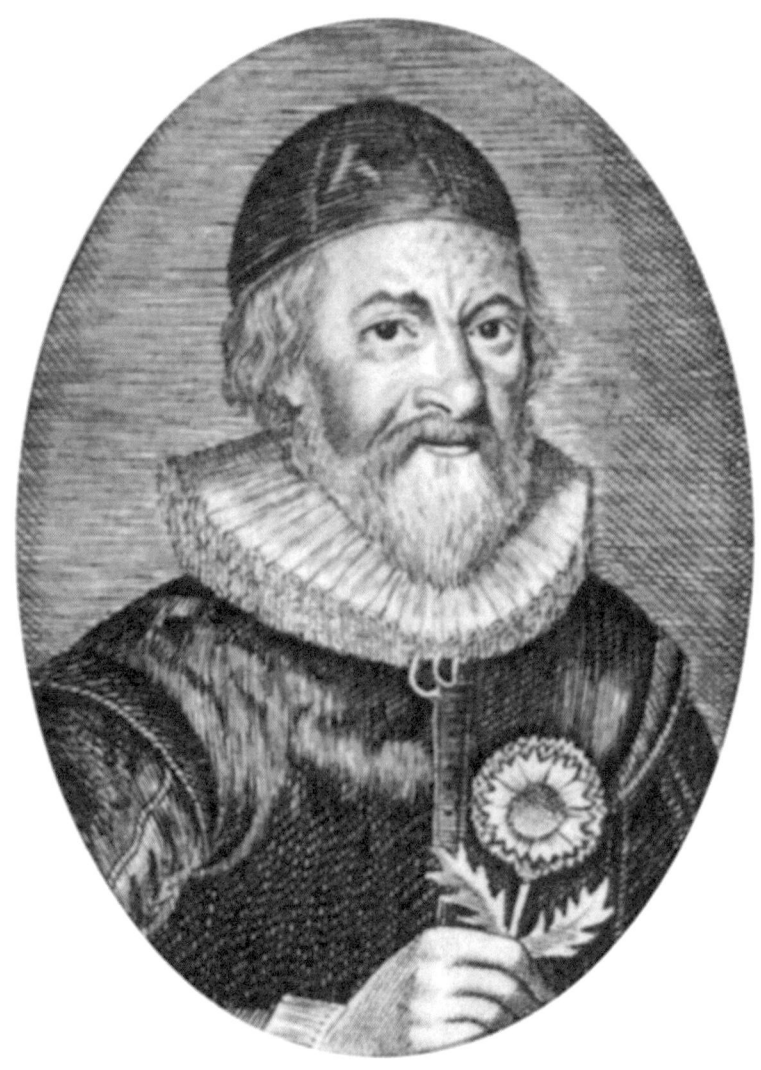

John Parkinson

It has been suggested that as a child, Charles had rickets in his earlier years. His daughter, Princess Elizabeth, also died with rickets, so perhaps the cause in this family was different from most cases at that time. Galen was a physician, surgeon and philosopher in the Roman Empire who influenced the development of anatomy, physiology, philosophy, and logic. Whether the extracts of thistle had any benefit to children remains unknown.

The first clear description of rickets was when Daniel Whistler submitted a thesis for the degree of Doctor of Medicine in Leiden in 1645, when, during the Battle of Naseby in the English Civil War, 12,000 Royalist forces were beaten by 15,000 Parliamentarian soldiers. Whistler was a founding fellow of the Royal Society and president of the College of Physicians of London.

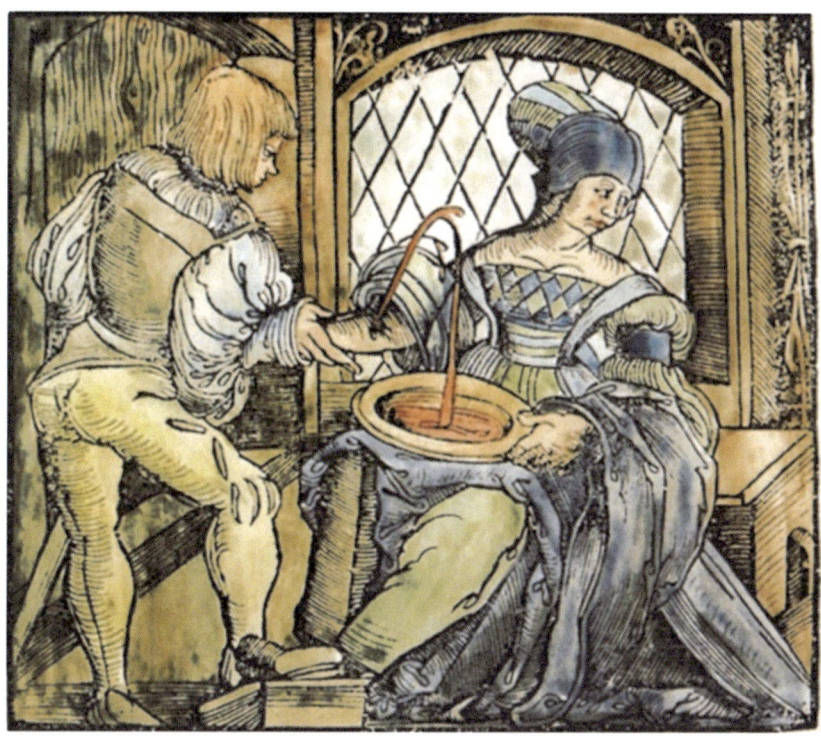

Blood Letting; A doctor bleeding the right forearm of a woman. From the Rostock Shepherd's Calendar of 1523

The second description was published in 1649 by a Dutch doctor called Arnold Boot who worked in Dublin. The most detailed account of this disease by far was the book published by Glisson in 1650. Both Whistler and Glisson believed that rickets was a 'new' disease and performed post-mortems on the patients involved. They thought it was related to the damp climate in England, but this was unlikely as it was found in the skeletons of the Medici children buried in a family vault in Florence, 1547-1602.

Bloodletting

Suggestions about treatment were along the lines of all therapies at the time for all diseases. Venesection seemed popular, especially from a vein on the lobe of the ear. Bloodletting was based on an ancient system of medicine in which blood and other bodily fluids were regarded as 'humours' that had to remain in proper balance to maintain health. In Europe, the practice continued to be relatively common until the start of the nineteenth century. Even after the humoral system fell into disuse, the practice was continued by surgeons and barber-surgeons. Though the bloodletting was often recommended by physicians, it was carried out by barbers. This led to the distinction between physicians and surgeons. The red-and-white-striped pole of the barbershop, still in use today, is derived from this practice: the red symbolises blood while the white symbolises the bandages. Bloodletting was used to 'treat' a wide range of diseases, becoming a standard treatment for almost every ailment, and was practiced prophylactically as well as therapeutically.

The damaging effect of coal pollution

In 1661, John Evelyn published a thesis on *The Inconvenience of the Air and Smoke of London Dissipated*, in which he described the pollution and named its cause as the burning of sea coal brought from Newcastle in the north of England. He described how gardens grew better when there was a shortage of coal in 1644, when Newcastle was blockaded in the Civil War. Evelyn suggested to King Charles II to move the factories away from the centre of the city and preferably downwind. There is little doubt that the smoky atmosphere blocked vitamin D syntheses by UV irradiation of the skin.

William Harvey disproved the basis of the practice in 1628, but it remained popular in the US. George Washington asked to be bled heavily after he developed a throat infection from weather exposure. Within a ten-hour period, nearly four litres of blood were withdrawn prior to his death from a throat infection in 1799. It was the same year that New York passed a law aimed at gradually abolishing slavery in the state. Both Whistler and Glisson had included the use of rooks' and frogs' livers as a possible treatment. It was also suggested that patients should have their abdomen exposed to sunlight as a source of heat, which provided a source of vitamin D.

The benefits of cod liver oil

In 1728, as Voltaire ended his exile in England, Moore wrote on the effectiveness of shark liver ointment in the treatment of rickets. Then other doctors, including Schenk and Schutte, wrote that cod liver oil taken daily for five weeks could cure rickets. In 1822, a Polish doctor called Sniadeki wrote:

'The sun must be regarded as the most efficient methods for the prevention and cure of rickets. Today, a growing body of doctors and scientists believe in the benefits of moderate sun exposure, and this is causing a different perception of sun/UV as it relates to human health.

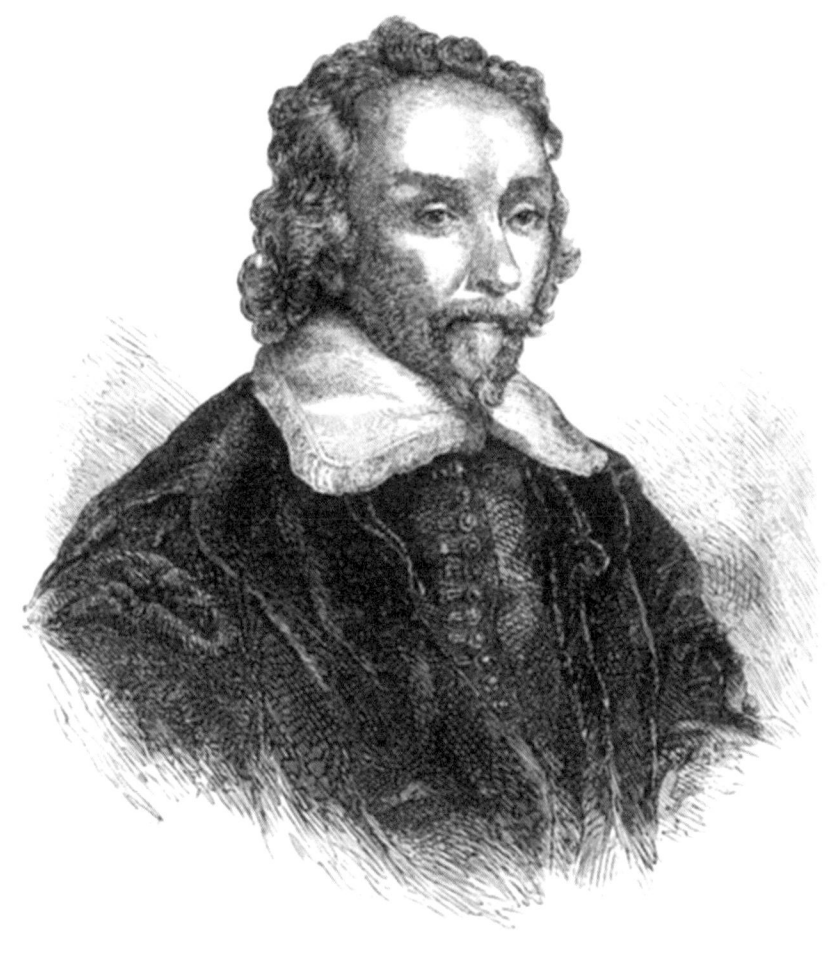

William Harvey

It is reasonable now to suggest that vitamin D deficiency was a major cause of the rickets described in the middle of the seventeenth century. In 1928, an American doctor, Huldschinski, from New Jersey, advocated ultraviolet light as a treatment for rickets.

The beneficial effect of sunlight

At the same time, across the Hudson in New York, Hess showed that cod liver oil could prevent and cure rickets in Afro-American children. At the end of World War I, doctors from Britain discovered the benefit of sunlight and cod liver oil while investigating an outbreak of rickets amongst children in Vienna.

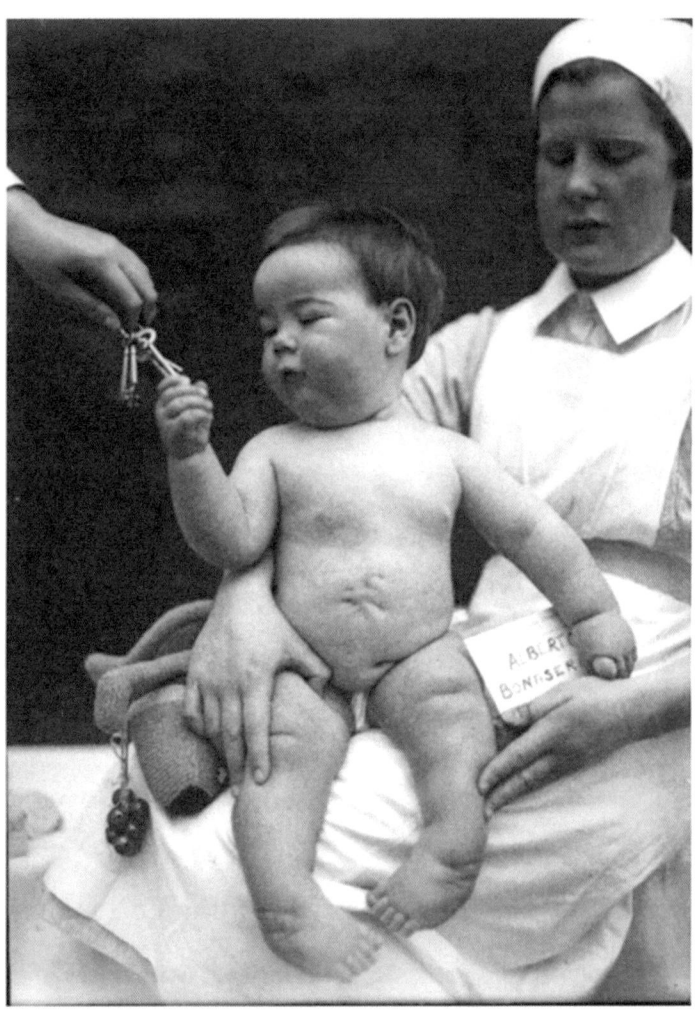

Child with rickets being treated at Lord Mayor Treloar Hospital in Hampshire 1925

However, it was not clear at that time whether the effectiveness of cod liver oil was due to vitamin A, discovered in 1913, or to vitamin D in 1921.

The Discovery of Vitamin A

The discovery of vitamin A by McCollum and Davis in 1913 ushered in the era of accessory food substances culminating in the achievement of that goal. It included the discovery of vitamin D and its production in skin caused by ultraviolet light. Although rickets, scurvy, beriberi, and other such diseases were known for centuries, the cause of them, as demonstrated above, remained elusive

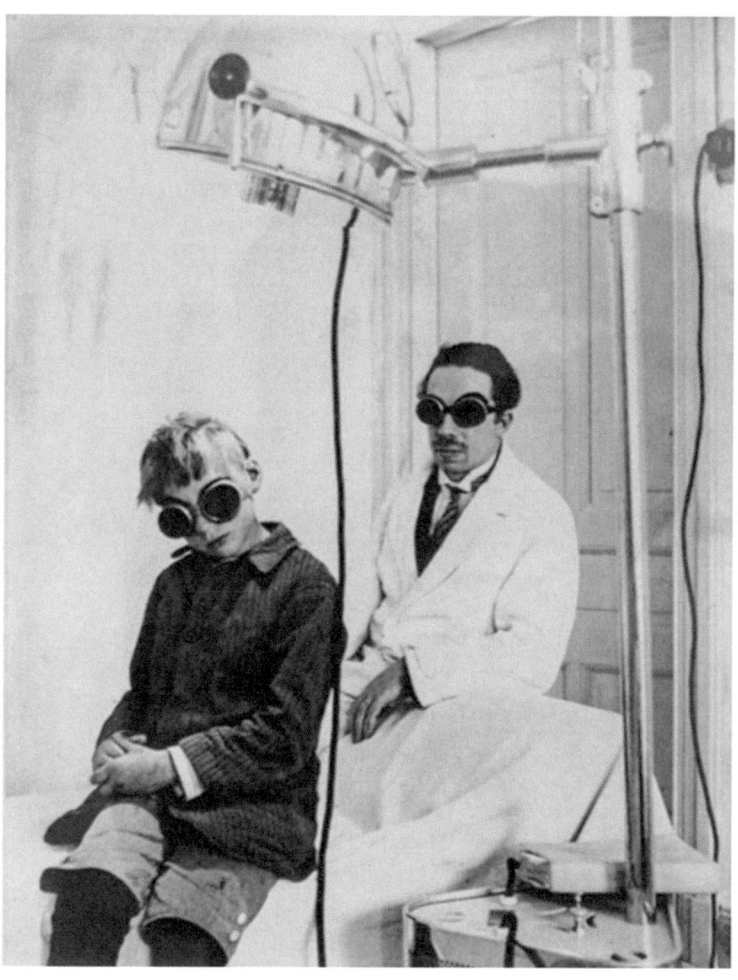

1930 photograph showing doctor and child patient with goggles during lighttherapy / phototherapy session

until the twentieth century. German investigators fed purified dietary components to animals with rickets and found that the animals failed to survive. Clearly, something was missing from these purified materials required for survival. Just before that, Eijkman was studying the high incidence of beriberi among prisoners in the Dutch East Indies if they were fed predominantly a diet of polished rice. Eijkman found that providing the hulls of rice solved the beriberi problem. Hoist and Frohlich found that scurvy experienced by seamen could be prevented or cured by citrus fruits or a substance found therein. Sir Edward Mellanby in Great Britain had been genuinely concerned with the extremely high incidence of rickets in the UK, especially in Scotland.

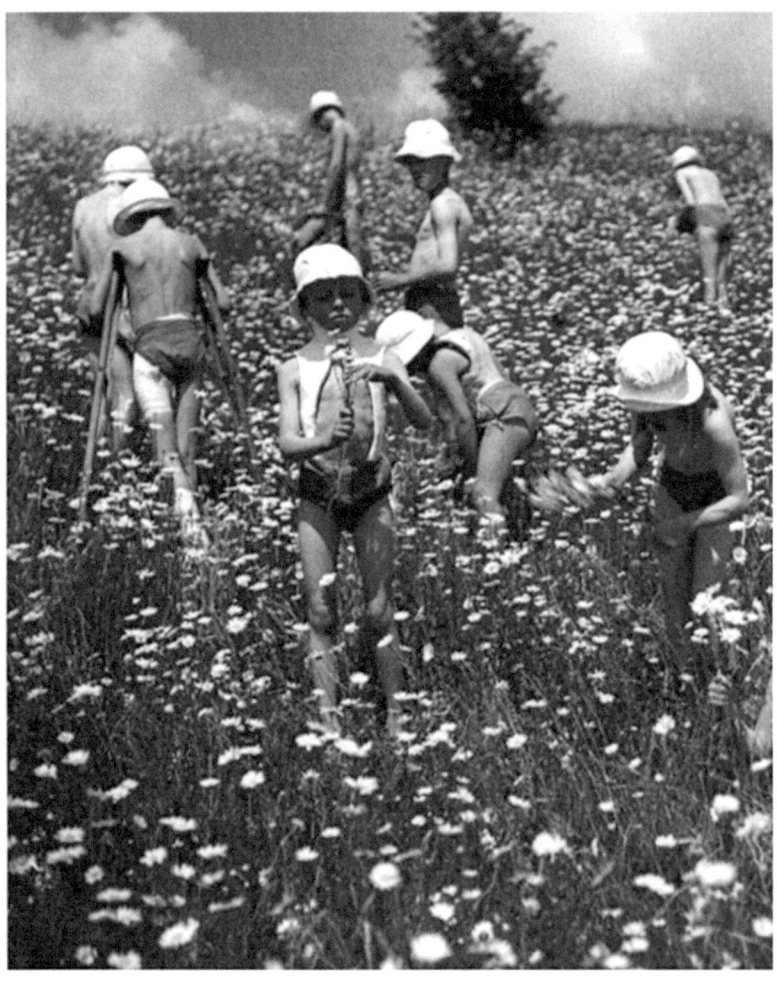

Children with Rickets being treated at a sanitorium in Hampshire England areexposed to sunlight in 1925

In fact, the disease became known as 'the English Disease'. After working as a research student from 1905 to 1907, Mellanby studied medicine at St Thomas's Hospital in London and, in 1913, became a medical doctor. It was the same year that New York City's Grand Central Terminal, having been rebuilt, reopened as the world's largest railroad station when Mellanby discovered that feeding caged dogs a diet of porridge induced rickets, which could then be cured with cod liver oil and concluded that rickets was caused by a dietary factor.

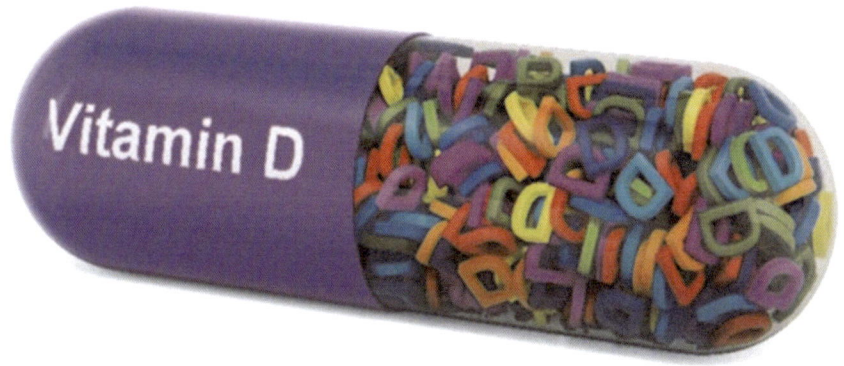

Rickets as a Dietary Disease

Sir Mellanby was taken by the work of two American scientists who were feeding animals on different diets and decided that rickets might be a dietary deficiency disease. One was Professor Babcock who carried out his experiments on a dairy herd at Wisconsin. The outcome was quite dramatic. Cows fed the corn diet did very well, reproduced and were able to produce large amounts of milk, whereas those on the wheat diet did poorly and, in fact, failed to survive. This led others at the University of Wisconsin to begin a series of experiments to test this hypothesis. Professor Elmer McCollum noted the same effect in white rats.

Mellanby decided to use the oatmeal diet consumed by the Scottish (who had the highest incidence of rickets) on dogs that he kept indoors and away from sunlight. They developed rickets, which was identical to the human disease. In 1925, McCollum published a paper entitled, *Vitamin D*, to Mellanby's *Accessory factor* in 1922, suggesting the existence of 'a vitamin which promotes calcium deposition'. As previously mentioned, in 1920, Huldshinsky, a physician in Vienna, and Chick in England, found that children suffering from rickets could be cured by exposing them to summer sunlight or artificially produced UV light.

Hess and Unger also noted that sunlight could cure rickets. Then, in 1916, a Professor Harry Steenbock, a professor of biochemistry at the University of Wisconsin-Madison, began working with goats. Steenbock was born in Charlestown, Wisconsin, and grew up on a model farm outside New Holstein, Wisconsin.

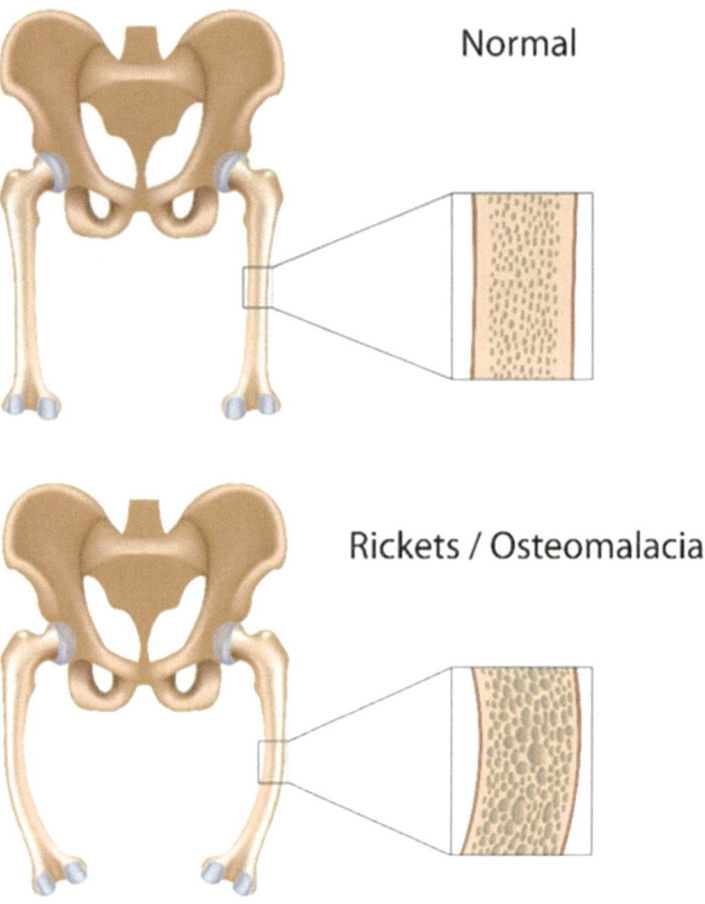

Normal

Rickets / Osteomalacia

The professor found that when they were kept in summer sun outdoors, they were in positive calcium balance but when kept indoors in the winter in the absence of sunlight, they went into negative calcium balance. In a flash of inspiration, Steenbock made a connection between sunlight and calcium retention. He then went on to irradiate rats in their cages with UV light. In 1923, he demonstrated that irradiation by ultraviolet light increased the vitamin D content of foods and other organic materials. He demonstrated this by irradiating rodent food and demonstrating that the rats were cured of rickets.

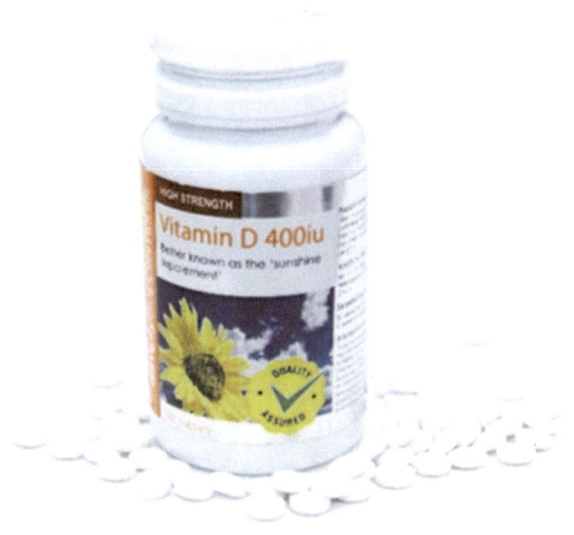

Vitamin D

Using $300 of his own money, Steenbock patented his invention, and his irradiation technique was used for foodstuffs, most memorably for milk. After receiving his patent, the Quaker Oats company offered $1 million (approximately $10 million today) for Steenbock's vitamin D technology. Steenbock thought twice about the offer. Instead of quickly selling his rights to a commercial company, Steenbock believed the money should be returned to the university. In 1927, he completed his first licensing agreement with the Quaker Oats company, permitting the company to fortify its breakfast cereals with vitamin D.

The effect of additions of fluorine to the diet of the rat on the quality of the teeth: 1925. Studies on experimental rickets. XXI. An experimental demonstration of the existence of a vitamin that promotes calcium deposition: 1922. The effect of additions of fluorine to the diet of the rat on the quality of the teeth. 1925.

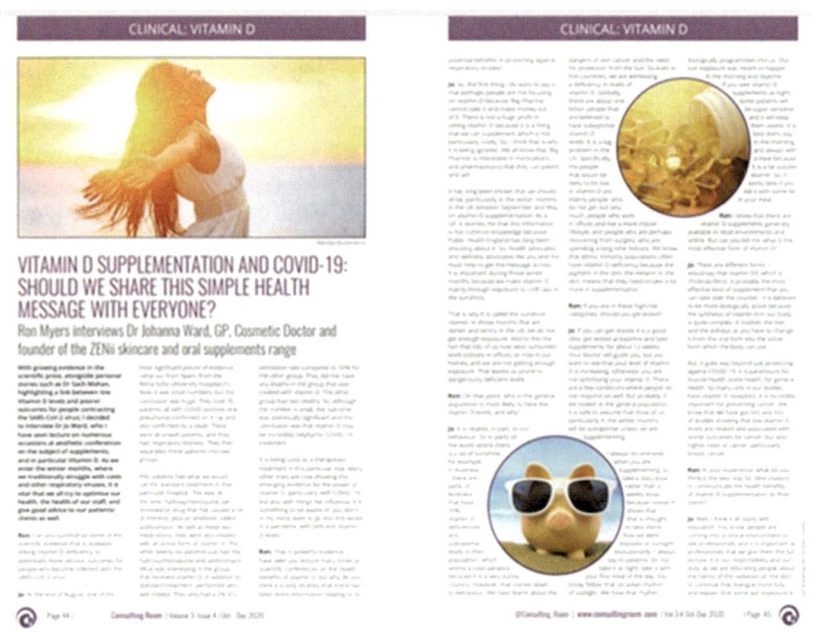

Article by Dr Johanna Ward in Consulting Room Magazine

Coronavirus disease (COVID-19) and Vit D

To date, there is no proven curative treatment for this virus; as a result, prevention remains to be the best strategy to combat infection. Currently available data suggest that sufficient Vitamin D level in serum is associated with a significantly decreased risk of COVID-19 infection. Not only does vitamin D enhance our innate immune systems, but it also prevents our immune systems from becoming dangerously overactive. This suggests that having healthy levels of vitamin D could protect patients against severe complications, including death, from COVID-19.

By analysing publicly available patient data from around the globe, Backman and his team discovered a strong correlation between vitamin D levels and cytokine storm – a hyperinflammatory condition caused by an overactive immune system – as well as a correlation between vitamin D deficiency and mortality.

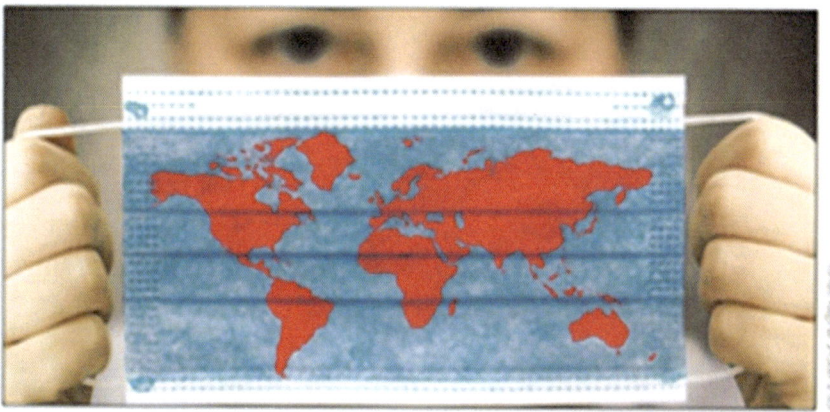

CUTANEOUS MANIFESTATIONS OF COVID-19

Dr Patrick Treacy outlines the clinical data and reports on skin lesions from COVID-19 which aesthetic practitioners may see in their clinics

The appearance of skin lesions or cutaneous manifestations of an illness is not uncommon with global pandemics, we saw this with HIV, Syphilis, and SARS too. The difficulty comes with knowing which manifestations are related to the

and low sensitivity of diagnostic tests available at the time, the investigators accepted patients with confirmed disease through nasopharyngeal swabs, as well as those diagnosed with clinical disease of COVID-19, ie those with respiratory distress who

children with meningitis.

By July 2020, we had forty six articles within PubMed which discussed a total of 997 patients from nine countries with skin manifestations related to COVID-19. To my mind, this proves

Article by the author on Covid and skin in Consulting Room Magazine

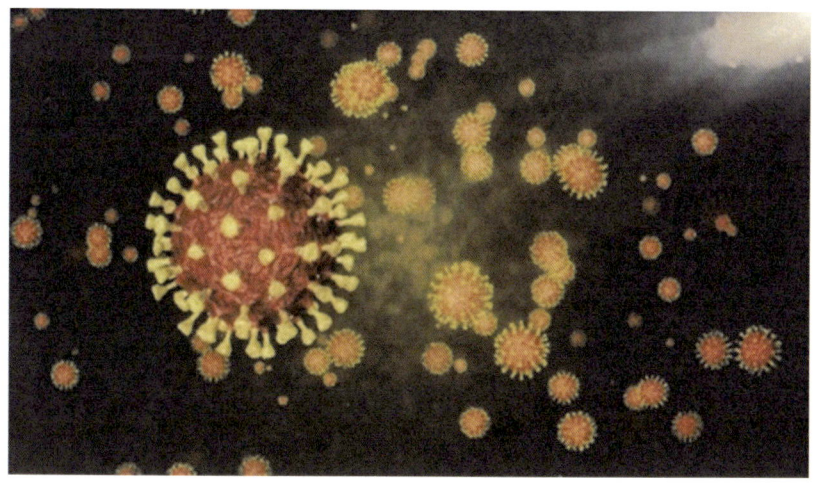

Letter: Vitamin D and Covid-19

By Contributor ⊙ 10th December 2020

Time to add some sunshine to our lives

Dear Editor,

Data from all over the world show that more than 80 per cent of patients hospitalised with Covid-19 are vitamin D deficient compared with the general population.

In a small study by Drs Jose Manuel Quesada Gomez and Luis Manuel Entrenasa in Spain, they showed high-dose vitamin D appeared to reduce the severity of Covid-19.

More recently, a consensus is emerging amongst doctors that we should all take vitamin D supplements, especially as many of our female patients are blocking out the sun with the widespread use of sun protection factor (SPF) in cosmeceuticals. This is even more important as Ireland gets a few sunny days anyway.

To address this long-standing problem, free vitamin D supplements will be sent to over two million clinically vulnerable people in England this winter. However, research shows that a third of people do not take the pills they are given.

It is now time both Ireland and the United Kingdom go further and fortify basic food such as flour and milk with vitamin D, which is common practice in Canada, Sweden, Finland and Australia. Taking vitamin D reduces the risk of fractures, improves muscle function, and reduces the risk of death from cancer.

I am aware that there may be a counterargument that this may violate the freedom of some people and excess vitamin D can cause other minor problems. However, fortifying essential food with sensible amounts of vitamin D is a cheap intervention that would have an important health benefit during this present Covid-19 pandemic.

Dr Patrick Treacy
Medical Director,
Ailesbury Clinics Ltd,
Clonskeagh, Co Dublin

Letter to the Irish Medical Times by the author advocating the use of Vit D during the Covid pandemic

Chapter 15: The Sun

The western world's restrictive guidance against sun exposure over the past 4 decades may be particularly ill-advised. People are probably using it to be out longer in the sun. Patients with more pigmentation should stop avoiding sunshine, as many people in India, for instance, follow guidelines like those in the western world. And because melanomas are rare among women with darker skin, benefit goes up in those populations when weighing sun exposure's risk against benefits.

Research from the Karolinska Institute, Sweden

Non-smokers who stayed out of the sun had a life expectancy like smokers who soaked up the most rays, according to researchers who studied nearly 30,000 Swedish women over 20 years. This indicates that avoiding the sun 'is a risk factor for death of a similar magnitude as smoking', write the authors of the article published on 21 March, 2016 in the *Journal of Internal Medicine*. Compared with those with the highest sun exposure, life expectancy for those who avoided sun dropped by 0.6 to 2.1 years. The researchers studied sun exposure as a risk factor for all-cause mortality for 29,518 women with no history of malignancy in a prospective 20-year follow-up of melanoma in Southern Sweden cohort. The women were recruited from 1990 to 1992 when they were 25 to 64 years old. Detailed information was available at baseline on sun-exposure habits and potential confounders such as marital status, education level, smoking, alcohol consumption and number of births.

When smoking was factored in, even smokers at approximately 60 years of age with the most active sun-exposure habits had a 2-year longer life expectancy during the study period compared with smokers who avoided sun exposure, the researchers noted. The authors did, however, acknowledge some major limitations.

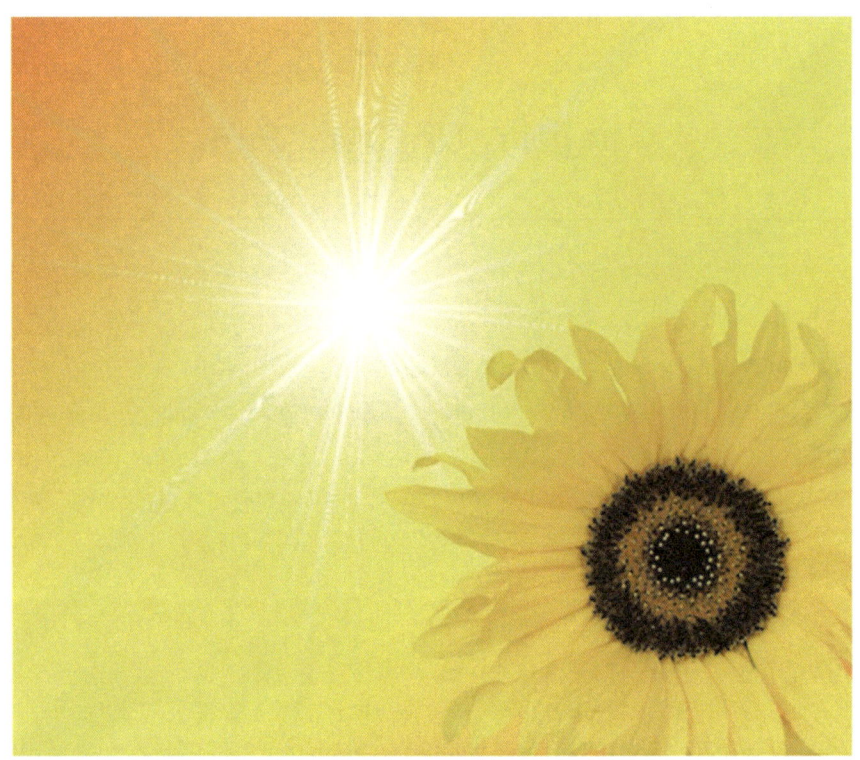

Among them, it was impossible to differentiate between active sun-exposure habits and a healthy lifestyle, and they did not have access to exercise data. There can be no doubt that a relation exists between UV radiation and melanoma of the skin. Also, there is no doubt that UV radiation is a form of electromagnetic radiation that is capable of damaging cells in different ways. The depletion of the ozone layer over the last decades has become a cause for concern regarding skin and eye melanoma. But no strong increase in UV radiation due to ozone depletion was noticed as early as 1955. I wrote a sentinel paper on the increasing level of malignant melanoma between the period 1950-85 back in the Mayo Clinic in 1989. Consequently, there must be something else that suddenly accelerated the transformation of damaged cells into skin cancer.

Research by Örjan Hallberg

Research by Örjan Hallberg and Olle Johansson shows no evidence that increased travel is the main cause of increased mortality in malignant melanoma since 1955. We found, however, a strong connection between the start of FM broadcasting and increased mortality from malignant melanoma of the skin in all investigated countries. The fact that melanoma mortality starts to increase earlier than the incidence implies that an environmental factor other than sunshine affects the survival probability of melanoma patients. This is further underscored by the fact that melanoma deaths can show peaks of the kind noticed in France during 1968. The results add to the longstanding debate on the role of vitamin D in health and the amount of it that people need, but this study does not resolve the question. Whether the positive effect of sun exposure demonstrated in this observational study is mediated by vitamin D, another mechanism related to ultraviolet radiation such as the release of nitrous oxide, or by unmeasured bias cannot be determined. From Irish studies, we know that vitamin D deficiency makes melanomas more malignant. This agrees with our results; melanomas of (those not exposed) to the sun had a worse prognosis.

****

This study was supported by the Clintec at the Karolinska Institute; ALF (Faculty of Medicine, Lund University, Region Skane); the Swedish Cancer Society; and the Swedish Medical Research Council. Funding was also received from Lund University Hospital; the Gustav V Jubilee Fund; the Gunnar Nilsson Foundation; the Kamprad Foundation; and the European Research Council. The authors declared no relevant financial relationships.

J Intern Med. Published online, 16 March 2016.

Although sun exposure can have positive effects on mood and stimulates production of vitamin D, exposure to UV radiation also damages DNA and cell functions, and that damage can lead to cancer. Excessive UV exposure can damage the immune system; cause premature skin aging, including wrinkling, mottled pigmentation, and loss of elasticity; increase the risk of actinic keratoses, which can progress to SCC. Treatment of precancerous lesions and cutaneous carcinoma should be tailored towards the individual patient scenario and the best clinical outcome.

Research from the Faculty of Medicine, Lund University; the Swedish Cancer Society; and the Swedish Medical Research Council.

Type of Skin Cancer

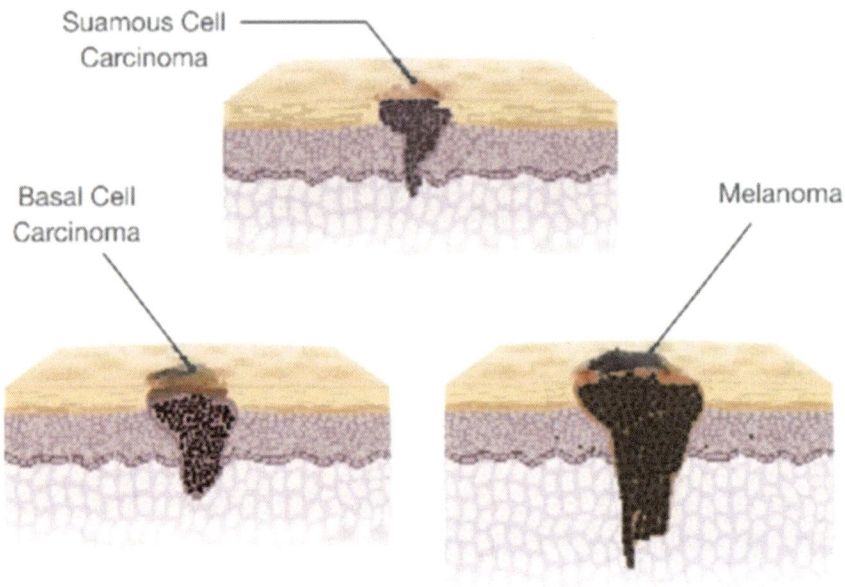

The sun's rays certainly can make us feel good, and in the short term, make us look good. Exposure to sun causes most of the wrinkles and age spots on our faces. We often associate a glowing complexion with good health, but skin colour obtained from being in the sun – or in a tanning booth – accelerates the effects of aging and increases your risk for developing skin cancer.

Chapter 16: Skin

Skin is the largest organ in the body and covers the body's entire external surface. It is made up of three layers, the epidermis, dermis, and the hypodermis, all three of which vary significantly in their anatomy and function. The skin's structure is the body's initial barrier against pathogens, UV light, and chemicals, and mechanical injury. It also regulates temperature and the amount of water released into the environment.

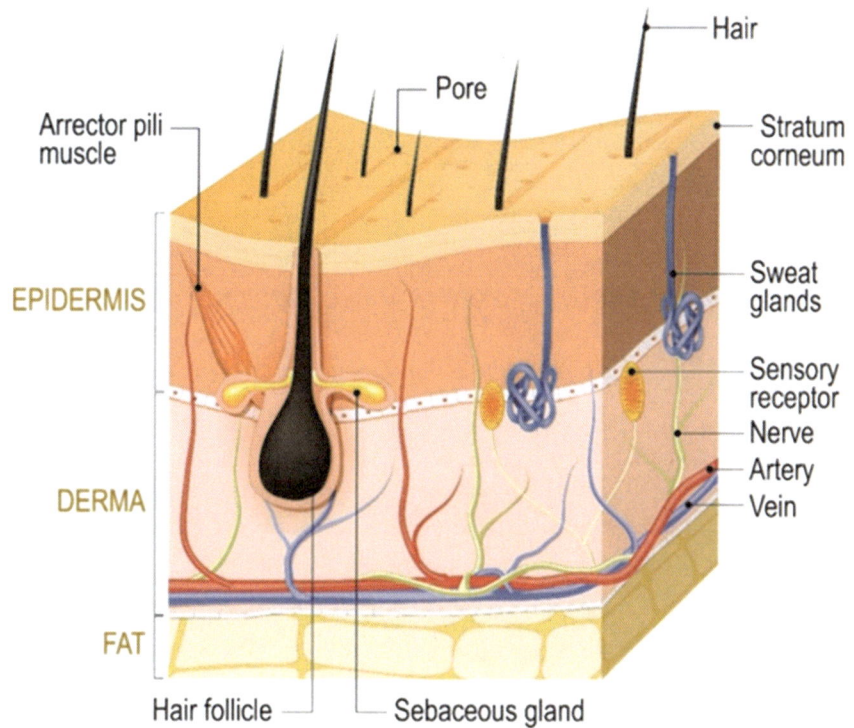

The skin has many functions. It serves as a barrier to water, invasion by microorganisms, mechanical and chemical trauma, and damage from UV light. The epidermal water barrier established by the cell envelop, a layer of insoluble proteins on the inner surface of the plasma membrane. The keratinocytes contain the enzymes needed to convert vitamin D to its active form of 1, 25 dihydroxy vitamin D.

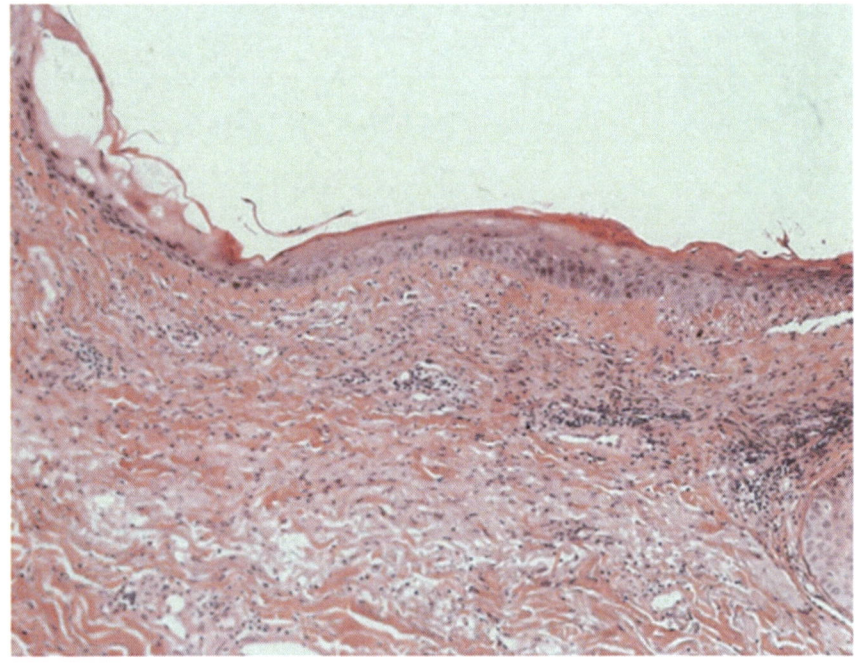

Courtesy of Prof. Kieran Sheahan, Consultant Histopathologist, St. Vincent's University Hospital, Elm Park, Dublin 4.

Layers of the Skin

Epidermis

The layers of the epidermis include the stratum basale (the deepest portion of the epidermis), stratum spinosum, stratum granulosum, stratum lucidum, and stratum corneum (the most superficial portion of the epidermis).

Stratum corneum is the uppermost layer, made up of keratin and horny scales made up of dead keratinocytes, known as anucleate squamous cells. Within this layer, the dead keratinocytes secrete defensins which are part of our first immune defense. Keratinocytes are the predominant cell type of epidermis and originate in the basal layer, produce keratin, and are responsible for the formation of the epidermal water barrier by making and secreting lipids. Keratinocytes also regulate calcium absorption by the activation of cholesterol precursors by UVB light to form vitamin D.

Melanocytes produce melanin, which is responsible for the pigment of the skin. UVB light stimulates melanin secretion, which is protective against UV radiation, acting as a built-in sunscreen. Melanin is produced during the conversion of tyrosine to DOPA by the enzyme tyrosinase. Melanin then travels from cell to cell by a process that relies on the long processes extending from the melanocytes to the neighboring epidermal cells. Langerhans cells are the skins first line defenders and play a significant role in antigen presentation. Merkel cells serve a sensory function as mechanoreceptors for light touch, and are most populous in fingertips, though also found in the palms, soles, oral, and genital mucosa.

Dermis

The dermis is connected to the epidermis at the level of the basement membrane and consists of two layers of connective tissue, the papillary and reticular layers which merge together without clear demarcation. The papillary layer is the upper layer, thinner, composed of loose connective tissue and contacts epidermis. The reticular layer is the deeper layer, thicker, less cellular, and consists of dense connective tissue/ bundles of collagen fibres. The dermis houses the sweat glands, hair, hair follicles, muscles, sensory neurons, and blood vessels. Blood vessels and lymphatic vessels are found in the dermal layer of the skin. These vessels are important for temperature regulation. The mechanism by which the body regulates temperature through the skin is very effective and works by increased blood flow to the skin, transferring heat from the body to the environment. The changes in blood flow are controlled by the autonomic nervous system, sympathetic stimulation resulting in vasoconstriction (heat retention) and while vasodilation results in heat loss.

Hypodermis

The hypodermis is deep to the dermis and is also called subcutaneous fascia. It is the deepest layer of skin and contains adipose lobules along with some skin appendages like the hair follicles, sensory neurons, and blood vessels.

What is the Skin Microbiome?

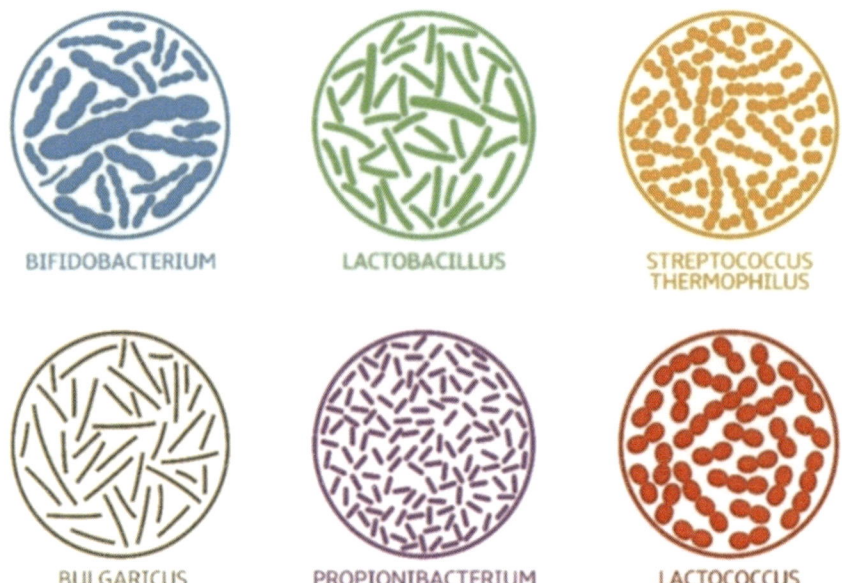

BIFIDOBACTERIUM

LACTOBACILLUS

STREPTOCOCCUS
THERMOPHILUS

BULGARICUS

PROPIONIBACTERIUM

LACTOCOCCUS

The Microbiome

The skin is the human body's largest organ, colonised by a diverse milieu of microorganisms, most of which are harmless or even beneficial to their host. Colonization is driven by the ecology of the skin surface, which is highly variable depending on topographical location, endogenous host factors and exogenous environmental factors. As the largest organ of the human body, skin is colonised by many beneficial microorganisms, which also serve as a physical barrier to prevent the invasion of pathogens. Our skin is home to millions of bacteria, fungi and viruses that compose what is called the skin 'microbiota'. The human gut microbiota consists of trillions of microbes which form a complex ecosystem. Although, some researchers have suggested that the number of microbes in the human gut is tenfold the total number of human somatic cells, a recent estimate has calculated that the numbers are of the same order, with the total number of bacteria in the human body being around 38 trillion microorganisms, mostly bacteria, living in and on the body. Many of these microorganisms reside in our gastrointestinal tract, but many others live in other places, like our mouth and on our skin. The microbiome is the ecosystem of the skin and compromises all the microorganisms that are living in or on our skin.

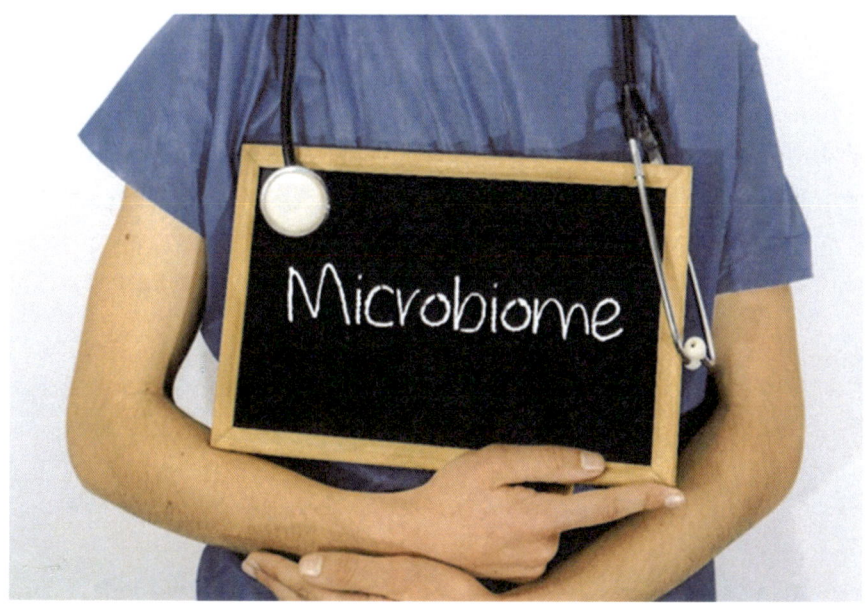

Microbiomes and Immunology

The microbiota plays a fundamental role on the induction, training, and function of the host immune system. In return, the immune system has largely evolved to maintain the symbiotic relationship of the host with these highly diverse and evolving microbes. Maintenance of tissue homeostasis is an imperative to host survival. This fundamental process relies on a complex and coordinated set of innate and adaptive responses that selects and calibrates responses against self, food, commensals, and pathogens in the most appropriate manner. In the gut, the formidable challenge represented by the exposure to the microbiota, food derived antigens, metabolites and pathogens requires a highly complex network of regulatory pathway which is only beginning to be understood. Tissues that are natural habitats of the microbiota such as the skin, the GI tract or the lung are also the portals by which pathogens access the host and often the primary site of infections. The initial encounter of pathogens with the immune system occurs in an environment conditioned and regulated by its endogenous microbiota. Autoimmune and inflammatory diseases, all associated with dysregulated immune responses have been rising dramatically over the past few decades. The mammalian immune system encompasses a complex network of innate and adaptive components in all tissues and plays a vital role in host defense against various potentially harmful external agents and endogenous perturbations of homeostasis. In westernized countries, the overuse of antibiotics, changes in the diet and elimination of chronic parasitic infections, has selected for a microbiota that may lack the resilience required for the establishment of balanced immune responses. As well, changes in diet have caused the disappearance of critical components of the human microbiota. The first indication that the commensal microbiota could drive cancer was provided by the observation that stomach ulcers and subsequent stomach cancer were caused by the presence of a single type of bacteria Helicobacter pylori.

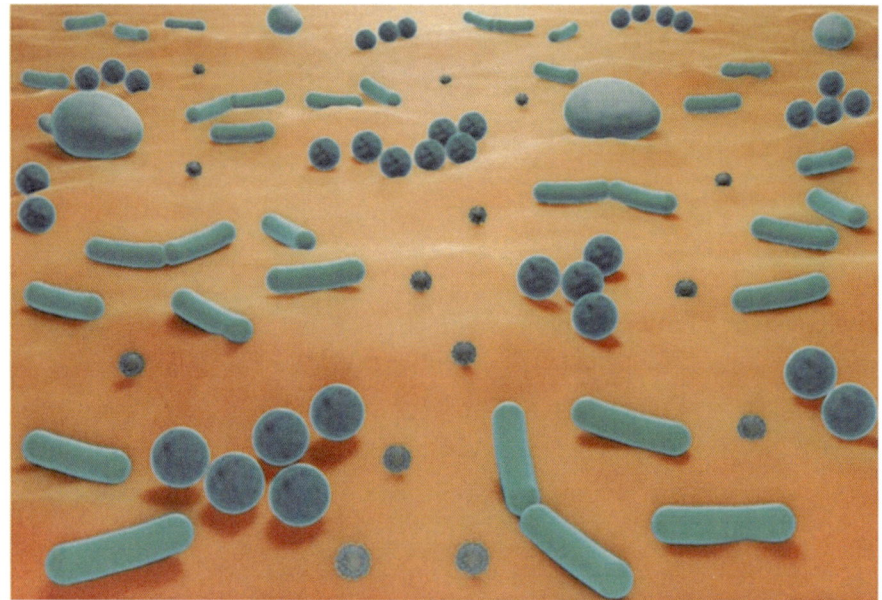

Skin Microbiome

The gut microbiota changes dramatically during pregnancy and intrinsic factors (such as stress), in addition to extrinsic factors (such as diet, and drugs) influence the composition and activity of the gut microbiome throughout life. Probiotics may restore the composition of the gut microbiome and introduce beneficial functions to gut microbial communities, resulting in amelioration or prevention of gut inflammation and other intestinal or systemic disease phenotypes.

Microbiomes and Skin

The skin is the human body's largest organ, colonized by a diverse milieu of microorganisms, most of which are harmless or even beneficial to their host. Colonization is driven by the ecology of the skin surface, which is highly variable depending on topographical location, endogenous host factors and exogenous environmental factors.

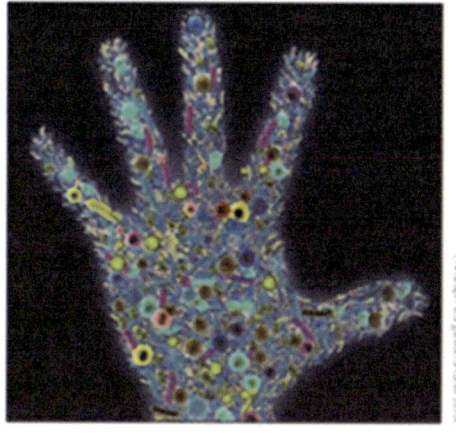

AESTHETIC: MICROBIOME-FRIENDLY SKINCARE

UNDERSTANDING SKIN MICROBIOME WHEN CHOOSING SKINCARE

Medical Aesthetician, Rebecca McMahon and Dr Patrick Treacy discuss the impact of skincare products on skin and the skin microbiome

Pharmaceuticals & cosmeceuticals

the skin. One can achieve proper skin health by using products that are clinically and scientifically proven and tested at different concentrations to achieve the optimal effect. It is also

Examples of types of cosmeceutical ingredients include

- Anti-oxidants
- Anti-inflammatories

Article by the author and Rebecca McMahon in Consulting Room Magazine

The harsh physical landscape of skin, particularly the desiccated, nutrient-poor, acidic environment, also contributes to the adversity that pathogens face when colonizing human skin. Despite this, the skin is colonized by a diverse microbiota. A rapidly growing body of evidence now also indicates that the microbiota acts as a metabolically active organ, capable of interacting with several host systems beyond the gastrointestinal tract, including the brain, urogenital tract, and respiratory tract.

Maintaining a Healthy Microbiome

The co-evolution of the microbiota and immune system has forged a mutually beneficial relationship. This relationship allows the host to maintain the balance between active immunity to pathogens and vaccines and tolerance to self-antigens and food antigens. I feel the microbiota is an intrinsic regulator of all immune responses, and we need to understand more the role of these communities of microbes, and the link between some of these components and disease states in humans. The microbiome plays a critical role in training both our innate and adaptive immune system. This also leads to the maintenance of a host-microbe symbiosis.

Chapter 17: Skin Cancer

Skin cancers are cancers that arise from the skin. They are due to the development of abnormal cells that can invade or spread to other parts of the body. They are the most common form of cancer and are generally classified as nonmelanoma skin cancer (NMSC), or melanoma. There are three main types of skin cancers: basal-cell skin cancer (BCC), squamous-cell skin cancer (SCC) and melanoma.

I have had a long history in dealing with skin cancer, particularly cutaneous malignant melanoma, since I was a student in the Mayo Clinic in Rochester, Minnesota, in 1985, where I researched and published my first paper on it. The sentinel paper on the increasing level of malignant melanoma in the Rochester, Minnesota, population in the period 1950-85 at the Mayo Clinic was published in 1989. I presented an article of my experiences with this condition at the 56th meeting of the (RCSI) Biological Society, earning me an award.

In 1996, as news emerged that Dolly the sheep was the first mammal to be successfully cloned, I emigrated to Australia, first to work with the Flying Doctors in Broken Hill. While there, I decided to try and find work in Toowoomba, Queensland, which had the highest melanoma incidence in the world. Toowoomba was a university town of about 150,000 people situated in the Darling Downs. The job that attracted me was mostly general practice with theatres dealing with skin cancer management. While there, I noted that many of my patients were part of the melanoma vaccine study by Brisbane's Princess Alexandra Hospital.

Australia was a wonderful place to learn dermatology, especially as Queensland had the unfortunate distinction of having the highest rate of melanoma skin cancer in the world (75 cases per 100,000); however, it also meant I was dealing with new melanoma cases every day.

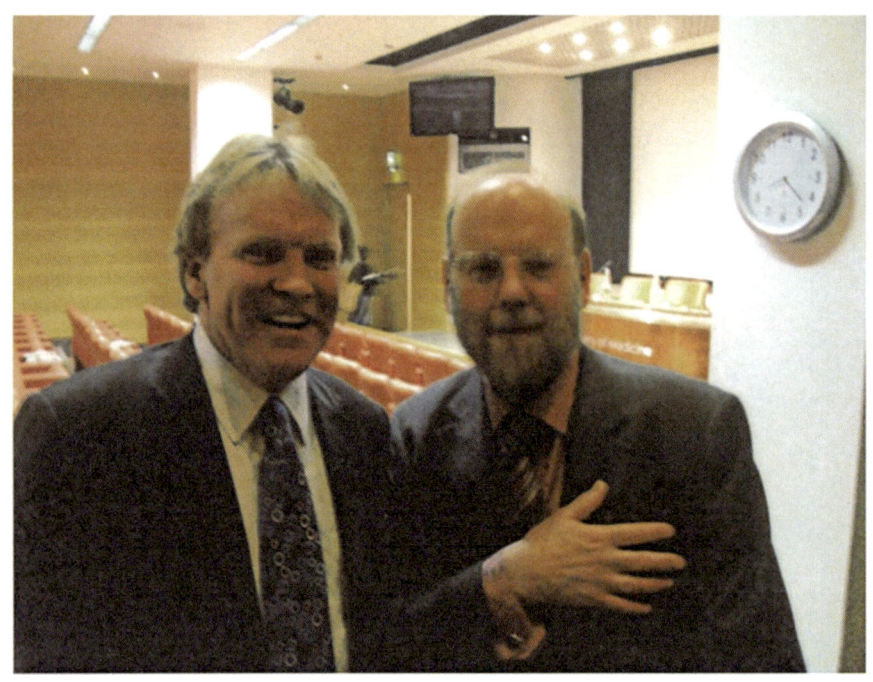

Lecturing with Sir Ian Wilmut at Royal Society of Medicine Congress 2015

As mentioned, many of my Toowoomba patients were part of a melanoma vaccine study at the Princess Alexandra Hospital in Brisbane, and I was disappointed when the result did not show as much benefit as we had hoped I was chastened one day when one of my patients from my Flying Doctor days drove 700 kilometres from Dubbo with his family to see me and be included in the melanoma vaccine program. He was not included as part of the Brisbane study, but his condition had spread, and even with the administration of the vaccine, there was little that could be done for the poor man. Such was the nature of malignant melanoma: once the tumour cells start to move into the deeper dermal layers of the skin, their behaviour changes dramatically and the patient has an extremely poor prognosis.

On another occasion, I was examining a truck driver, when I noticed what at first appeared like a recent blood blister under one of his thumbnails. Despite his protestation that it was a jacking injury, I took off part of his nail to have a closer look. There was no blood, just dark pigment. As I had suspected, it was a subungual malignant melanoma; my perseverance in obtaining a diagnosis probably saved his life. He left the hospital later that week dressed in bandages. They had taken no chances and removed the last part of his thumb above the joint.

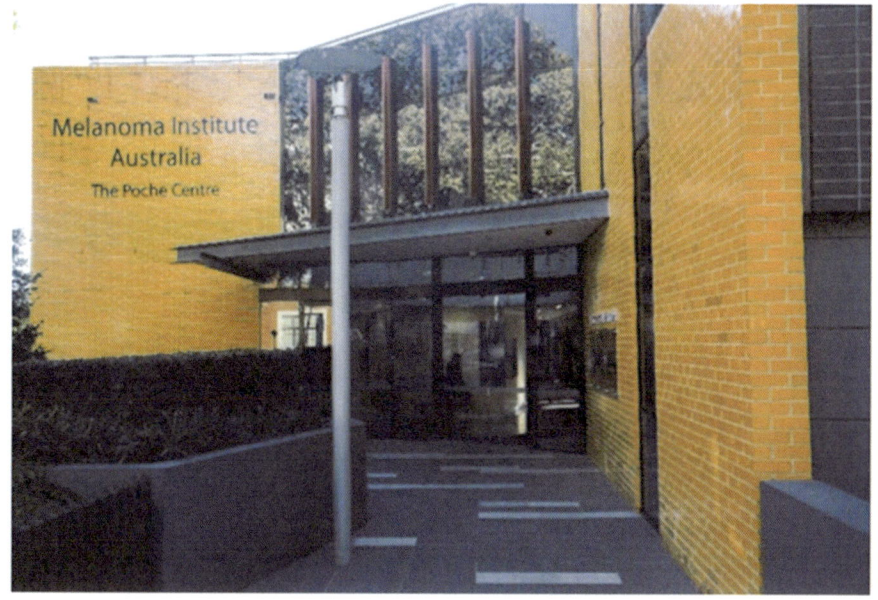

The Melanoma Institute in Sydney

On my return to Dublin, I worked with the Irish Medical Times and wrote many articles concerning malignant melanoma. I surmised if solar radiation was the primary risk factor for malignant melanoma, then it would be reasonable to conclude that reducing sun exposure via topical sunscreen use would be associated with reduced disease risk. However, the available epidemiological data was contradictory. Some studies even suggested that sunscreen use was associated with an increased melanoma risk. Epidemiological evidence from Lindqvist and Epstein at the Karolinska Institute suggested that sun avoidance and exposure advice was too restrictive in many countries with low solar intensity and indeed might even be harmful to women's health. In other words, cardiac disease is much more prevalent than skin cancer, and we should take this into account, especially as high-level SPF was being put into every cosmeceutical sold in Ireland – a nation that ranks amongst the lowest sunshine levels in the world! Ireland gets typically about 1,250 hours of sunshine each year, while many other cities around the world are nearly three times this level. The

Karolinska Institute is one of the world's foremost medical universities and is Sweden's single largest centre of medical academic research.

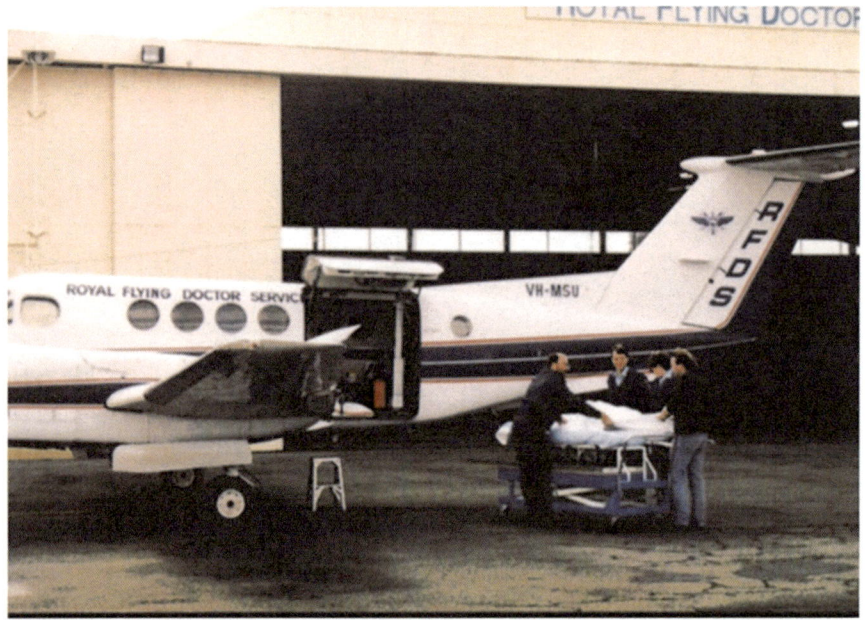

Working with the Royal Flying Doctor Service

In 2017, I was invited by Dr Federico W. von Son de Fernex, CCME Congress, to attend a stem cell conference in Playa del Carmen in Riviera Maya, Mexico. Federico wished me to talk about a new technique, which I was implementing to restore necrotic skin after dermal filler vascular occlusion.

During the conference, I met Dr Diego Correa, assistant professor at the University of Miami, Miller School of Medicine, who is one of the top mesenchymal stem cell researchers in the world. He had spent over eighteen years of basic and translational research experience in the areas of adult stem cell biology and regenerative medicine, with emphasis on Adult Mesenchymal Stem Cell (MSC) biology.

Diego and his wife and family came with me to visit Tulum, the site of a pre-Columbian Mayan walled city about one hour down the coast from Playa Del Carmen.

On route, we chatted about the melanoma vaccine and the progress he was having with research on it in Miami. It was now twenty years since I had been involved in the trials in Queensland. Sometimes, asking the correct questions from nature takes quite a bit of time. Skin cancer remains the most common malignancy in the UK and Ireland. And of these, malignant melanoma is the deadliest cutaneous neoplasm. It is because of my interest in this field for many years that I decided to include a case and how we tend to deal with it.

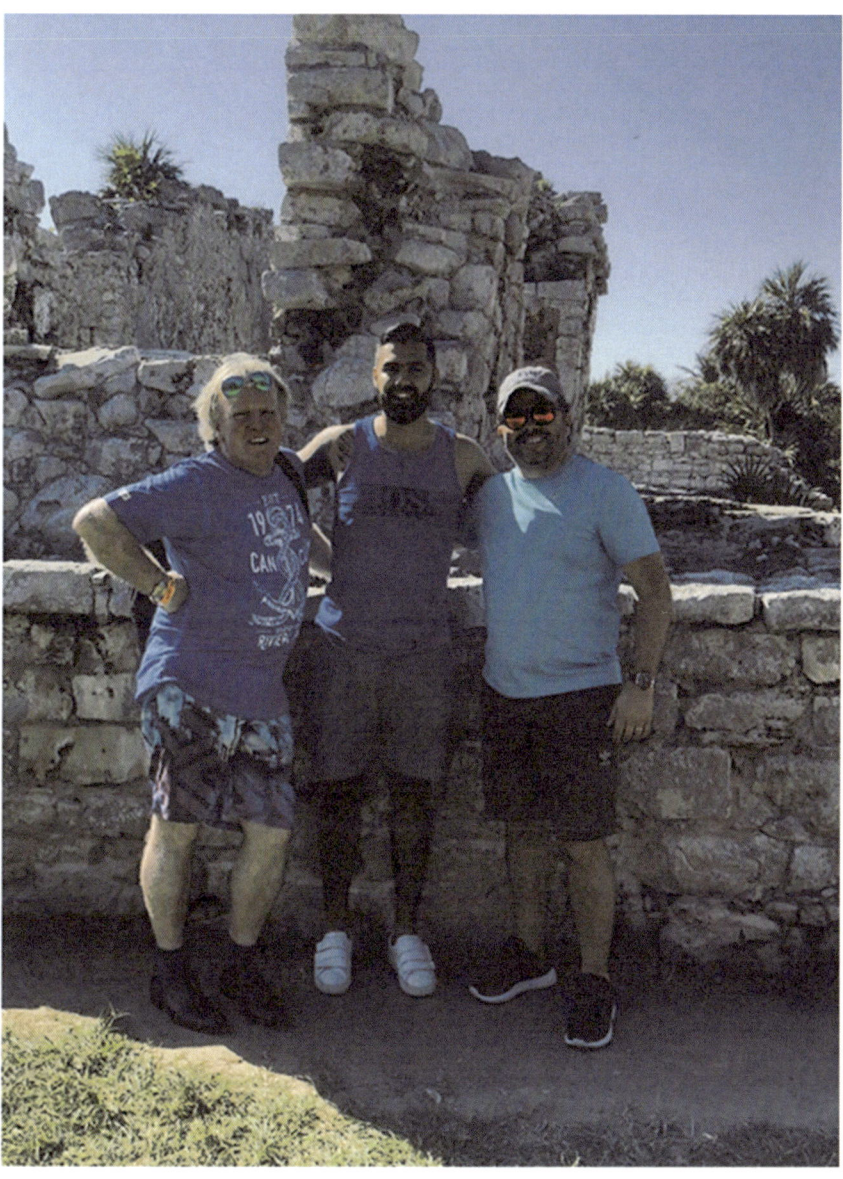

The author with Dr Federico W. von Son de Fernex and Mesenchymal Stem Cell (MSC) expert, Dr Diego Correa at CCME Congress, Playa del Carmen in Riviera Maya, Mexico

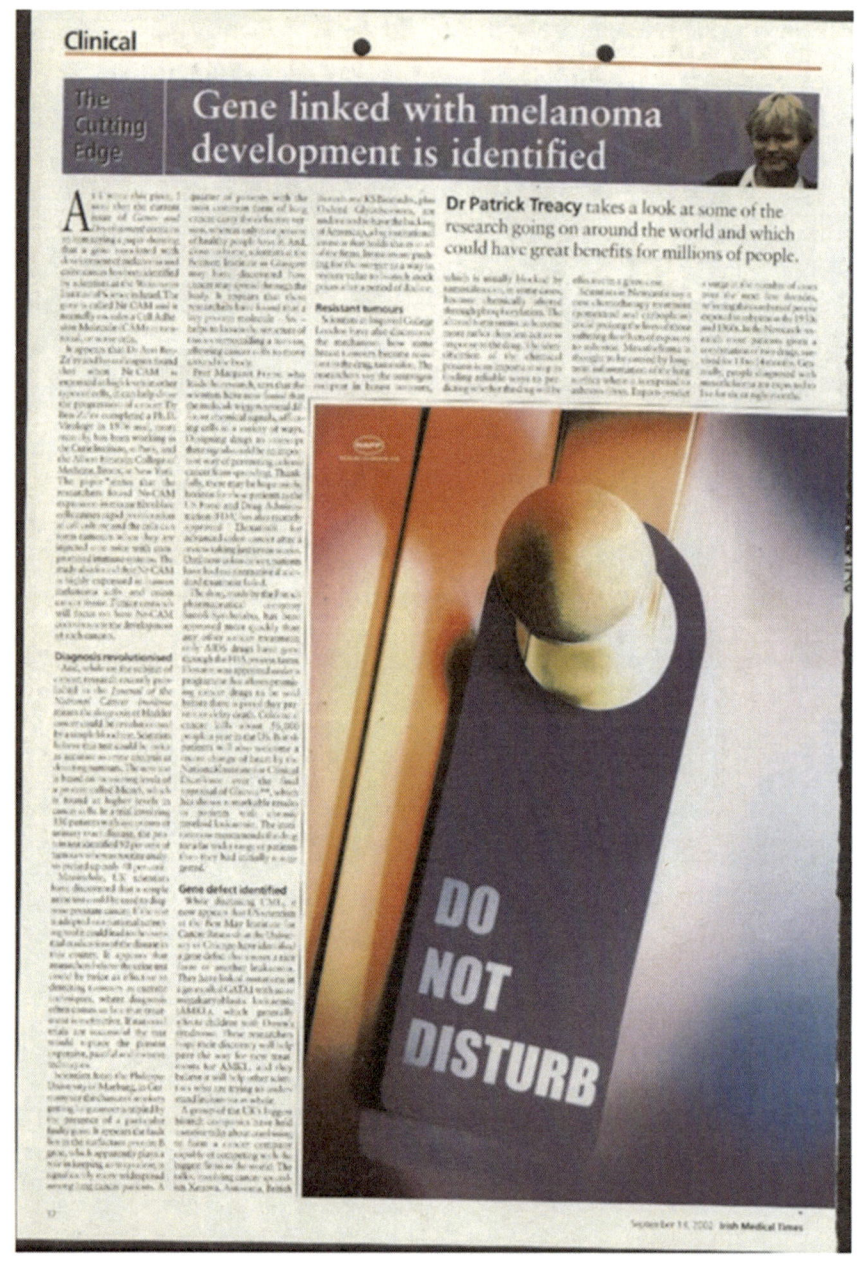

Article by the author on malignant melanoma from The Irish Medical Times circa 2001

Unlike vaccines for flu, pneumonia and other illnesses, melanoma vaccines do not prevent melanoma. Two small clinical trials show that a vaccine may help to prevent surgically removed melanoma tumours from returning. Results from a new study show that, in patients with melanoma, a personalized treatment vaccine generated a robust immune response against the cancer and may have helped to prevent it from returning.

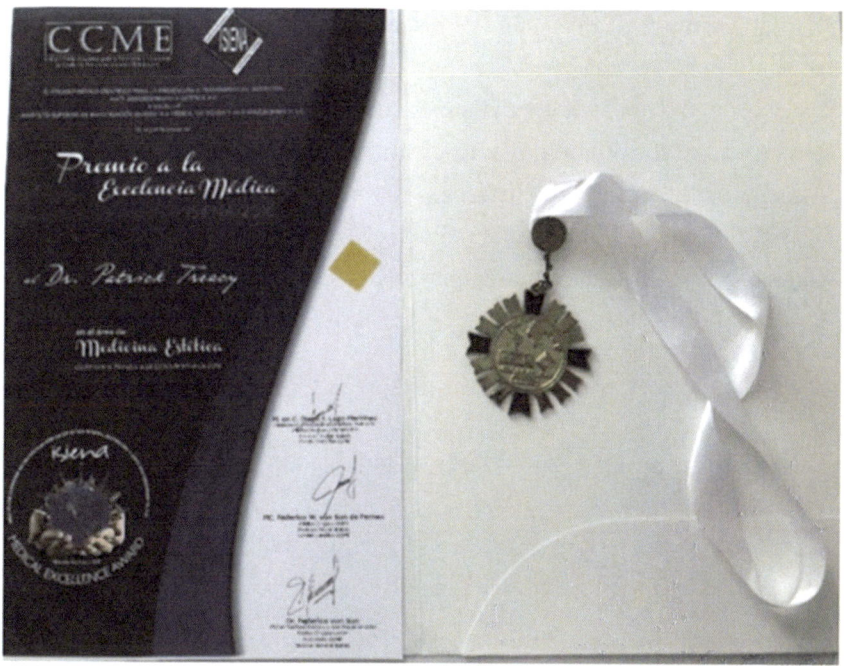

Award from CCME Congress in Mexico 2016

CASE 'Treating Malignant Melanoma

Melanomas are the most aggressive. Signs include a mole that has changed in size, shape, and colour, has irregular edges, has more than one colour, is itchy or bleeds. Sun exposure is the most important modifiable risk factor associated with the development of NMSC and melanoma. Sunlight is made up of different types of electromagnetic radiation, mostly infrared, visible and UV. Exposure to sunlight has both positive and negative effects.

In 2009, a 23-year-old female patient presented to Ailesbury Clinic with a changing lesion on her abdomen. The patient stated that the lesion had been present for about two years and had started off from within a freckle, which started to grow larger and somewhat darken in appearance. It had the clinical appearance of a melanoma and the dermoscopy 3-point checklist (designed to allow non-experts not to miss detection of melanomas) was used to determine whether this had a high likelihood of malignancy. It included asymmetry, colour and structure in one or two perpendicular axes, an atypical pigment network with irregular holes and thick lines and there was some evidence of a blue-white veil and regression structures.

It was decided that the likely diagnosis was a superficial spreading melanoma and to remove the lesion with a 1-cm clearance and work in association with a multi-disciplinary team. The histology report on the patient confirmed the diagnosis and included comments about cell type and its growth pattern, invasion of blood vessels or nerves, inflammatory response, regression and whether there

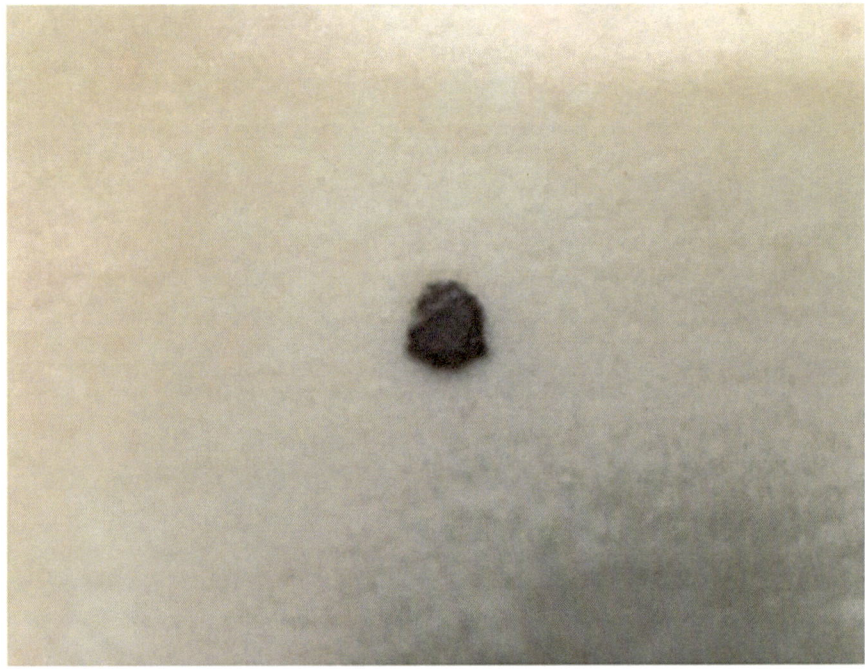

is associated in-situ disease. Because I was so used to dealing with melanomas over many years, I thought it might be worthwhile looking at the work-up, interpretation of data and decision of treatment. However, I must first stress that it is recommended that a patient who presents with signs and symptoms suggestive of melanoma should immediately be referred to a consultant dermatologist or consultant plastic surgeon and lesions suspicious of melanoma should not be removed in primary care. In this instance, the pathologist's report (below) included a macroscopic description (the naked eye view) of the specimen and a microscopic description. The pathology team sends us the following data with features that allow one to suggest the severity of an invasive melanoma.

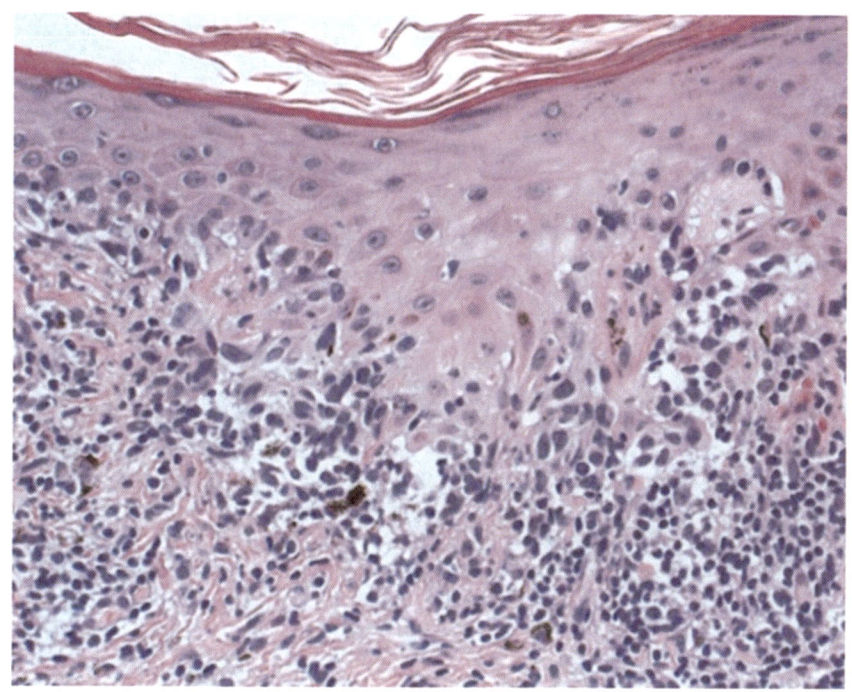

Patient histopathology report: Microscopy: Skin, left inframammary, skin ellipse: malignant melanoma, superficial spreading subtype: Clark level III. Breslow thickness: 1 mm. No regression identified. Lymphovascular invasion is not identified. Perineural invasion is not identified. Mitotic rate is 2 per 10. Microsatellite lesions are not identified. Melanoma arises in the naevus. Margins: Closest margin (radial): 1 cm. Deep margin: 4 mm Prof K Sheahan, St Vincent's University Hospital.

Types of Melanomas

Melanomas are described according to their appearance and behaviour. Those that start off as flat patches (i.e., have a horizontal growth phase) include:

1) Superficial spreading melanoma (SSM) – 70% of all melanomas Lentigo malignant melanoma (sun-damaged skin of face, scalp, and neck)

2) Acral lentiginous melanoma (on soles of feet, palms of hands or under the nails) (*subungual melanoma)

These include primary diagnosis, Breslow thickness, Clark level of invasion, the margins of excision – i.e., the normal tissue around the tumour – the mitotic rate, which is a measure of how fast the cells are proliferating, and whether there is ulceration.

These superficial forms of melanoma tend to grow slowly, but at any time, they may begin to thicken up or develop a nodule (i.e., progress to a vertical growth phase).

ABCDE
rule for the early
detection of melanoma

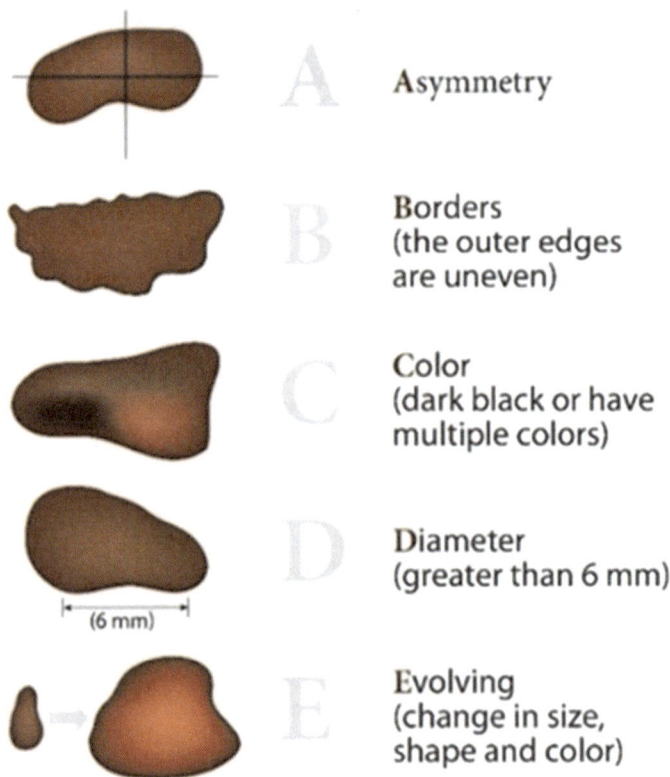

A   Asymmetry

B   Borders
(the outer edges
are uneven)

C   Color
(dark black or have
multiple colors)

D   Diameter
(greater than 6 mm)

(6 mm)

E   Evolving
(change in size,
shape and color)

Breslow thickness is reported for invasive melanomas. It is measured vertically in millimetres from the top of the granular layer (or base of superficial ulceration) to the deepest point of tumour involvement. It is a strong predictor of outcome; the thicker the melanoma, the more likely it is to metastasize.

Clark level indicates the anatomic plane of invasion. The deeper the Clark level, the greater the risk of metastasis. It is useful in predicting outcome in thin tumours and less useful for thicker ones.

Clark Level 1	Involves only the epidermis (in situ melanoma). Not an invasive lesion.
Clark Level 2	Melanoma has invaded papillary dermis. Has not reached papillary-reticular interface.
Clark Level 3	Melanoma has filled papillary dermis but not the reticular dermis.
Clark Level 4	Melanoma has invaded reticular dermis but not the subcutaneous tissue.
Clark Level 5	Melanoma has invaded the subcutaneous tissue.

Melanomas that quickly invade deeper tissues include:

1) Nodular melanoma (presenting as a rapidly enlarging lump) 15-30% of all melanomas
2) Spitzoid melanoma (a nodule that resembles a Spitz naevus)
3) Mucosal melanoma (arising on lips, eyelids, vulva, penis, and anus)
4) Neurotropic and desmoplastic melanoma (fibrous tumour with a tendency to nerves)

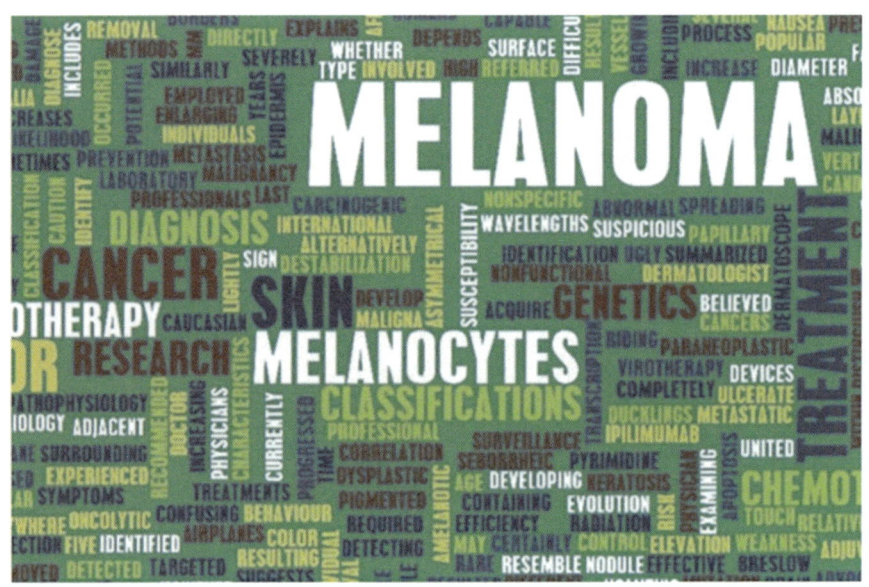

Three types of melanoma

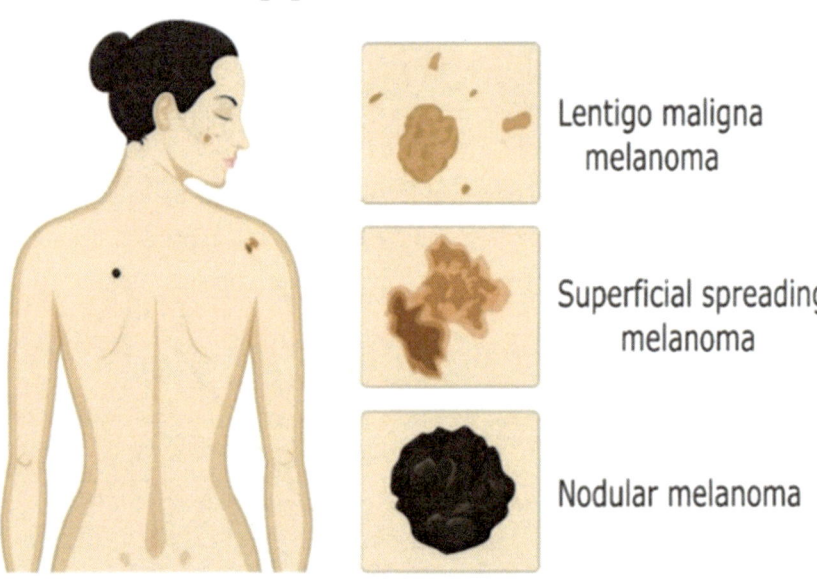

Lentigo maligna melanoma

Superficial spreading melanoma

Nodular melanoma

Staging

The American Joint Committee on Cancer (AJCC) has designated staging by TNM (tumour, node, metastasis) classification to define melanoma. Melanoma staging means finding out if the melanoma has spread from its original site in the skin. The stages are:

Stage	Characteristics
Stage 0	In situ melanoma
Stage 1	Thin melanoma <2 mm in thickness
Stage 2	Thick melanoma >2 mm in thickness
Stage 3	Melanoma spread to involve local lymph nodes
Stage 4	Distant metastases have been detected

Who is At Risk of Melanoma?

The main risk factors for developing superficial spreading melanoma include:

- Affluence, increasing age, female
- Fair skin that burns easily, red or light-coloured hair
- Blue eyes and light-coloured skin (Anglo-Celtic) (Gandini S. et al., 2005)
- Multiple (>5) atypical naevi (moles that are histologically dysplastic) (Garbe C. et al., 1994)
- Many benign melanocytic naevi person (Ferrone CR. et al., 2005)
- Giant congenital melanotic naevi ≥20 cm in diameter
- Previous invasive melanoma or melanoma in situ (Goggins WB. et al., 2003)
- Family history of melanoma, two first-degree relatives affected (Florrell Sr. et al., 2005)

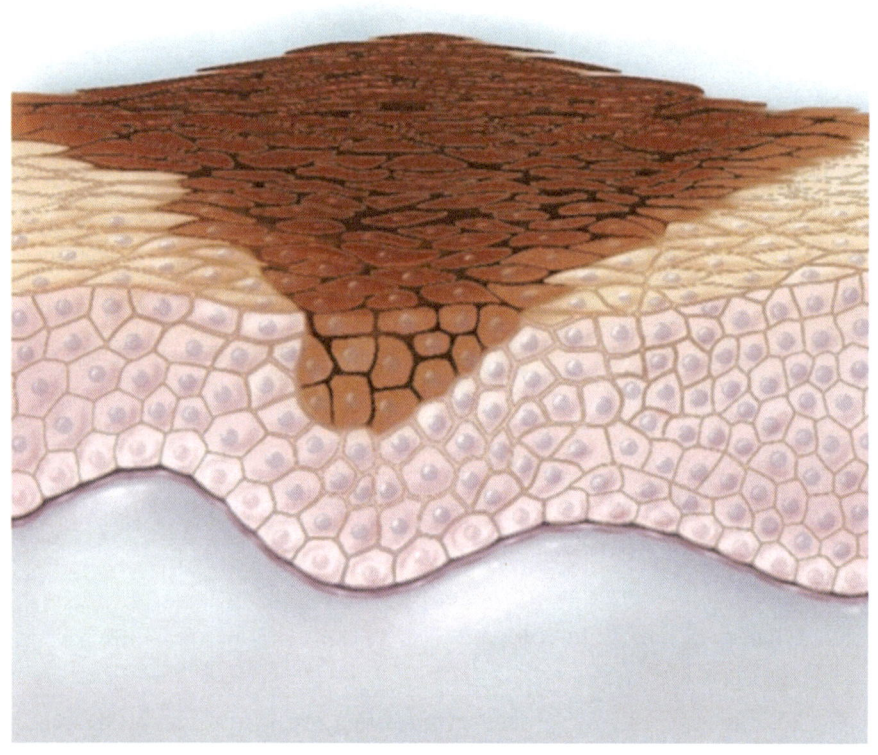

UVB (280-320 nm) solar radiation (causing sunburn) is the principal cause of melanoma. UVA may be involved in the pathogenesis of melanoma (Wang SQ. et al., 2001).

Treatment

Surgical excision remains the primary modality for treating melanoma. Cutaneous melanomas that have not spread beyond the site at which they developed are highly curable. Surgical margins of 5 mm are currently recommended for melanoma in situ, and margins of 1 cm are recommended for melanomas ≤1 mm in depth. For tumours of intermediate thickness (1-4 mm Breslow depth), randomised prospective studies show that 2-cm margins are appropriate, although 1-cm margins have been proven effective for tumours of 1- to 2-mm thickness. Margins of 2 cm are recommended for cutaneous melanomas greater than 4 mm in thickness (high-risk primaries) to prevent potential local recurrence in or around the scar site.

Lymphatic mapping and Sentinel Lymph Node Biopsy (SLNB) can be considered to assess the presence of occult metastasis in the regional lymph nodes of patients with primary tumours larger than 1 to 4 mm, potentially identifying individuals who may be spared the morbidity of regional lymph node dissections and individuals who may benefit from adjuvant therapy. Numerous adjuvant therapies have been investigated for the treatment of localised cutaneous melanoma following complete surgical removal. Adjuvant interferon (IFN) alfa-2b is the only adjuvant therapy approved by the US FDA for high-risk melanoma. While early-stage melanomas can often be cured with surgery, more advanced melanomas can be much harder to treat. But in recent years, newer types of immunotherapy and targeted therapies have shown a great deal of promise and have changed the treatment of this disease.

Drugs that block CTLA-4: Ipilimumab targets CTLA-4, a protein that normally suppresses the T-cell immune response, which helps melanoma cells survive. Ipilimumab has been shown to help people with advanced melanomas live longer. However, ipilimumab has significant toxicity at therapeutic dose. Combining ipilimumab with GM-CSF is better than using ipilimumab alone. The combination has fewer serious side effects.

Drugs that block PD-1 or PD-L1: Melanoma cells also use pathways in the body to avoid being detected, and a protein called PD-L1 on their surface helps them evade the immune system. Two drugs that block PD-1, pembrolizumab (Keytruda) and nivolumab (Opdivo), are now approved to treat advanced melanoma. Large, randomised trials with the newer drugs (nivolumab and pembrolizumab) and with combination signal transduction inhibitors (dabrafenib plus trametinib) demonstrate a clinically significant impact on relapse-free survival (RFS) with less toxicity than with ipilimumab.

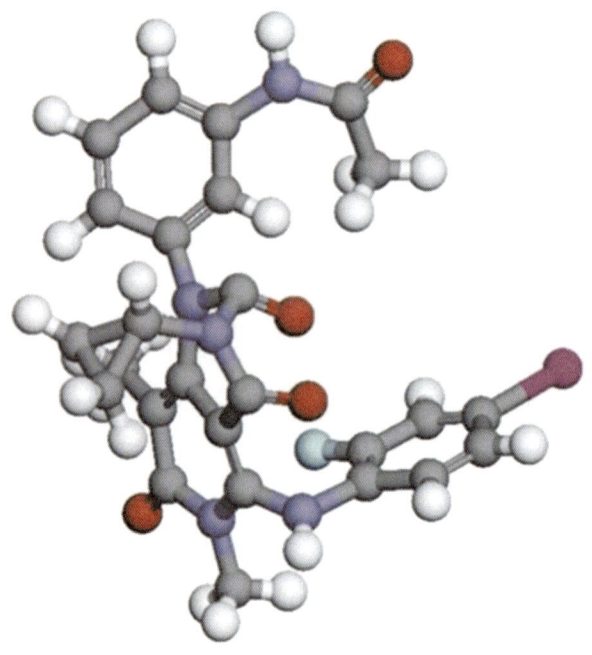

Trametinib melanoma cancer drug, molecule

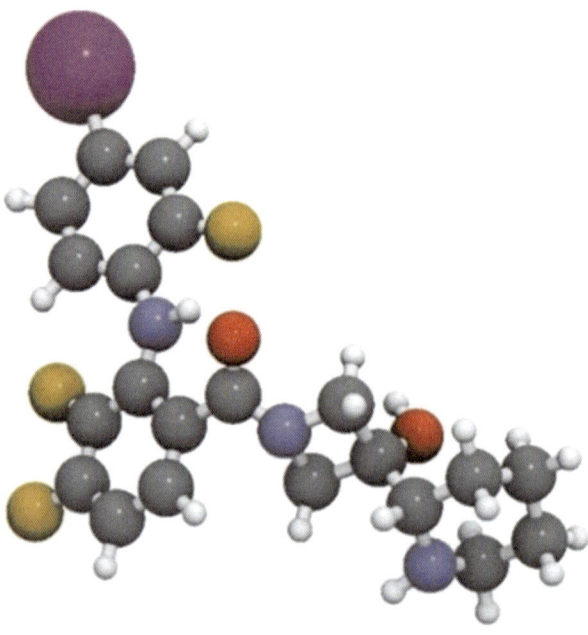

Cobimetinib melanoma drug molecule

Melanoma Vaccines

These are experimental therapies that have not yet been proven to be helpful. Anti-tumour therapeutic vaccines tend to aim at priming an effector immune response able to recognise and kill tumour cells. Metastatic advanced melanoma has been a model disease to test novel advances in vaccine design due to the intrinsic immunogenicity of this tumour and the accessibility to melanoma lesions to monitor the immune response. Despite many clinical trials, clinical benefit remains elusive.

Although sun exposure is a risk factor for melanoma, cutaneous melanomas can also arise in areas of the body not exposed to the sun. Sun exposure in childhood and having more than one blistering sunburn in childhood are associated with an increased risk of melanoma. Most melanomas arise as superficial tumours confined to the epidermis. The prognosis for melanoma is closely related to the thickness of the tumour.

To effectively treat melanomas, drugs that target proteins that normally suppress the T-cell immune response or block ones that help them evade the immune system provide the best chance for treating patients with advanced melanoma. In early studies, combination drugs have shrunk tumours in about one half of patients with melanoma.

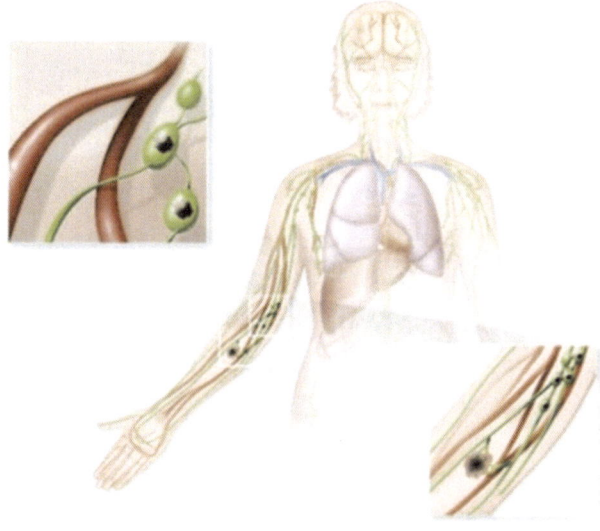

Melanoma invading the lymphovascular system

Sentinel paper written by the author while on a residency in the Mayo Clinic, Minnesota, during 1985 confirmed an increase in incidence of cutaneous malignant melanoma for both sexes, most notably in the past decade. Mayo Clin Proc., 1990 Oct; 65 (10):1293-302. DOI: 10.1016/s0025-6196(12)62140-5.

Cutaneous Malignant Melanoma in Rochester, Minnesota: Trends in Incidence and Survivorship, 1950 Through 1985. P. J. Treacy, N. A. Popescu, C. M. Beard, R. K. Winkelmann, P. C. O'Brien, L. T. Kurland

Abstract

In Rochester, Minnesota, 107 incidence cases of cutaneous malignant melanoma (in 46 male and 61 female patients) were diagnosed during the years 1950 through 1985. Overall crude incidence rates were 6.0 and 6.6 per 100,000 males and females, respectively. Age-specific rates suggested that the highest incidence occurs in the age groups of 50 to 59 years and 70 years or older for males and 40 to 49 years and 70 years or older for females. Lesions were most common in the head and neck area among males (P = 0.044) and on the lower extremities among females (P = 0.018). The most frequent histologic type was superficial spreading melanoma (61%). Five-year survival was diminished overall for patients with cutaneous malignant melanoma – 0.72 in comparison with 0.88 expected for the general population. Statistically significant risk factors for survival were depth of invasion of the lesion (Clark level), thickness of the lesion, histologic type, and age of the patient.

Conclusion

Our study in a defined population has confirmed an increase in incidence of cutaneous malignant melanoma for both sexes, most notably in the past decade. The most frequent sites for lesions in this series were the head and neck for males and the lower extremities for females. Although sample sizes were relatively small for evaluating multivariate associations of risk factors with survival, the best predictors of survival were histologic findings (including histologic type, Clark level and Breslow scale) and age of the patient. The most prevalent histologic type in our study was superficial spreading melanoma, which was also associated with the best survival rate; nodular melanoma, which was second in frequency, was associated with the worst survival rate.

Older patients with nodular melanoma had a poorer survival than did other subjects, as did males with lesions 3.0 mm or more in thickness. The value of this local population group as a means of evaluating trends in disease status has been reconfirmed, and the importance of melanoma as a local and a general health hazard has beenreemphasised, even though the reasons and causes for the increase in incidence remain obscure.

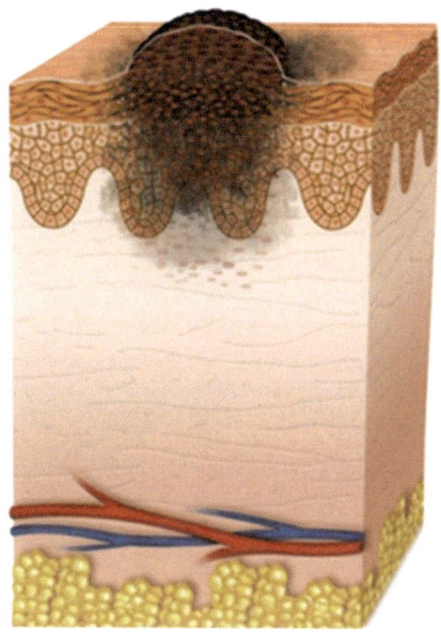

In view of high mortality rates due to metastatic melanoma, better understanding of the molecular pathogenesis of malignant melanoma is urgently needed.

Sentinel paper on cutaneous malignant melanoma by the Author 1990*

*Treacy Patrick J.; Popescu NA; Kurland LT; Cutaneous malignant melanoma in Rochester, Minnesota: trends in incidence and survivorship, 1950 through 1985, *Mayo Clin Proc.* 1990 Oct, 65(10):1293-302.

CASE 'Treating Squamous Cell Cancer'

A 64yo Irish male patient with a history of male pattern baldness and leukaemia was referred to Ailesbury with multiple scaly thickened reddened lesions on the area of his scalp and face. These lesions presented mostly on his nose, temples, and forehead with the largest collection along the vertex of his scalp. He had lived in South Africa for nearly twenty years. There were at least four lesions present on his face and scalp that would not heal and bled easily when traumatized. More recently his wife had become concerned because her friend had died of skin cancer.

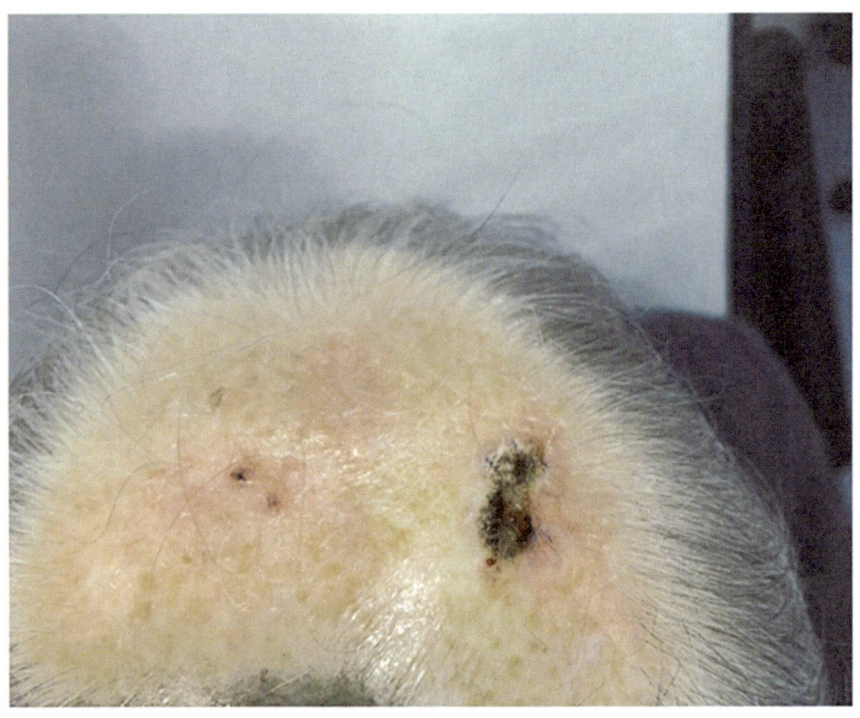

Treatment (Excisional Surgery)

After numbing the area with local anaesthesia, an 11 scalpel to remove the entire growth along with a surrounding border of normal skin as a safety margin. The skin around the surgical site is then closed with several stitches, and the excised tissue is sent to the laboratory for microscopic examination to verify that all the malignant cells have been removed.

Characteristic features of SCC tumours include the following:

- The clinical appearance of SCC is highly variable but usually presents as an ulcerated lesion with hard, raised edges or reddish skin plaque that is slow growing
- The lesion caused by SCC is often asymptomatic but may have intermittent bleeding, especially on the lip
- SCC may present as a hard plaque or a papule with tiny blood vessels
- The tumour commonly presents on sun-exposed areas (e.g., back of the hand, scalp, lip, and superior surface of pinna)

Histopathological types

SCC is a histologically distinct form of cancer that arises from the epithelium, from cells showing tissue architectural characteristics of squamous cell differentiation, such as the presence of keratin, tonofilament bundles, or desmosomes, structures involved in cell-to-cell adhesion. SCC typically initially occurs in the sixth decade of life (the 50s) but is most common in the eighth decade (the 70s). It is twice as prevalent in men as in women. People with darker skin are less at risk to develop SCC. Populations with fair skin, light hair, and blue/green/grey eyes are at highest risk of developing the disease. Most invasive cutaneous SCCs are due to exposure to ultraviolet radiation, which damages the DNA of fair-skinned individuals. SCCs most often arise within actinic keratoses, and less often within Bowen's disease. Other risk factors for invasive SSC include:

- Inherited predisposition to skin cancer.
- Smoking – especially SCC of the lip.
- Thermal burn scars.
- Longstanding leg ulcers.
- Immunosuppression from drugs such as ciclosporin or azathioprine, especially in organ transplant recipients.
- Infection with human papillomavirus (HPV causes carcinoma cuniculatum but rarely causes other forms of cutaneous SCC.

Treatment of invasive SCC

Squamous cell carcinoma is the second-most common cancer of the skin (after basal cell carcinoma but more common than melanoma). It usually occurs in areas exposed to the sun. Sunlight exposure and immunosuppression are risk factors for SCC of the skin, with chronic sun exposure being the strongest environmental risk factor. The treatment for SCC depends upon its size and location, the number to be treated, and the preference or expertise of the doctor. Patients with larger or aggressive lesions, or one in a difficult site, may first require imaging with ultrasound, CT, or MRI to determine the extent of the tumour and to look for metastases in the regional lymph nodes or elsewhere (3) Surgery Invasive SCCs are usually excised by a full thickness surgical procedure to cut out the lesion completely. Mohs micrographic surgery may be necessary for large, ill-defined, deep, or recurrent tumours. After excising a large tumor, the dermatologic surgeon or plastic surgeon may create a flap or graft to repair the defect.

Radiotherapy

Radiotherapy is sometimes used for high-risk primary skin cancers on the face and for metastatic disease.

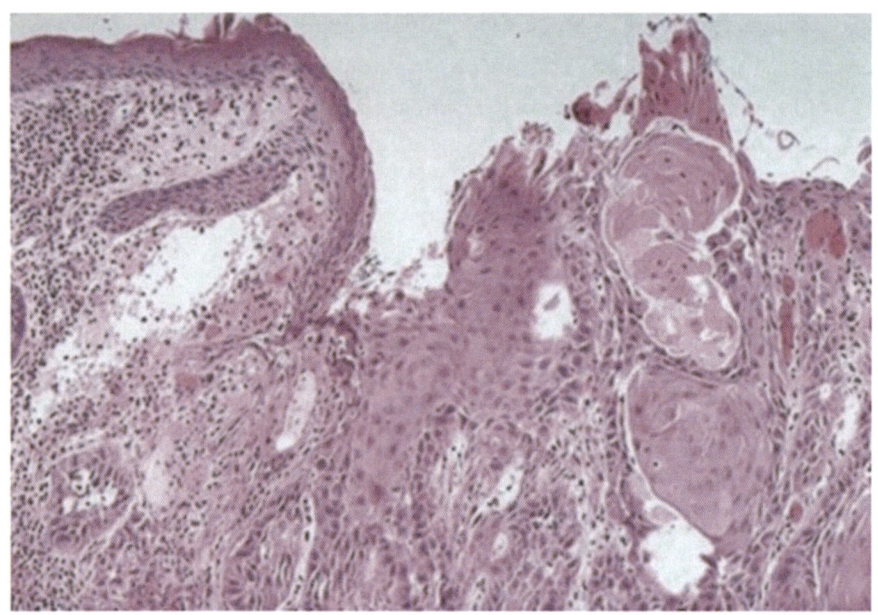

Squamous Cell Cancer

Histology

CLINICAL DETAILS: History of Squamous cell carcinoma. Leukaemic patient. MICROSCOPY: A: Skin, left zygoma, excision: Specimen corresponds to a squamous cell carcinoma, well differentiated. Maximum dimension = 2mm. Depth of invasion = 1.1mm Clark level 4. Lymphovascular invasion not identified. Perineural invasion not identified. Margins: Closest margin = 2mm. Deep margin = uninvolved. Pathological stage (TNM 7'h edition): pTl. The second described specimen corresponds to actinic keratosis. *Prof. Kieran Sheahan, Consultant Histopathologist, St. Vincent's University Hospital, Elm Park, Dublin 4.*

CASE REPORT 'Treating Basal Cell Cancer'

A 43yo Irish male patient was referred to Ailesbury with a slowly enlarging lesion on the right side of his neck that would not heal and bled when traumatized. The patient described it as an acne lump that had appeared around a year before and he felt in the beginning that he could express some pus or fluid from it from time to time. More recently he had become concerned because a course of antibiotics from his GP had failed to make any impact on the lesion. The patient gave a history of occupational sun exposure as he worked in the construction industry. There was no relevant medical history, and the patient did not have any clinical evidence of autoimmune or allergic diseases.

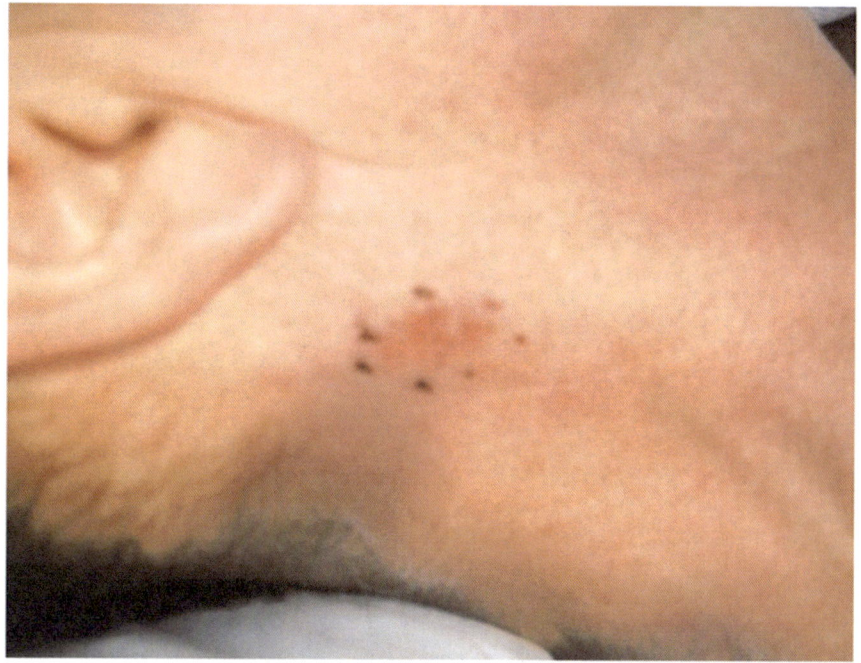

On examination the lesion appeared eroded and ulcerated and bled easily when traumatized. There was some crusting at the anterior margins. The presence of rolled borders, pearly edges and telangiectases gave a clinical suspicion of basal cell carcinoma and a decision was made to proceed to removal rather than do a biopsy. The author feels that any doctor should consider BCC in any patient with a history of a sore or skin anomaly that does not heal within 4-6 weeks and occurs on sun-exposed skin, especially if it is dimpled in the middle. These tumours may take many months or years to reach even 1 cm in diameter.

- Clinical Details: Rule out basal cell carcinoma.
- Macroscopy: Labelled, skin neck 3 x 4 cm excisional biopsy of cream skin. All embedded. 1/1.
- Microscopy: Basal cell carcinoma below the epidermis. Nuclear palisading at the peripheral layer of the tumour. Infiltrating, with a depth of invasion of 1.8 mm.
- Medical Codes ** T01000 - Skin M80003 - Neoplasm, malignant M80903 - Basal cell carcinoma Pathologists: Prof. Kieran Sheahan, Dr Linda Mulligan.

Prof. Kieran Sheahan, Consultant Histopathologist, St. Vincent's University Hospital, Elm Park, Dublin 4. Dr Linda Mulligan, Pathology Registrar, St. Vincent's University Hospital, Elm Park, Dublin 4.

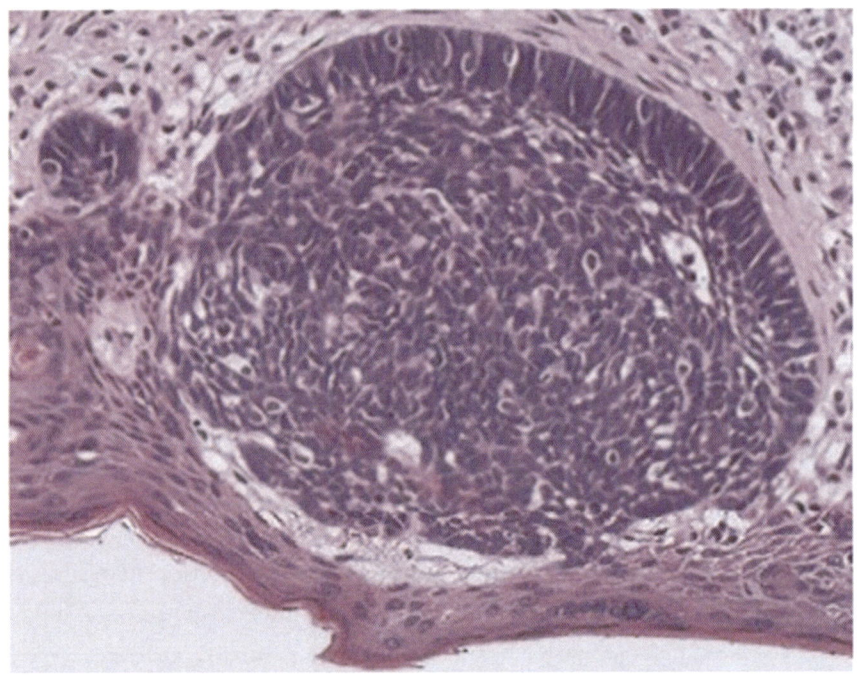

Basal cell carcinoma below the epidermis

Treatment (Excisional Surgery)

After numbing the area with local anaesthesia, an 11 scalpel to remove the entire growth along with a surrounding border of normal skin as a safety margin. The skin around the surgical site is then closed with several stitches, and the excised tissue is sent to the laboratory for microscopic examination to verify that all the malignant cells have been removed. People who sunburn are more likely to develop skin cancer than those who do not; however, sunlight damages the skin with or without sunburn. History of any prior treatment to the index tumour should be elicited, as well as history of any prior non-melanoma skin cancer. In patients with recurrent tumours, deeper invasion should be expected. Recurrence following radiation therapy is often biologically more aggressive.

Characteristic features of BCC tumours include the following:

- Slow growing (0.5 cm in 1-2 y)
- Erosion or ulceration, often central
- Telangiectases over the surface
- Rolled (raised) border
- Waxy papules with central depression
- Pearly appearance
- Bleeding, especially when traumatized
- Crusting
- Translucency

BCC seldom causes regional or distant metastasis. Attention should be taken for lymph node metastasis to suboccipital, and upper cervical groups of lymph nodes.

Histopathological types

There are several different histopathological types of BCC exist, each with distinct clinical presentation.

- Nodular - Cystic, pigmented, keratotic
- Infiltrative
- Micronodular
- Morpheaform

- Superficial

Nodular basal cell carcinoma

Nodular basal cell carcinoma is the most common type of basal cell carcinoma and usually presents as a round, pearly, flesh-coloured papule with telangiectases. More than 60% of BCCs belong to this subtype. As it enlarges, it frequently ulcerates centrally, leaving a raised, pearly border with telangiectases, which aids in making the diagnosis. The tumour may present as a cyst or pigmented with brown-black macules making it like a melanoma. Keratotic BCC is a variant of nodular BCC and is usually clinically indistinguishable from nodular BCC histologically.

Infiltrative basal cell carcinoma: With this variant of BCC, tumour infiltrates the dermis in thin strands between collagen fibres, making tumour margins less clinically apparent. Mohs micrographic surgery is the treatment of choice for infiltrative basal cell carcinoma. Because of its growth pattern, electrodessication and curettage has a significantly higher recurrence rate when used to treat infiltrative BCC compared to the treatment of nodular BCC; other treatment methods should be sought.

Micronodular basal cell carcinoma: This aggressive BCC subtype has the typical BCC distribution. It is not prone to ulceration, it may appear yellow-white when stretched, and it is firm to the touch. It may have a seemingly well-defined border.

Morpheaform (sclerosing) basal cell carcinoma: Morpheaform basal cell carcinoma is an uncommon variant in which tumour cells induce a proliferation of fibroblasts within the dermis and an increased collagen deposition (sclerosis) that clinically resembles a scar. This form accounts for 10% of lesions. Such lesions appear as flat or slightly depressed, fibrotic, and firm. The morpheaform (sclerosing) type of basal cell carcinoma is often the most difficult type to diagnose, as it bears little resemblance to the typical nodular BCC. Ulceration, bleeding, and crusting are uncommon, and these tumours are commonly mistaken for scar tissue.

Superficial basal cell carcinoma: Superficial basal cell carcinomas are seen mostly on the upper trunk or shoulders. This type of BCC grows slowly, has minimal tendency to be invasive, and appears clinically as an erythematous, well-circumscribed patch or plaque, often with a whitish scale. Occasionally, minute eschars may appear within the patch or plaque. The tumour often appears multicentric, with areas of clinically normal skin intervening among clinically involved areas.

Gorlin syndrome or basal cell nevus syndrome: Basal cell carcinoma (BCC) is also a feature of basal cell nevus syndrome (Gorlin syndrome) (2) an autosomal dominant inherited condition. The gene responsible for this syndrome is located on arm 9q, and chromosome abnormalities develop in some patients. Multiple BCCs begin to appear after puberty on the face, trunk, and extremities. In many cases, the tumours are highly invasive and may involve areas around the eyes and nose.

Basal Cell Cancer Treatments

- BCC is commonly treated with surgical excision, curettage, carbon dioxide (CO_2) laser ablation or cryotherapy, depending on the tumour depth and the histological subtype of the BCC.
- The effectiveness of excisional surgery does not match that of Mohs but produces cure rates around 90 percent.
- Photodynamic therapy (PDT) has been widely used for the treatment of superficial BCC in preference to excision due to its minimal invasiveness and satisfactory cosmetic results. However, the efficacy of this treatment modality is limited in the treatment of deeper lesions and the more aggressive subtypes of BCC. Retreatment and recurrences of the disease are frequent if the tumour depth is >2 mm.
- The gold standard of treatment is Mohs surgical excision with histological control of excision margins, which has a 5-year recurrence rate of less than 3% on the face.
- For superficial BCC, approved medications such as imiquimod (total remission rate, 82-90%) and topical 5-fluorouracil (80%) are available, as is photodynamic therapy (71-87%).

- Conventional cryotherapy following PDT additionally kills the remaining cancer cells by interrupting vital metabolic cycles, destabilizing cell membranes, creating an adverse hyperosmolar environment and forming water crystals.

Radiotherapy is an alternative treatment for invasive, inoperable BCC. Recently, drugs that inhibit an intracellular signalling pathway have become available for the treatment of locally advanced or metastatic BCC tissue.

Chapter 18: Pregnancy

Dr Patrick Treacy became guest editor for LVBX Magazine in 2018. The topic he covered was 'Aesthetic Medicine and Pregnancy'. Pregnancy causes many changes in a woman's body. The growing foetus causes mechanical changes by stretching skin, muscle and fascia. The amount of physiological change during pregnancy varies among women but often persists long after the post-partum period despite the best efforts of the patient regarding exercise and diet. Many women find it difficult to deal with these major body changes and humanoid females are almost unique amongst species in accumulating fat in the lower abdomen midriff, while males seem more prone to develop visceral fat around their organs. During pregnancy, human skin often stretches out of shape and loses the ability to spring back into shape, forming sagging breasts and stretch marks in the period. His answers are not to promote one product over another and reflect the author's own experience.

Q: What is the most beneficial treatment for a woman looking to reduce the appearance of stretch marks post pregnancy?

A: In this physiological state, the dermal tissue of the abdomen has been distended and sometimes left with long-term 'stretch marks'. Stretch marks occur during pregnancy and are caused by rapid stretching of the dermal tissue of the abdomen during the distension and weight gain of pregnancy. It is thought that nearly 85% of women will develop some degree of stretch marks during their pregnancy and these usually appear after prolonged weakening of the dermal tissues about the beginning of the third trimester. This is also a period of sustained distension.

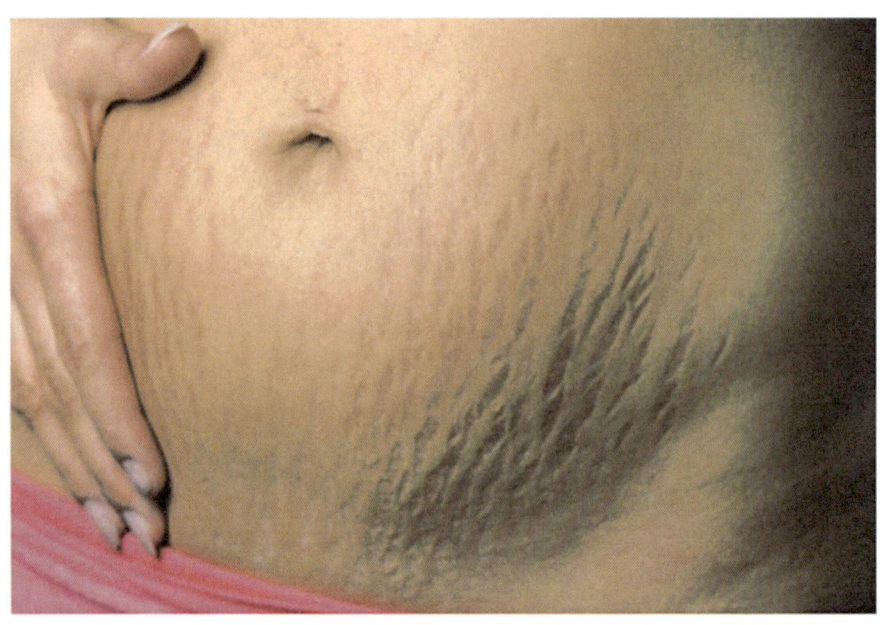

Stretch marks post pregnancy

Various treatments are available for improving the appearance of existing stretch marks, including radiofrequency, laser treatments, microneedling, dermabrasion, carboxytherapy and prescription retinoids. Many patients ask if there are any topical creams to help with stretch marks, either during their formation or after they have occurred. There are no proper control studies, but some research suggests a daily application of a cream containing Gotu Kola extract, vitamin E and collagen hydrolysates are associated with fewer stretch marks during pregnancy. Carboxytherapy is a simple and proven technique that can dramatically improve the appearance of stretch marks by improving local tissue metabolism and perfusion. Treatments are rapid, comfortable, and effective for a high percentage of patients. Also great for treating stretch marks is BTL Exilis Elite, which uses radiofrequency to lightly heat your skin, encouraging collagen production for cell replenishment. This smooths out and contours the area, tightening it in the process. It's an extremely safe procedure, with temperature control based on your skin's temperature. The number of sessions will depend on the severity of your stretch marks; however, four sessions are usually required for the desired effect.

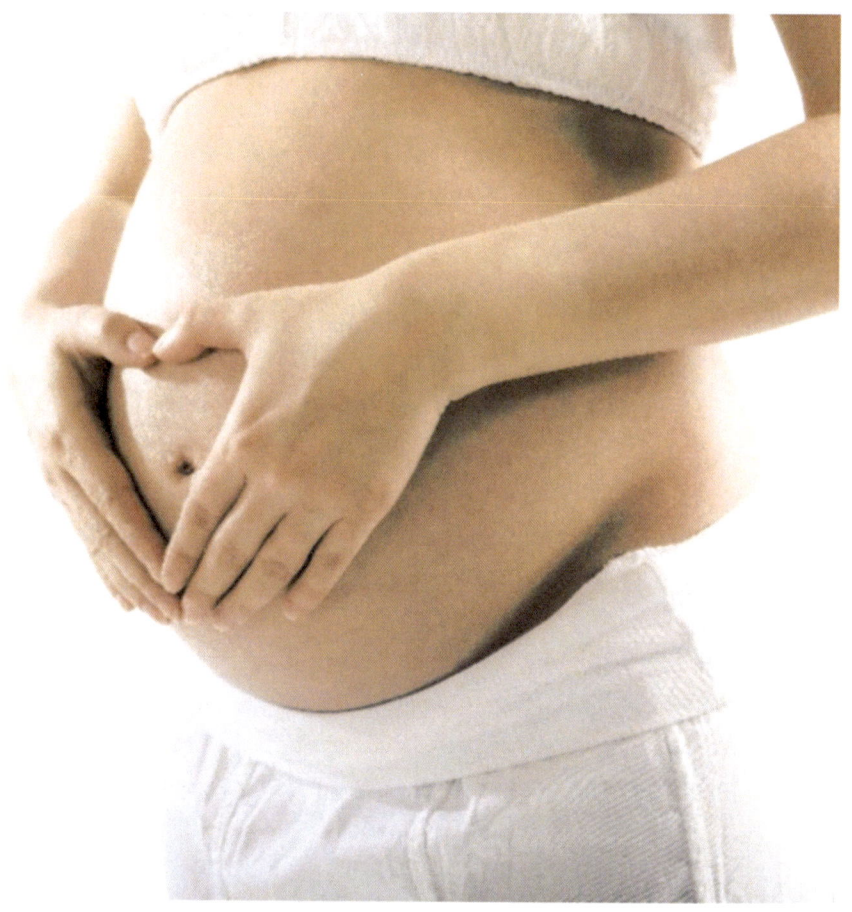

Q: Are there any treatments safe to receive during pregnancy; if so, which are the best ones to opt for?

A: The safety of cosmetic procedures in patients who are pregnant and/or lactating is a complex clinical question surrounded by uncertainty. It probably goes without saying everyday hair washing, makeup, bathing and showering are perfectly fine. The physician involved in giving the treatment will usually be well versed in whether the procedure is safe or not. However, we shall look at some of the aesthetic procedures in more detail.

Temperature: Do not raise your core body temperature above 39 degrees centigrade. This is considered the maximum temperature one should reach to keep both mother and baby healthy.

Facials: Be careful about using only natural products. Do not use any chemical peels (including retinoids) directly on your skin as they may be absorbed into the mother's bloodstream, whose developing baby also depends on that blood. A mother's skin is more sensitive during the stages of pregnancy. Peels: With respect to chemical peels, glycolic and lactic acid peels are deemed safe; however, trichloroacetic and salicylic acid peels should be avoided or used with caution. Again, retinol can damage a developing baby.

Botox: Although safety data on Botulinum toxin A is insufficient, the procedure may be safe because systemic absorption and placental transfer are negligible.

Sclerotherapy can be safe during pregnancy but must be avoided during the first trimester and after week 36 of the pregnancy. Consider also the differing sclerosing agents and question the physician.

Dental work while pregnant, such as cavity fillings and crowns, should be treated to reduce the chance of infection. If dental work is done during pregnancy, the second trimester is preferable. It is best to avoid this dental work while pregnant and avoid exposing the developing baby to any risks, even if they are minimal.

Massages: A massage is beneficial to help a mother relax and reduce stress. It willalso help those pregnancy aches and pains.

Acupuncture is generally considered safe. Manicures and pedicures are usually safe.

Q: How can women enhance their breasts post childbirth? If breastfeeding, what is the typical wait period for any producers?

A: The 'post-baby' body type with fat now distributed subcutaneously, especially in the buttocks and thigh area. There are breast volume changes with sagging, especially if the female has breastfed her infant. Breast volume may increase but usually, we get shrinkage.

Q: When one refers to the 'Mommy Makeover', what are the most typical kinds of treatments related to this post-childbirth makeover? What are women most likely looking to treat or enhance post birth?

A: Most of these makeovers are related to the removal of fat. Liposuction has been the mainstay of this quite recently. This is a cosmetic surgery operation that removes fat from the abdomen, thighs, and buttocks and elsewhere. There are many differing mechanisms of liposuction. Conventional liposuction is mostly performed under general anaesthesia, and largely practiced by plastic surgeons. The whole procedure lasts 2-3 hours. It is possible to remove large amounts of fat, often 8-10 litres, quickly in 1-2 hours. However, it has many disadvantages, including the fact that the patient must be hospitalised, which adds significantly to the cost. Recovery time is slow, as after any procedure under general anaesthesia. More recently, it can be combined with other procedures (i.e., radiofrequency) that involve a level of skin retraction. The result is affected by the age of the patient, quality of skin, presence of underlying disease or smoking and the presence of previous skin damage such as those caused by childbirth and surgery. The risks, financial costs and lengthy downtime associated with surgical procedures for fat reduction have led to the development of several non-invasive techniques.

By maintaining a healthy diet and exercise, you can expect long-term results. None of these procedures are recommended during pregnancy. With any of the procedures, it takes about ninety days for new collagen to form so after that, you can expect results to last approximately two years.

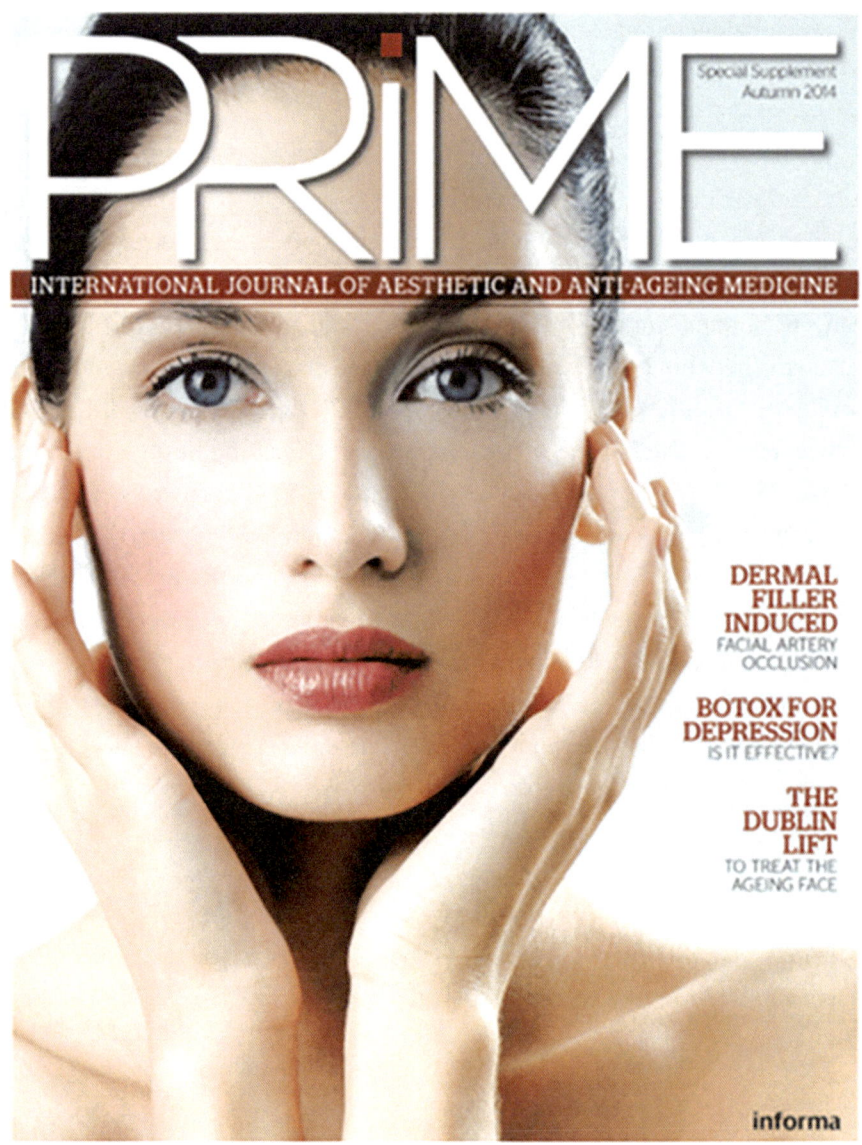

Articles from the author in peer reviewed PRIME Magazine

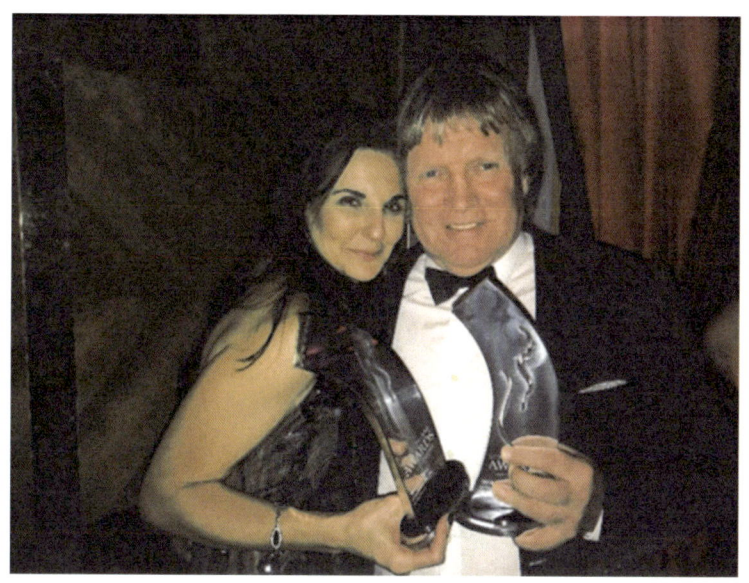

With Dr Beatriz Molina at MyFaceMyBody Awards London 2017

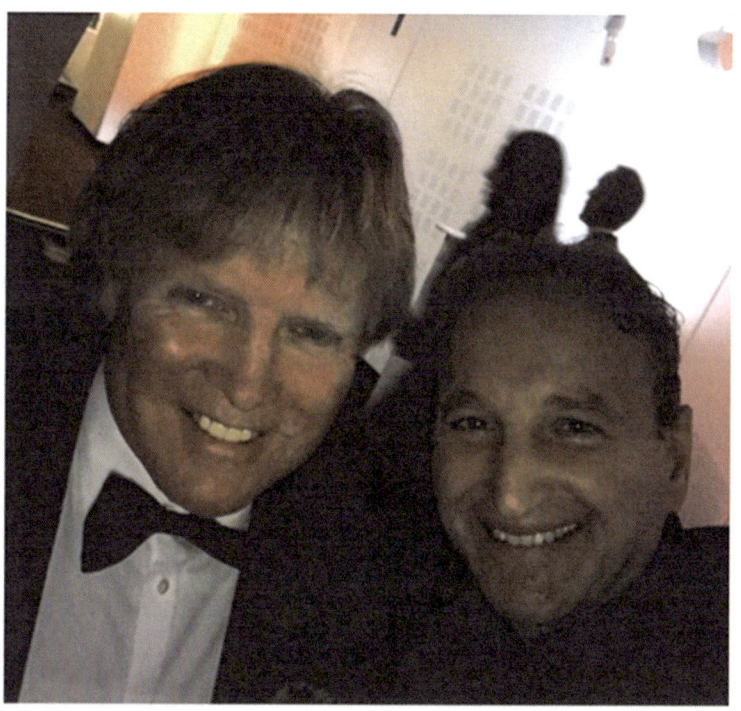

With Dr Steven Dayan at IMCAS Conference Paris 2019

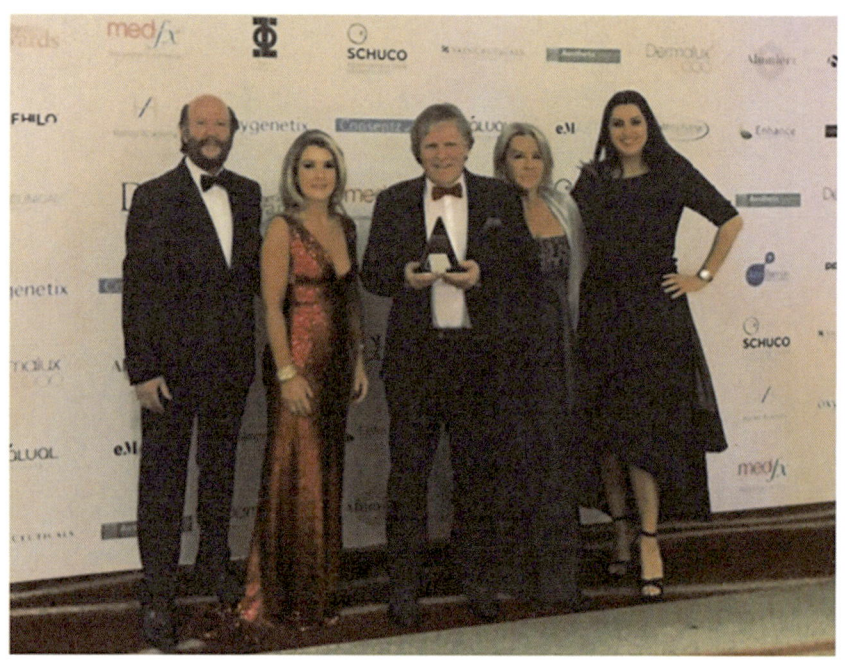

Top Aesthetic Clinic UK & Ireland Aesthetic Awards London 2017

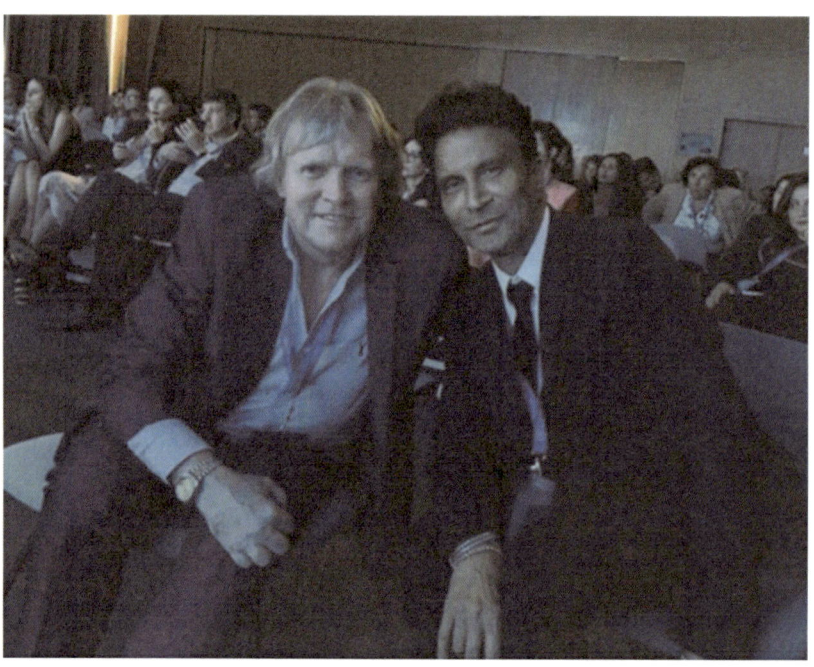

With Dr Raj Kanodia (Beverly Hills) TAMC Conference Dubrovnik 2019

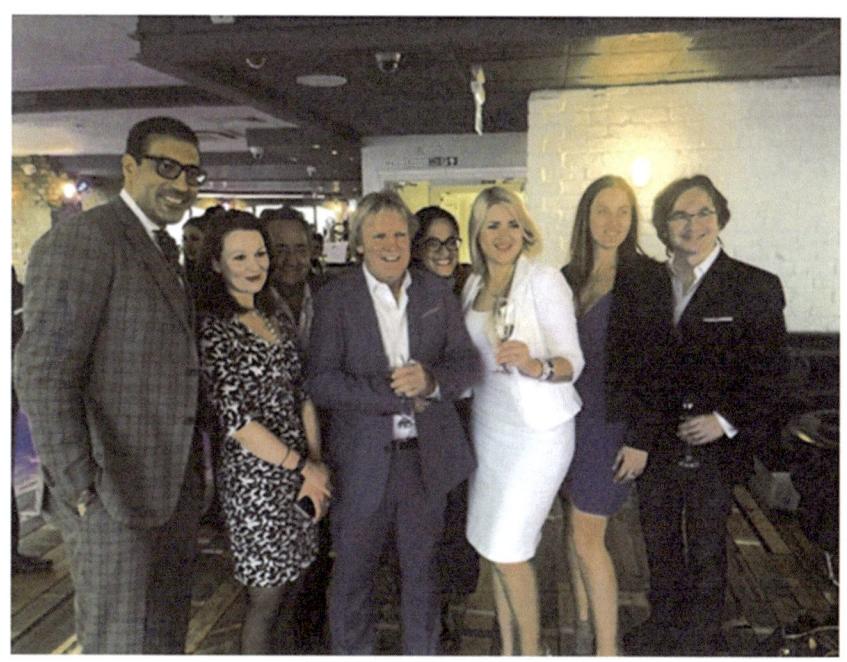

FACE Conference in London 2016

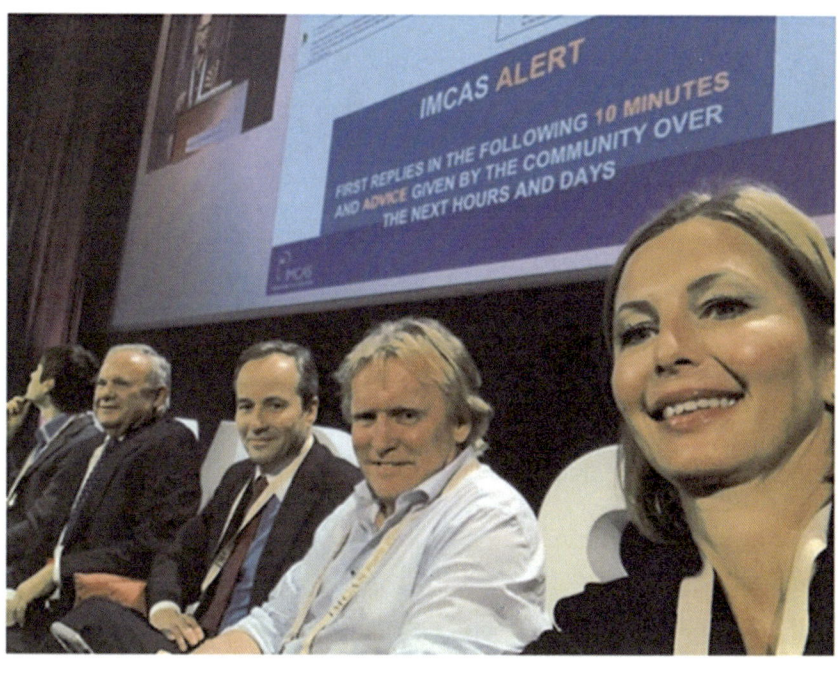

With medical colleagues AMWC Conference Monaco 2018

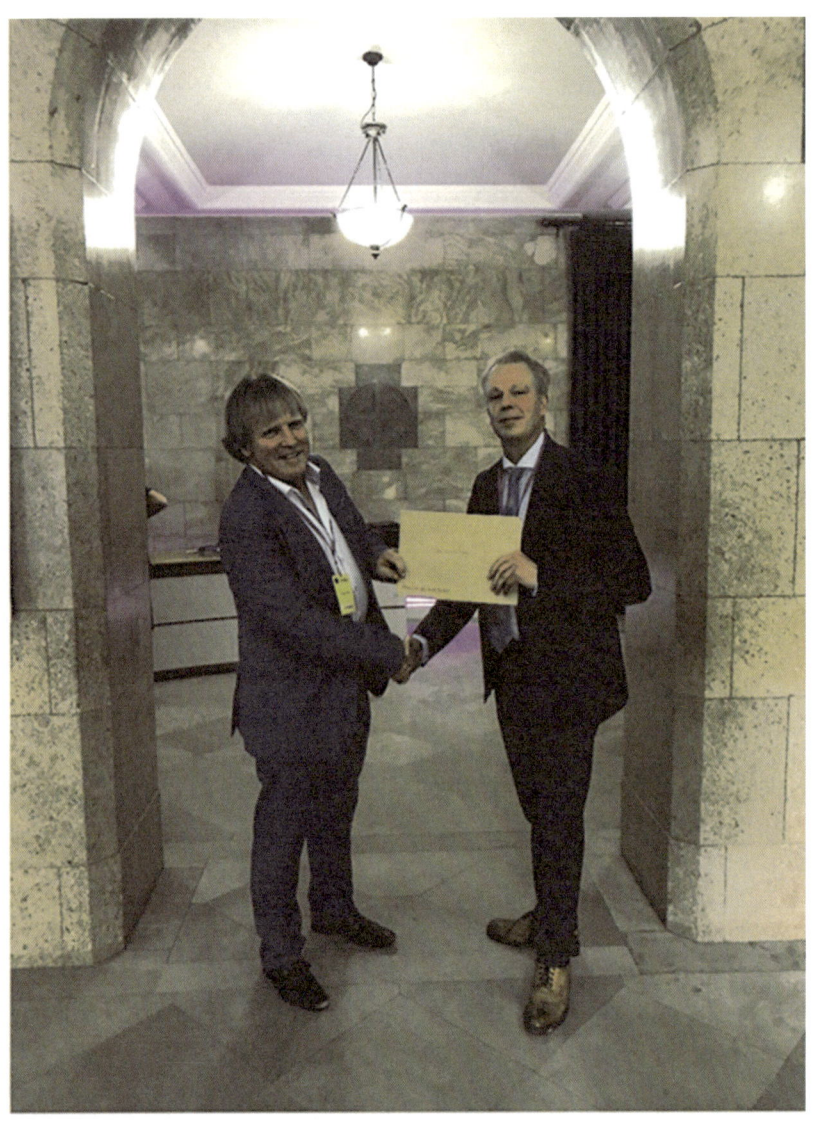

The author receiving British College of Aesthetic Medicine Award London 2017

Award for inventing the HELPIR technique, which was formulated to treat dermal filler vascular occlusion. This is an acronym for: H = Hyperbaric oxygen; E = Epithelial stimulation; L = Low level (light) laser (633nm). P = Platelet rich plasma (PRP); I = Intense pulsed light (IPL); R = Resurfacing laser.

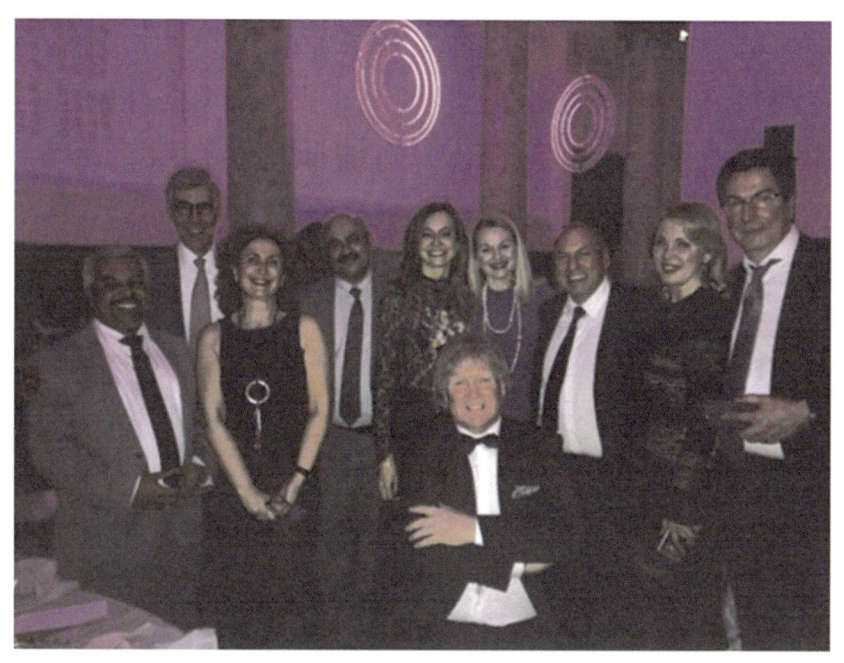

With medical colleagues Euromedicom Conference Monaco 2018

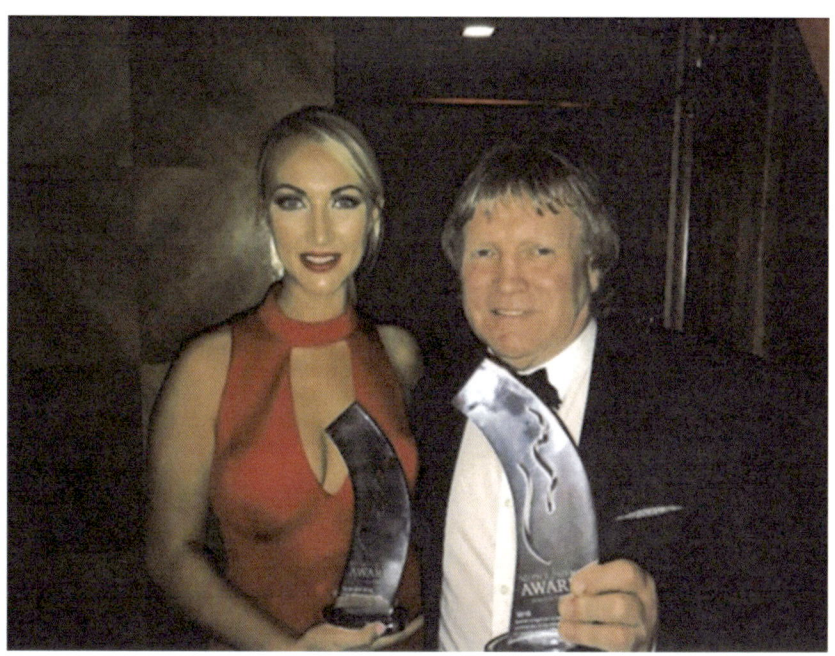

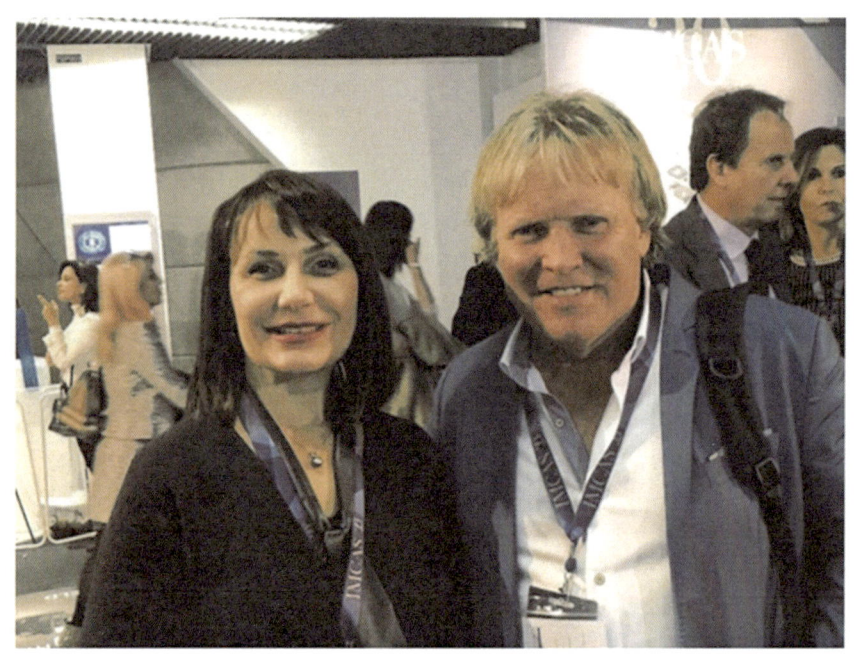

With Dr Irene Gubanova (Moscow) at IMCAS Conference Paris 2018

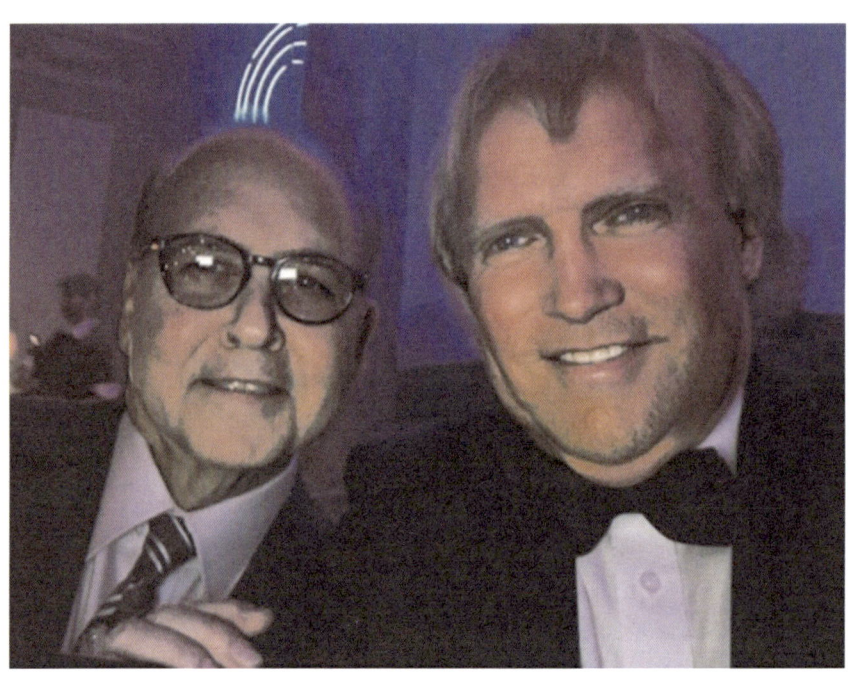

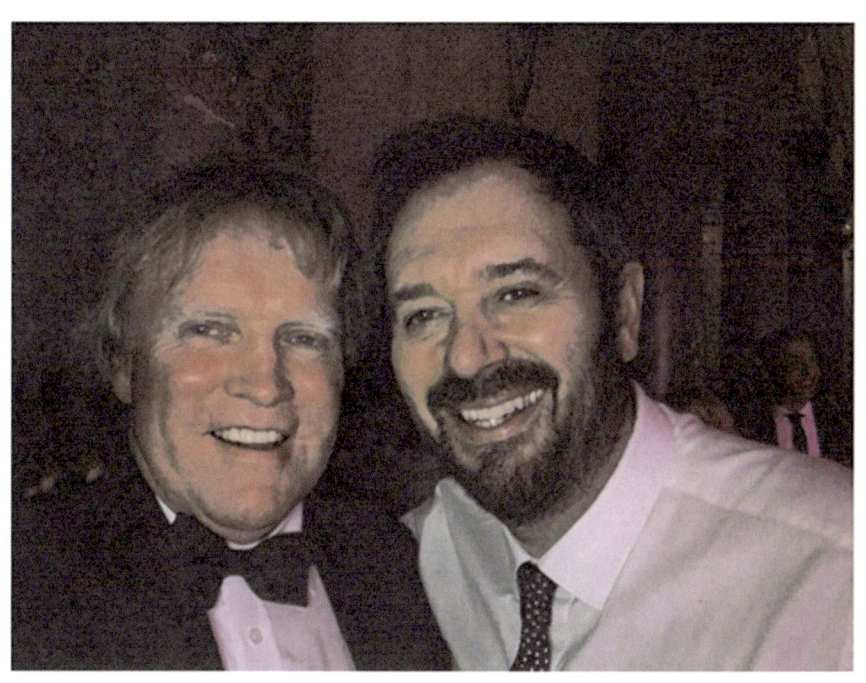

With Dr Hughes Cartier (Paris) at IMCAS Conference Paris 2019

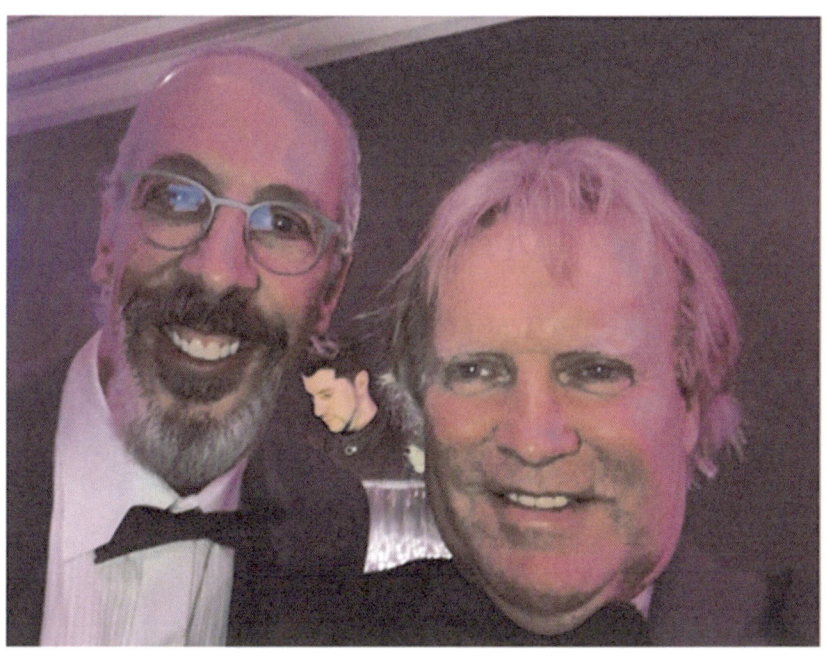

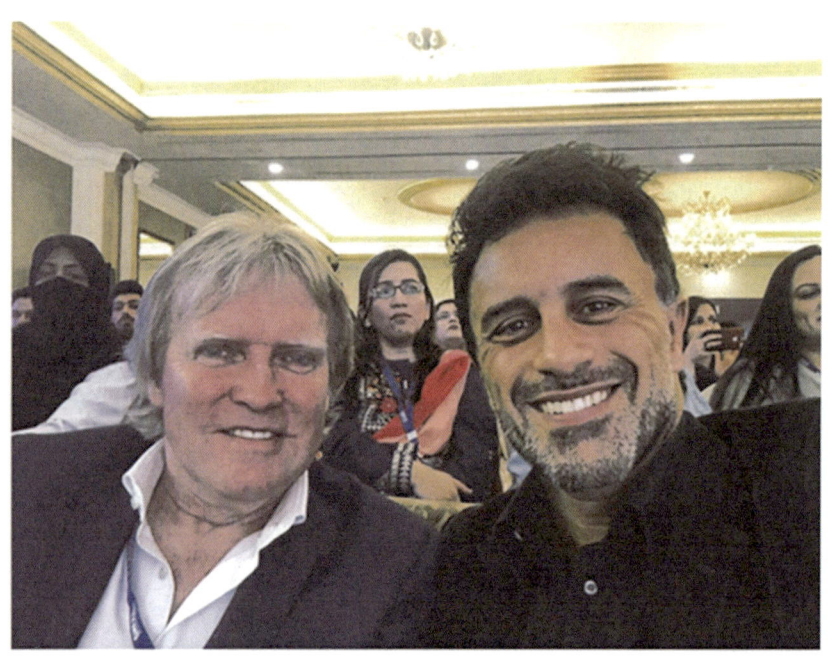

With Dr Matt Stefanelli (Paris) at PAADS Conference Karachi Pakistan 2019

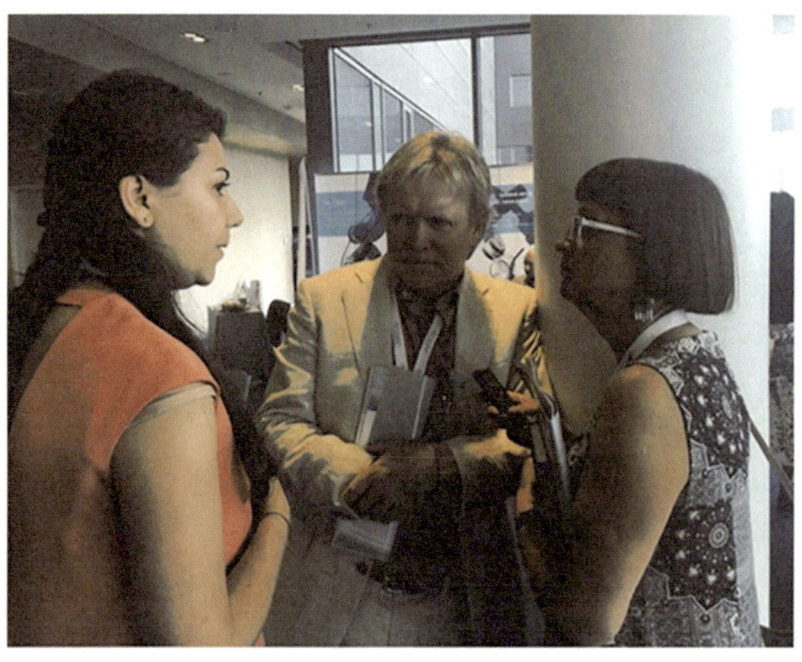

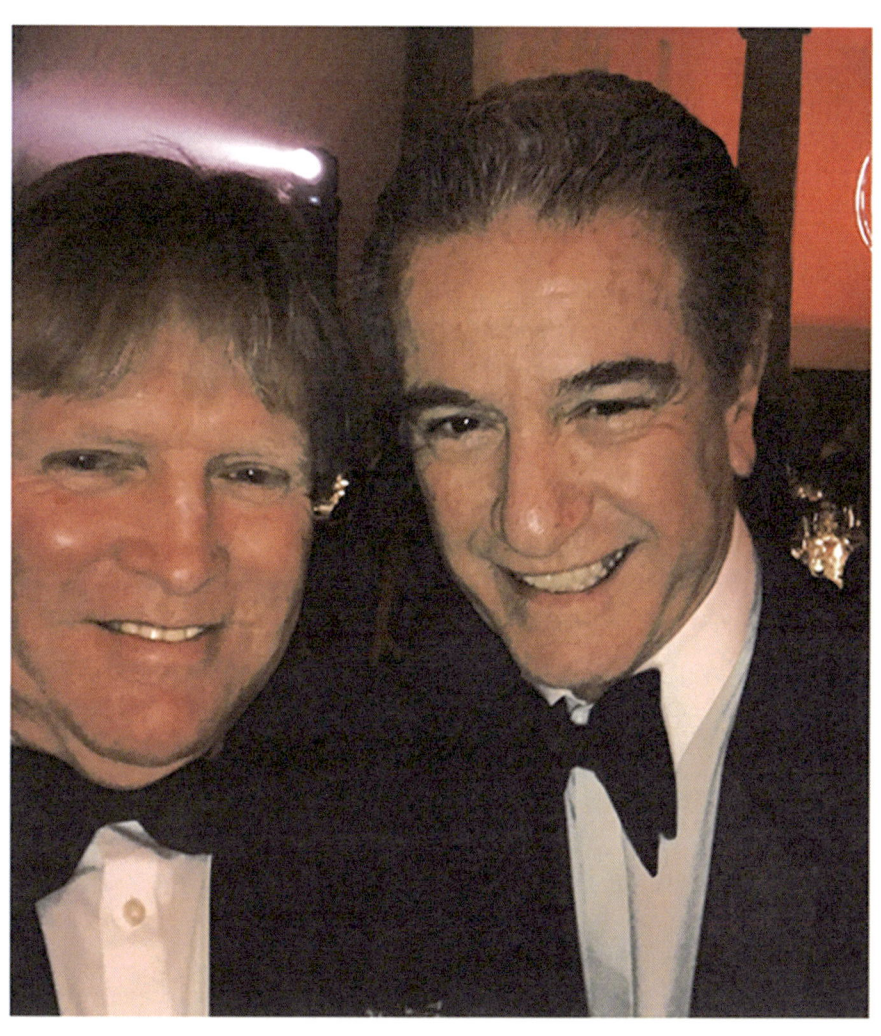

With Dr Benjamin Ascher at IMCAS Conference Paris 2019

References

Chapter 1: The Discovery of Botox

Clin Cosmet Investig Dermatol (2019) 12: 223-8. Published online 10 April 2019. DOI: 10.2147/CCID.S202919 PMCID: PMC6489637 Botulinum toxin A (Botox) for reducing the appearance of facial wrinkles: a literature review of clinical use and pharmacological aspect: Bagus Komang Satriyasal.

Grusser O-J Die ersten systematischen Beschreibungen and teirexperimentellen Untersuchungen des Botulismus.

Van Ermengne E. Uber einen neuen anaeroben Bacillus und seine Beziehungen zum Botulismus Z Hygeine Infectionskrankh.

Burgen, A. S. V., Dickens, F. and Zatman, L. J. (August 1949) 'The action of Botulinum toxin on the neuro-muscular junction', *The Journal of Physiology* (University of Chicago Press) 109 (1-2): 10-24.

Clark, R. P. and Berris, C. E. (August 1989) 'Botulinum toxin: a treatment for facial asymmetry caused by facial nerve paralysis', *Plastic and Reconstructive Surgery*, 84, 2, 353-5. DOI:10.1097/01.

Carruthers, J. D. and Carruthers, J. A. (January 1992) 'Treatment of glabellar frown lines with C. Botulinum-A exotoxin', *The Journal of Dermatologic Surgery and Oncology*, 18, 1, 17-21.

Walsh, S. (15 October 2010) 'FDA approves Botox® to treat chronic migraine'. Heckmann, M., Teichmann, B., Schröder, U., Sprengelmeyer, R. and Ceballos-Baumann, A. O. (2003) 'Pharmacologic denervation of frown muscles enhances baseline expression of happiness and decreases baseline expression of anger, sadness and fear', *Journal of the American Academy of Dermatology*, 49, 213-6.

Hennenlotter, A., Dresel, C., Castrop, F., Ceballos-Baumann, A. O., Wohlschläger, A. M. and Haslinger, B. (2009) 'The link between facial feedback and neural activity within central circuitries of emotion – new insights from Botulinum toxin-induced denervation of frown muscles', *Cerebral Cortex*, 19, 537-42.

Larsen, R. J., Kasimatis, M. and Frey, K. (1992) 'Facilitating the furrowed brow: an unobtrusive test of the facial feedback hypothesis applied to unpleasant affect', *Cognition Emotion*, 6, 321-38.

Neal, D. T. and Chartrand, T. L. (2011) 'Embodied emotion perception: amplifying and dampening facial feedback modulates emotion perception accuracy', *Social Psychological and Personality Science*, 1948550611406138.

Wollmer, M. A., de Boer, C., Kalak, N., Beck, J., Götz, T., Schmidt, T. and Hodzic, M. (2012) 'Facing depression with Botulinum toxin: a randomised controlled trial', *Journal of psychiatric research*.

Carruthers, A., Kiene, K. and Carruthers, J. (1996) 'Botulinum A exotoxin use in clinical dermatology', *Journal of the American Academy of Dermatology*, 34, 5 I, 788-97.

Jankovic, J. and Brin, M. F. (1991) 'Therapeutic uses of Botulinum toxin', *The New England Journal of Medicine*, 324, 17, 1186-94.

Klein, A. W. (2004) 'The therapeutic potential of Botulinum toxin', *Dermatologic Surgery*, 30, 3, 452-5.

Chapter 1a: Botulinum Toxin and Neuropathic Pain

Bagheri, S. C., Farhidvash, F. and Perciaccante, V. J. (2004) 'Diagnosis and treatment of patients with trigeminal neuralgia', *Journal of the American Dental Association*, 135, 12, 1713-7.

Dufour, S. K. (2002) 'An unusual case of stabbing eye pain: a case report and review of trigeminal neuralgia', *Optometry*, 73, 10, 626-34.

Various treatment modalities for trigeminal neuralgia include medicinal management, peripheral nerve injection of local anaesthetic or alcohol, peripheral neurectomies, alcohol injection of trigeminal ganglion and intracranial neurosurgical procedures.

Woolf, C. J. and Costigan, M. (1999) 'Transcriptional and posttranslational plasticity and the generation of inflammatory pain', *Proceedings of the National Academy of Sciences of the United States of America*, 96, 14, 7723-30.

Borodic, G. E. and Acquadro, M. A. (2002) 'The use of Botulinum toxin for the treatment of chronic facial pain', *Journal of Pain*, 3, 1, 21-7.

Acquadro, M. A. and Borodic, G. E. (1994); Treatment of myofascial pain with Botulinum A toxin', *Anesthesiology*, 80, 3, 705-6.

Aurora, S. (2006) 'Botulinum toxin type A for the treatment of migraine', *Expert Opinion on Pharmacotherapy*, 7, 8, 1085-95.

Mense, S. (2004) 'Neurobiological basis for the use of Botulinum toxin in pain therapy', *Journal of Neurology*, 251, 1, 1-7.

Woolf, C. J. and Mannion, R. J. (1999) 'Neuropathic pain: aetiology, symptoms, mechanisms and management', *Lancet*, 353, 9168, 1959-64.

Carlton, S. M., Hargett, G. L. and Coggeshall, R. E. (1995) 'Localisation and activation of glutamate receptors in unmyelinated axons of rat glabrous skin', *Neuroscience Letters*, 197, 1, 25-8.

Durham, P. L., Cady, R. and Blumenfeld, A. J. (2004) 'Regulation of calcitonin gene-related peptide secretion from trigeminal nerve cells by Botulinum toxin type A: implications for migraine therapy', *Headache*, 44, 1, 35-43.

Rapp, D. E., Turk, K. W., Bales, G. T. and Cook, S. P. (2006) 'Botulinum toxin type a inhibits calcitonin gene-related peptide release from isolated rat bladder', *Journal of Urology*, 175, 3, 1138-42.

Wu, C. J., Lian, Y. J., Zheng, Y. K., et al. (2012) 'Botulinum toxin type A for the treatment of trigeminal neuralgias: results from a randomised, double-blind, placebo-controlled trial', *Cephalgia*, 32, 6, 443-50.

Borodic, E. and Acquadro, M. A. (2002) 'The use of Botulinum toxin for the treatment of chronic facial pain', *Journal of Pain*, 3, 1, 21-7.

Borodic, G. E., Acquadro, M. and Johnson, E. A. (2001) Botulinum toxin therapy for pain and inflammatory disorders: mechanisms and therapeutic effects', *Expert Opinion on Investigational Drugs*, 10, 8, 1531-44.

Türk, Ü., Ilhan, S., Alp, R. and Sur, H. (2005) 'Botulinum toxin and intractable trigeminal neuralgia', *Clinical Neuropharmacology*, 28, 4, 161-2.

Piovesan, E. J., Teive, H. G., Kowacs, P. A., Della Coletta, M. V., Werneck, L. C. and Silberstein, S. D. (2005) 'An open study of Botulinum-A toxin treatment of trigeminal neuralgia', *Neurology*, 65, 8, 1306-8.

Zúñiga, C., Díaz, S., Piedimonte, F. and Micheli, F. (2008) 'Beneficial effects of Botulinum toxin type a in trigeminal neuralgia', *Arquivos de Neuro-Psiquiatria*, 66, 3 A, 500-3.

Wu, C. J. Lian, Y. J., Zheng, Y. K., et al. (2012) 'Botulinum toxin type A for the treatment of trigeminal neuralgias: results from a randomised, double-blind, placebo-controlled trial', *Cephalgia*, 32, 6, 443-50.

Bagus Komang Satriyasal (2019) 'Botulinum toxin (Botox) A for reducing the appearance of facial wrinkles: a literature review of clinical use and pharmacological aspect', *Clin Cosmet Investig Dermatol*, 12, 223-8. Published online: 10 April 2019. DOI: 10.2147/CCID.S202919 PMCID: PMC6489637.

Chapter 1b: Botulinum Toxin and Depression

Treacy, P. (May 2013) 'The Botox paradox: is it effective for depression?' *PRIME Journal*.

Beck, A. T. (1972). *Depression: Causes and Treatment*, Philadelphia: University of Pennsylvania.

E. Finzi, E. Wasserman Treatment of depression with botulinum toxin A: a case series Dermatologic Surgery, 32 (2006), pp. 645-649

M. Heckmann, B. Teichmann, U. Schröder, R. Sprengelmeyer, A.O. Ceballos-Baumann Pharmacologic denervation of frown muscles enhance baseline expression of happiness and decreases baseline expression of anger, sadness, and fear Journal of the American Academy of Dermatology, 49 (2003), pp. 213-216

Hennenlotter, C. Dresel, F. Castrop, A.O. Ceballos-Baumann, A.M. Wohlschläger, B. Haslinger. The link between facial feedback and neural activity within central circuitries of emotion–new insights from botulinum toxin-induced denervation of frown muscles Cerebral Cortex, 19 (2009), pp. 537-542

Facing depression with botulinum toxin: a randomized controlled trial. Journal of psychiatric research May 2012 Wollmer MA, de Boer C, Kalak N, Beck J, Götz T, Schmidt T, Hodzic M

Chapter 1c: Botulinum Toxin and Axillary Hyperhidrosis

Li, C., Wu, F., Zhang, Q., Gao, Q., Shi, Z. and Li, L. Cochrane Database Syst Rev. 17 March 2017, 17;3:CD009959. DOI: 10.1002/14651858.CD009959.pub2. Interventions for the treatment of Frey's syndrome.

Mund Kiefer Gesichtschir (2004) 8(6):369-75. Epub: 29 Oct 2004. 'Botulinum toxin for treatment of gustatory sweating. A prospective randomised study'.

Eckardt, A. and Kuettner, C. (2003) 'Treatment of gustatory sweating (Frey's syndrome) with Botulinum toxin', *Head Neck*, 8, 624-8.

Choi, Hyo Geun; Kwon, Sae Young; Won, Jung Youn; Yoo, Seung Woo; Lee, Min Gu; Kim, Si Whan and Park, Bumjung (2013) 'Comparisons of three indicators for Frey's syndrome: subjective symptoms, Minor Starch-Iodine test and infrared thermography', *Clinical and Experimental Otorhinolaryngology*, 6, 4, 249. DOI:10.3342/ceo.2013.6.4.249. ISSN 1976-8710.

Ann Vasc Surg. (2013) 27(4):447-53. DOI: 10.1016/j.avsg.2012.05.026. Epub: 11 Feb 2013.

Sciuchetti, J. F., Corti, F., Ballabio, D. and Angeli, M. C. 'Results, side effects and complications after thoracoscopic sympathetic block by clamping. The Monza clinical experience', Clin Auton Res. (2008) 18(2):80-3. DOI: 10.1007/s10286-008-0460-5.

de Andrade Filho, L., Kuzniec, S., Wolosker, N., Yazbek, G., Kauffman, P. and Milanez de Campos, J. R. 'Technical difficulties and complications of sympathectomy in the treatment of hyperhidrosis: an analysis of 1731 cases'.

Pomprasit, M. and Chintrakarn, C. (2007) 'Treatment of Frey's syndrome with Botulinum toxin', *J Med Assoc Thai*, 11 2397-402.

Ada Regina Trindade de Almeida and Suelen Montagner (2014) 'Botulinum toxin for axillary hyperhidrosis', *Dermatol Clin.*, 32(4):495-504. DOI: 10.1016/j.det.2014.06.013. Epub: 15 July 2014.

Chapter 2: The Discovery of Hyaluronic Acid Fillers

Mikhail A. Selyanin, Petr Ya. Boykov and Vladimir N. Khabarov (2015) *Hyaluronic Acid: Preparation, Properties, Application in Biology and Medicine*, First Edition, John Wiley & Sons, Ltd.

Mikhail A. Selyanin, Petr Ya. Boykov and Vladimir N. Khabarov (2015) *The History of Hyaluronic Acid Discovery, Foundational Research and Initial Use*, John Wiley & Sons, Ltd.

Meyer, K. and Palmer, J. (1934) 'The polysaccharide of the vitreous humor', *Journal of Biological Chemistry*, 107, 629-34.

Levene, P. A. and Lopez-Suarez, J. (1918) 'Mucin and mucoids', *Journal of Biological Chemistry*, 36, 105-26.

Kendall, F. E., Heidelberger, M. and Dawson, M. H. (1937) 'A serologically inactive polysaccharide elaborated by mucoid strains of group A hemolytic streptococcus', *Journal of Biological Chemistry*, 118, 61-9.

Balazs, E. A. and Piller, L. (1943) 'The formation of the synovial fluid', *Magyar Orvosi Arch*, 44, 1-11.

Ragan, C. and Meyer, K. (1949) 'The hyaluronic acid of synovial fluid in rheumatoid arthritis', *Journal of Clinical Investigations*, 28, 56-9.

Dorfman, A. (1948) 'The kinetics of the enzymatic hydrolysis of hyaluronic acid', *Journal of Biological Chemistry*, 172, 2, 377-87.

Ogston, A. G. and Stanier, J. I. (1951) 'The dimensions of the particle of hyaluronic acid complex in synovial fluid', *Biochemical Journal*, 49, 585-99.

Linker, A. and Meyer, K. (1954) 'Production of unsaturated uronides by bacterial hyaluronidases', *Nature*, 174, 1192-4.

Roseman, S., Moses, F. E., Ludowieg, J. and Dorfman, A. (1953) 'The biosynthesis of hyaluronic acid by group A Streptococcus. Utilisation of 1-C14-glucose', *Journal of Biological Chemistry*, 203, 213-25.

Warren, G. H. and Gray, J. (1959) 'Isolation and purification of streptococcal hyaluronic acid', *Proceedings of the Society of Experimental Biology and Medicine*, 102, 125-7.

DeAngelis, P. L., Papaconstantinou, J. and Weigel, P. H. (1993) 'Isolation of a Streptococcus pyogenes gene locus that directs hyaluronan biosynthesis in acapsular mutants and in heterologous bacteria', *Journal of Biological Chemistry*, 268, 14568-71.

Radaeva, I. F., Kostina, G. A. and Zmievski, A. V. (1997) 'Hyaluronic acid: biological role, structure, synthesis, isolation, purification and application' (in Russian), *Applied Biochemistry and Microbiology* (Prikladnaya biokhimiyai mikrobiologiya), 33, 133-7. Радаева И.Ф., Костина Г.А., Змиевский А.В. (1997) Гиалуроновая кислота: биологическая роль, строение, синтез, выделение, очистка и применение. Прикладная биохимия и микробиология. **33**, 2, 133-7.

Garg, H. G. and Hales, C. A. (2004), *Chemistry and Biology of Hyaluronan*, Elsevier, Amsterdam.

Chapter 2a: Hyaluronic Acid use in Ophthalmology

Balazs, E. A., Miller, D. and Stegmann, R. (1979) 'Viscosurgery and the use of Na-Hyaluronate in intraocular lens implantation'. Presented at the International Congress and Film Festival on Intraocular Implantation, Cannes, France.

Higashide, T. and Siguyama, K. (2008) 'Use of viscoelastic substance in ophthalmic surgery – focus on sodium hyaluronate', *Journal of Clinical Ophthalmology*, 2, 1, 21-30.

Fraser J. R., Laurent, T. C., Pertoft, H. and Baxter, E. (1981) 'Plasma clearance, tissue distribution and metabolism of hyaluronic acid injected intravenously in the rabbit', *Biochemical Journal*, 200, 415-24.

Miller, D. and Stegmann, R. (1982) 'The use of healon in intraocular lens implantation', *Int OphthalmolClin*.22,2,177-87.DOI:10.1097/00004397-198202220-00011.

C.R. Darwin The expression of emotion in man and animals Murray, London (1872)

Chapter 2b: Hyaluronic Acid use in Aesthetic Medicine

Markovitz, A., Cifonelli, J. A. and Dorfman, A. (1959) 'The biosynthesis of HA by group A Streptococcus. VI. Biosynthesis from uridine nucleotides in cell-free extracts', *Journal of Biological Chemistry*, 234, 9, 2343-50.
Lansing, M., Lellig, S., Mausolf, A., et al. (1993) 'Hyaluronate synthase: cloning and sequencing of the gene from Streptococcus sp', *Biochemical Journal*. 289, 179-84.

Van de Rijn, I. and Drake, R. R. (1992) 'Analysis of the streptococcal hyaluronic acid synthase complex using the photoaffinity probe 5-azido-UDP-glucuronic acid', *Journal of Biological Chemistry*, 267, 24302-6.

Kuo, J. W. (2005) *Practical Aspects of Hyaluronan-Based Medical Products*, New York: CRC Press.

Necas, J., Bartosikova, L., Braune, P. and Kolar, J. (2008) 'Hyaluronic acid (hyaluronan): a review', *Veterinarni Medicina*, 53, 8, 397-411.

Balazs, E. A., Hargittai, I. and Hargittai, M. (2011) *Hyaluronan: From Basic Science to Clinical Application*, New Jersey: PubMatrix Inc., Edgewater.

Karol A. Gutowski (2016) 'Hyaluronic Acid Fillers: Science and Clinical Uses', *Clin Plast Surg*, 43, 3, 489-96. DOI: 10.1016/j.cps.2016.03.016. Epub: 5 May 2016.

Chapter 2c: Treating Pectus Excavatum Medically with Hyaluronic Acid Filler

de Oliveira Carvalho, P. E., da Silva, M. V., Rodrigues, O. R. and Cataneo, A. J. (2014) 'Surgical interventions for treating pectus excavatum', *Cochrane Database Syst Rev*.

Pasrija, C., Wehman, B., Singh, D. P. and Griffith, B. P. (2014) 'Recurrent pectus excavatum repair via Ravitch technique with rib locking plates', *Eplasty*. No abstract available.

Aizawa, T., Togashi, S., Domoto, T., Sasaki, K., Kiyosawa, T. and Sekido, M. (2014) 'Modification of the Nuss procedure: the single-incision technique', *Plast Reconstr Surg Glob Open*, 2, 11:e256.

Park, H. J., Kim, K. S., Lee, S. and Jeon, H. W. (2014) *A Next-Generation Pectus Excavatum Repair Technique: New Devices Make a Difference*, Ann Thorac Surg. pii: S0003-4975(14)01727-5.

Kim, J. J., Park. H., Park, J., Cho, D. and Moon, S. J. (2014) 'A study about the costoclavicular space in patients with pectus excavatum', *Cardiothorac Surg.*, 9, 1, 189.

Chapter 2d: Complications in Breast Augmentation using Hyaluronic Acid Filler

Cheng, N. X., Wang, Y. L., Wang, J. H., Zhang, X. M. and Zhong, H. (2002) 'Complications of breast augmentation with injected hydrophilic polyacrylamide gel', *Aesthetic Plast Surg.*, 26, 375-82.

Ann Chir Plast Esthet. (2011) 'Macrolane®, a too premature indication in breast augmentation', 56, 3, 171-9. DOI: 10.1016/j.anplas.2011.04.002. Epub: 2 June 2011.

Cheng, N. X., Xu, S. L., Deng, H., et al. (2006) 'Migration of implants: a problem with injectable polyacrylamide gel in aesthetic plastic surgery', *Aesthetic Plast Surg.*, 30, 215-25.

Christensen, L. H., Breiting, V. B., Aasted, A., Jorgensen, A. and Kebuladze, I. (2003) 'Long-term effects of polyacrylamide hydrogel on human breast tissue', *Plast Reconstr Surg.*, 111, 1883-90.

Rubin, J. P. and Yaremchuk, M. J. (1997) 'Complications and toxicities of implantable biomaterials used in facial reconstructive and aesthetic surgery: a comprehensive review of the literature', *Plast Reconstr Surg.* 100, 1336-53.

Tokuya Omil and Kayoko Numanol (2014) 'The role of the CO_2 laser and fractional CO_2 laser in dermatology', *Laser Ther.*, 23, 1, 49-60. DOI: 10.5978/islsm.14-RE-01.

Gold, M. H. (2007) 'Lasers and light sources for the removal of unwanted hair', Clinics in Dermatology, 25, 5, 443-53.

Manstein, D., Herron, G. S., Sink, R. K., Tanner, H. and Anderson, R. R. (2004) *Lasers Surg Med.*, 34, 5, 426-38.

Hantash, B. M., Bedi, V. P., Sudireddy, V., Struck, S. K., Herron, G. S. and Chan, K. F. (2006) *J Biomed Opt.*, 11, 4, 041115.

Bedi, V. P., Chan, K. F., Sink, R. K., Hantash, B. M., Herron, G. S., Rahman, Z., Struck, S. K. and Zachary, C. B. (2007) *Lasers Surg Med.*, 39, 2, 145-55.

Hantash, B. M., Bedi, V. P., Chan, K. F. and Zachary, C. B. (2007) *Lasers Surg Med.*, 39, 2, 87-95.

Hantash, B. M., Bedi, V. P., Kapadia, B., Rahman, Z., Jiang, K., Tanner, H., Chan, K. F. and Zachary, C. B. (2007) *Lasers Surg Med.*, 39, 2, 96-107.

Moran, M. L. (2013) 'Office-based periorbital rejuvenation', *Facial Plast Surg.*, 29, 1, 58-63. DOI: 10.1055/s-0033-1333834. Epub: 20 Feb 2013.

Roberts, 3rd T. L. (1998) 'Laser blepharoplasty and laser resurfacing of the periorbital area', *Clin Plast Surg.*, 25, 1, 95-108.

Treacy, P. (2012) 'Combining therapies for the ageing face: the DUBLiN Lift', *PRIME Aesthetic Journal*.

Matteo Tretti Clementoni a; Patricia Gilardino a; Gabriele F. Muti a; Daniela Beretta b and Rossana Schianch (2007) 'Non-sequential fractional ultrapulsed

C0$_2$ resurfacing of photoaged skin', *Journal of Cosmetic and Laser Therapy*, 9, 4, 218-25.

Manuskiatti, W., Fitzpatrick, R. E. and Goldman, M. P. (1999) 'Long-term effectiveness and side effects of carbon dioxide laser resurfacing for photoaged facial skin', *J Am Acad Dermatol*, 40, 401-11.

Taylor, C. R., et al. (1990) 'Photoaging/photodamage and photoprotection', *J Am Acad Dermatol*, 22, 1.

Chapter 3a: The History of Aesthetic Lasers -CO2

Lavker, R. M. (1995) *Cutaneous Ageing: Chronological Versus Photoaging in Photodamage*, edited by Gilchrest BA. Cambridge: MA, Blackwell Science.

Fitzpatrick, R. E., Goldman, M. P., Satur, N. M. and Tope, W. D. (1996) 'Pulsed carbon dioxide laser resurfacing of photoaged facial skin', *Arch Dermatol*, 132, 395-402.

Hamilton, M. M. (2004) 'Carbon dioxide laser resurfacing', *Facial Plast Surg Clin North Am.*, 12, 289-95.

Fitzpatrick, R. E. (2001) 'CO$_2$ laser resurfacing', *Dermatol Clin.*, 19, 443-51. Nanni, C. A. and Alster, T. S. (1998) 'Complications of carbon dioxide laser resurfacing: an evaluation of 500 patients', *Dermatol Surg.*, 24, 315-20.

Hruza, G. J. and Dover, J. S. (196) 'Laser skin resurfacing', *Arch Dermatol*, 132, 451-5.

Bernstein, L., Kauvar, A., Grossman, M. and Geronemus, R. (1997) 'The short- and long-term side effects of carbon dioxide laser resurfacing', *Dermatol Surg.*, 23, 519-25.

Epstein, E. H. Jr. and Oren, M. E. (1970) 'Popsicle panniculitis', *N Engl J Med.*, 282, 17, 966-7.

Levene, P. A. and López-Suárez, J. (1916) 'The conjugated sulfuric acid of the Mucin of pig's stomach (Mucitin sulfuric acid)', *Biol. Chem.*, 25, 511.

Chapter 3b: Treating a Giant Cell Congenital Naevus

Wu, D., Wang, M., Wang, X., Yin, N., Song, T., Li, H., et al. (2011) 'Lack of BRAF (V600E) mutations in giant congenital melanocytic naevi in a Chinese population', *Am J Dermatopathol*, 33, 341-4.
Slutsky, J. B., Barr, J. M., Femia, A. N. and Marghoob, A. A. (2010) 'Large congenital melanocytic naevi: associated risks and management considerations', *Semin Cutan Med Surg.*, 29, 79-84.

Kovalyshyn, I., Braun, R. and Marghoob, A. (2009) 'Congenital melanocytic naevi', *Australas J Dermatol*, 50, 231-40.

Koot, H. M., de Waard-van der Spek, F., Peer, C. D., Mulder, P. G. and Oranje, A. P. (2000) 'Psychosocial sequelae in 29 children with giant congenital melanocytic naevi', *Clin Exp Dermatol*, 25, 589-93.

Marghoob, A. A., Bittencourt, F. V., Kopf, A. W. and Bart, R. S. (2000) 'Large congenital melanocytic naevi', *Curr Probl Dermatol*, 12, 146-52.

Slutsky, J. B., Barr, J. M., Femia, A. N. and Marghoob, A. A. (2010) 'Large congenital melanocytic naevi: associated risks and management considerations', *Semin Cutan Med Surg.*, 29, 79-84.

Arneja, J. and Gosain, A. (2009) 'Giant congenital melanocytic naevi', *Plast Reconstr Surg.*, 124, 1e-13e.

Marghoob, A. A., Borrego, J. P. and Halpern, A. C. (2007) 'Congenital melanocytic naevi: treatment modalities and management options', *Semin Cutan Med Surg.*, 26, 231-40.

Ana Carolina Leite Viana, Bernardo Gontijo and Flávia Vasques Bittencourt. (2013) 'Giant congenital melanocytic naevus', *An Bras Dermatol*, 88, 6, 863-78.

Zaal, L., Mooi, W., Sillevis Smitt, J. and van der Horst, C. (2004) 'Classification of congenital melanocytic naevi and malignant transformation: a review of the literature', *Br J Plast Surg.*, 57, 707-19.

Bittencourt, F., Marghoob, A., Kopf, A., Koenig, K. and Bart, R. (2000) 'Large congenital melanocytic naevi and the risk for development of malignant melanoma and neurocutaneous melanocytosis', *Pediatrics*, 106, 736-41.

Hale, E., Stein, J., Ben-Porat, L., Panageas, K., Eichenbaum, M., Marghoob, A., et al. (2005) 'Association of melanoma and neurocutaneous melanocytosis with large congenital melanocytic naevi – results from the NYU-LCMN registry', *Br J Dermatol*, 152, 512-7.

Zitelli, J. A., Grant, M. G., Abell, E. and Boyd, J. B. (1984) 'Histologic patterns of congenital nevocytic naevi and implications for treatment', *J Am Acad Dermatol*, 11, 402-9.

Michel, J. L. (2003) 'Laser therapy of giant congenital melanocytic naevi', *Eur J Dermatol*, 13, 57-64.

Bohn, J., Svensson, H. and Aberg, M. (2000) 'Dermabrasion of large congenital melanocytic naevi in neonates', *Scand J Plast Reconstr Surg Hand Surg.*, 34, 321-6.

Chapter 3a: The influence of Radiofrequency

Fritz K, Salavastru C. Ways of noninvasive facial skin tightening and fat reduction. Facial Plast Surg. 2016;32(3):276-282

Alster TS, Lupton JR. Nonablative cutaneous remodeling using radiofrequency devices. Clin Dermatol. 2007;25(5):487-491

Goldsmid, H. J., 2009, Introduction to Thermoelectricity, Springer, New York

Potekaev N, Zhukoval O. Evaluation of safety and efficacy of the maximus™ system for facial wrinkles. J Cosmet, Dermatol Sci Appl.2013;3:151–156

Elman M, Vider I, Harth Y, Gottfried V, Shemer A. Non-invasive therapy of wrinkles, lax skin using a novel multi-source phase-controlled radiofrequency system. J Cosmet Laser Ther. 2010;12: 81–86 Hantash BM, Ubeid AA, Chang H, Kafi R, Renton B. Bipolar fractional radiofrequency treatment induces neoelastogenesis and neocollagenesis. Lasers Surg Med. 2009;41

Kaplan H, Kaplan L. Combination of microneedle radiofrequency (RF), fractional RF skin resurfacing and multi-source non-ablative skin tightening for minimal-downtime, full-face skin rejuvenation. J Cosmet Laser Ther. 2016;18(8):438-441

Harth Y, Elman M, Ackerman E, Frank I. Depressed acne scars – effective, minimal downtime treatment with a novel smooth motion non-insulated microneedles radiofrequency technology. J Cosmet, Dermatol Sci Appl. 2014;4:212–218

Harth Y, Elman M, Ackerman E, Frank I. Depressed acne scars – effective, minimal downtime treatment with a novel smooth motion non-insulated microneedles radiofrequency technology. J Cosmet, Dermatol Sci Appl. 2014;4:212–218

Zip C. The impact of acne on quality of life. Skin Ther Lett.2007;12(10):7–9.

Moretti M. Skin tightening: Softening demand in a weak economy. Medical Insight Inc; 2008

Dierickx CC. The role of deep heating for noninvasive skin rejuvenation.Lasers Surg Med. 2006; 38:799–807.

Lolis MS, Goldberg DJ. Radiofrequency in Cosmetic Dermatology: AReview: Dermatol Surg. 2012;38(11):1765–1776.

Mulholland RS. Radio frequency energy for non-invasive and minimallyinvasive skin tightening. Clin Plast Surg. 2011; 8:437–448

Cameli N, Mariano M, Serio M, Ardigò M. Preliminary comparison of fractional laser with fractional laser plus radiofrequency for the treatmentof acne scars and photoaging. Dermatol Surg Off Publ Am Soc DermatolSurg Al. 2014;40(5):553–561.

Levy LL, Zeichner JA. Management of acne scarring, part II: a comparative review of non-laser-based, minimally invasive approaches.Am J Clin Dermatol. 2012;13(5):331–340.
Jacob CI, Dover JS, Kaminer MS. Acne scarring: A classification systemand review of treatment options. J Am Acad Dermatol. 2001;45(1):109–117.

Alexiades-Armenakas MR, Dover JS, Arndt KA. The spectrum of laser skin resurfacing: Nonablative, fractional, and ablative laser resurfacing. JAm Acad Dermatol. 2008;58(5):719–737.

Chapter 4: The History of Chemical Peels

Treatment of photoaging. Facial chemical peeling (phenol and trichloroacetic acid) and dermabrasion J M Stuzin 1, T J Baker, H L Gordon

Dermatol Clin 1995 Apr;13(2):263-76. Chemical peels. Trichloroacetic acid and phenol R G Glogau 1, S L Matarasso

Stuzin, J. M. Phenol peeling and the history of phenol peeling. Clin. Plast. Surg. 25: 1, 1998.

Rosner, F. (Ed.). Maimonides' Glossary of Drug Names. Philadelphia: The American Philosophical Society, 1979. P. 22.

Selwyn-Brown, A. The Physician throughout the Ages. New York: Capehart-Brown, 1928. P. 254.

Sayre, L. A. Three cases of lead palsy from the use of a cosmetic called "Laird's Bloom of Youth." Trans. Am. Med. Assoc. 20:563, 1869.

Van Scott, E. J., and Yu, R. J. Alpha hydroxy acids: Procedures for use in clinical practice. Cutis 43:222, 1989.

Parish, L. C. Cosmetics: A historical review. Clin Dermatol. 6: 1, 1988.

Hughes-Hallett, L. Cleopatra: Histories, Dreams and Distortions. New York: Harper & Row, 1990. P. 37.

Vail, G. A. A History of Cosmetics in America. New York: Toilet Goods Association, 1947. Pp. 74–139.

Rubinstein, H. My Life for Beauty. New York: Simon & Shuster, 1966. P. 41.

Paracelso, Botánica Oculta: Las Plantas Mágicas. Buenos Aires: Editorial Kier, 1937. P. 136.

Chapter 5: The History of Fat Removal

Elisa Bellini, Michele P. Grieco and Edoardo Raposio (2017) 'A journey through liposuction and liposculture', *Ann Med Surg (Lond)*, 24, 53-60. Published online 6 Nov 2017. DOI: 10.1016/j.amsu.2017.10.024.

Flynn, T. C., Coleman, W. P. 2nd, Field, L. M., Klein, J. A. and Hanke, C. W. (2000) 'History of liposuction', *Dermatol Surg.*, 26, 515-20.

Coleman, W. P. 3rd. (1999) 'The history of liposuction and fat transplantation in America', *Dermatol Clin.*, 17, 723-7.

Illouz, Y. (1983) 'Body contouring by lipolysis: a 5-year experience with over 3,000 cases', *Plast. Reconstr. Surg.*, 72, 511.

Illouz, Y. G. (1996) 'History and current concepts of lipoplasty', *Clin. Plast. Surg.*, 23, 721-30.

Fournier, P. and Otten, F. (1983) 'Lipodissection in body sculpturing: the dry procedure', *Plast. Reconstr. Surg.*, 75, 598.

Fischer, A. and Fischer, G. (1976) 'First surgical treatment for moulding body's cellulite with three 5-mm incisions', Bull. Int. Acad. Cosmet. Surg., 3, 35.

Newman, J. (1984) 'Liposuction surgery: past-present-future', *Am. J. Cosmet. Surg.*, 1, 19-20.

Klein, J. A. (1987) 'The tumescent technique for liposuction surgery', *Am. J. Cosmet. Surg.*, 4, 263-7.

Klein, J. A. (1993) 'Tumescent technique for local anaesthesia improves safety in large volume liposuction', *Plast. Reconstr. Surg.*, 92, 1085-98.

Klein, J. A. (1990) 'Tumescent technique for regional anaesthesia permits lidocaine doses of 35 mg/kg for liposuction', *J. Dermatol Surg. Oncol.*, 16, 248-63.

Lawrence, N. and Cox, S. E. (2000) 'The efficacy of external ultrasound-assisted liposuction: a randomised controlled trial', *Dermatol Surg.*, 26, 329-32.

Apfelberg, D., Rosenthal, S. and Hunstad, J. (1994) 'Progress report on multicentre study of laser-assisted liposuction', *Aesth. Plast. Surg.*, 18, 259-64.

Treacy, Patrick J. and Goldberg, D. (2006) 'Use of a BioPolymer filler for facial lipodystrophy in HIV-positive patients undergoing treatment with anti-retro viral drugs', *Journal of Dermatologic Surgery*, 32, 6, 804-8.

Field, L., Asken, S. and Caver, C. (1984) 'Liposuction surgery: a review', J. Dermatol Surg. Oncol., 10, 530-8.

Coleman, W. (1988) 'Non-cosmetic applications of liposuction', Dermatol Surg. Oncol., 14, 1085-90.

Chapter 6: The History of Hair Transplant

Harris, J. A. (2004) 'Follicular unit transplantation: dissecting and planting techniques', *Facial Plast Surg Clin North Am*, 12, 2, 225-32.

Konior, R. J. (2013) 'Complications in hair-restoration surgery', *Facial Plast Surg Clin North Am*, 21, 3, 505-20.

Kerure, A. S. and Patwardhan, N. (2018) 'Complications in hair transplantation', *J Cutan Aesthet Surg.*, 11, 4, 182-9.

Autografts in alopecia and other selected dermatological conditions.

ORENTREICH N Ann N Y Acad Sci., (1959) 83, 463-79.

Sasagawa, M. (1923) 'Hair transplantation' (in Japanese), *Jpn J Dermatol*, 30, 493.

Okuda, S. (1939) 'Clinical and experimental studies on transplanting of living hair' (in Japanese), *Jpn J Dermatol*, 46, 135-8.

Tamura, H. (1943) 'Pubic hair transplantation', *Jpn J Dermatol*, 53, 76.

Fujita, K. (1953) 'Reconstruction of the eyebrows' (in Japanese), *La Lepro*, 22, 364.

Limmer, R. (1991) 'Bob Limmer does it all one hair at a time', *Hair TransplantForum Int.*, 2, 8-9.

Andrew, B. (2015) 'C. Walton Lillehei and the origins of open-heart surgery', *Minnesota Historical Society*.

Chapter 6a: The History of Hair Transplant -FUE

Rassman, W. R., Bernstein, R. M., McClellan, R., Jones, R., Worton, E. and Uyttendaele, H. (2002) 'Follicular unit extraction: minimally invasive surgery for hair transplantation', *Dermatol Surg.*, 28, 8, 720-8.

Limmer, B. L. (1994) 'Elliptical donor stereoscopically assisted micrografting as an approach to further refinement in hair transplantation', *J Dermatol Surg Oncol.*, 20, 12, 789-93.

Bernstein, R. M., Rassman, W. R., Szaniawski, W. and Halperin, A. (1995) 'Follicular transplantation', *Int J Aesthetic Restorative Surg.*, 3, 119-32.

Aman Dua and Kapil Dua. (2010) 'Follicular Unit Extraction Hair Transplant', *J Cutan Aesthet Surg.*, 3, 2, 76-81. DOI: 10.4103/0974-2077.69015.

Bernstein, R. M. and Rassman, W. R. (1997) 'What is delayed growth?', *Hair Transplant Forum Intl.*, 7, 2, 22.

Bernstein, R. M. and Rassman, W. R. (1997) 'Wall-mounted placing stand', *Hair Transplant Forum Intl.*, 7, 4, 17-8.
Bernstein, R. M. and Rassman, W. R. (1997) 'Follicular transplantation: patient evaluation and surgical planning', *Dermatol Surg*, 23, 771-84.

Bernstein, R. M. and Rassman, W. R. (1997) 'The aesthetics of follicular transplantation', *Dermatol Surg*, 23, 785-99.

Chapter 7: The History of Facial Threads

James A. Greenberg, MD. and Randi H. Goldman, MD. (2013) Barbed suture: a review of the technology and clinical uses in obstetrics and gynaecology', *Rev Obstet Gynecol.*, 6, 3-4, 107-15.

Wu, W. (2004) 'Barbed sutures in facial rejuvenation: APTOS threads and the Woffles Lift', *Aesthet Surg.*, 24, 582-7. DOI: 10.1016/j.asj.2004.09.007. [PubMed] [CrossRef] [Google Scholar].

Wu, W. (2006) 'Innovative uses of Botox® and the Woffles Lift', Panfilov D, editor. Aesthetic surgery of the facial mosaic. Berlin: Springer; pp. 636-649. [Google Scholar].

Wu, W. (2013) 'Non-surgical facelifting with long barbed suture slings', *J Aesthet Chir.*

Isse, N. and Fodor, P. B. (2005) 'Elevating the midface with barbed polypropylene sutures', *Aesthet Surg J.*, 25, 301-3. DOI: 10.1016/j.asj.2005.03.007.

Kress, D. W. (2008) 'The history of barbed suture suspension: applications and visions for the future', In: Shiffman MA, Mirrafati SJ, Lam SM, editors. Simplified facial rejuvenation. New York: Springer; 2008. pp. 247-256

Alcamo, J. H. (1961) 'Surgeon's suturing device', US patent 2,988,028.Alcamo, J. H. (1964) 'Surgical suture', US patent 3,123,077.
Fukuda. (1984) 'Surgical barbed suture', US patent 4,467,805.

Ruff, G. L. (1994) 'Insertion device for a barbed tissue connector', US patent 5,342,376.
Buncke, H.J. (1999) 'Surgical methods using one-way suture', US patent 5,931,855.

Ruff, G. L. (2001) 'Barbed bodily tissue connector', US patent 6,241,747B1.
Chapter 7a: The History of Facial Threads -APTOS
Sulamanidze, M. A., Fournier, P. F., Paikidze, T. G. and Sulamanidze, G. M. (2002) 'Removal of facial soft tissue ptosis with special threads', *Dermatol Surg.*, 28, 367-71. DOI: 10.1046/j.1524-4725.2002.01297. x.

Sulamanidze, M. A. and Sulamanidze, G. M. (2005) 'Facial-lifting with APTOS threads: featherlift', *Otolaryngol Clin North Am*, 8, 1109-17. DOI: 10.1016/j.otc.2005.05.005.

Sasaki, G. H, Komorowska-Timek, E. D., Bennett, D. C. and Gabriel, A. (2008) 'An objective comparison of holding, slippage, and pullout tensions for eight suspension sutures in the malar fat pads of fresh-frozen human cadavers', *Aesthet Surg J.*, 28, 387-96. DOI: 10.1016/j.asj.2008.04.001.

Wu, W. (2003) 'Facial rejuvenation using APTOS and WAPTOS (the Woffles lift): a novel approach'. In: 13th International Congress of the International Confederation of Plastic and Reconstructive Surgery (IPRAS), Sydney, Australia.

Joachim, H. (Tr.). Papyros Ebers. Das Alteste Buch Uber Heilkunde. Aus dem Aegyptischen Zum Erstenmal Vollstandig Ubers. Berlin: Druck und Verlag von Georg Reimer, 1890. P. 77.

Bryan, C. P. (Tr.). Papyrus Ebers. New York: D. Appleton and Company, 1931. Pp. 151–160.
Sperber, P. A. Treatment of Skin Aging and Dermal Defects. Springfield, Ill.: Charles C Thomas, 1965. P. 3.
Woodforde, J. The History of Vanity. New York: St. Martin's Press, 1992. P. 55.
Humphries, R. (Tr.). Ovid: The Loves, the Art of Beauty, the Remedies for Love. Bloomington, Ind.: Indiana University Press, 1966. P. 159.

Ellis, A. The Essence of Beauty: A History of Perfume & Cosmetics. New York: Macmillan Press, 1960. P. 91.

Dirckx, J. H. Ovid's dermatologic formulary. Am. J. Dermatopathol. 2:327, 1980.

Brody, H. J. History of Chemical Peels. In H. J. Brody (Ed.), Chemical Peeling.St. Louis: Mosby-Yearbook, 1992.

Cavendish, M. L. Poems and Fancies. Facsimile Ed. Yorkshire: The Scolar Press Limited, 1972. P. 221

Stuttgen, G. Historical observations: Dermatology. Clin. Dermatol. 14:135, 1996.

Benjmain, M. Dangerous cosmetics. New Remedies 7:324, 1878.

Johnston, H. W. (Ed.). The Private Life of the Romans. New York: CooperSquare Publishers, 1973. P. 290.

Majno, G. The Healing Hand: Man and Wound in the Ancient World. Cambridge, Mass.: Harvard University Press, 1975. P. 313.

G. A. A History of Cosmetics in America. New York: Toilet Goods Association, 1947. Pp. 74–139.

Paracelso, Botánica Oculta: Las Plantas Mágicas. Buenos Aires: Editorial Kier, 1937. P. 136.

Delgado, A. (Ed.). Hernan Cortes: Cartas de Relación. Madrid: Editorial Castalia, 1993. P. 143.

McNutt, F. A. Fernando Cortes: His Five Letters of Relation to the Emperor Charles V (1519–1526), Vol, I. New Glorieta, Mexico: Rio Grande Press Inc., 1977. P.

Obermayer, M. E. Mexican dermatology of the pre-Columbian period. Int. J. Dermatol. 13:293, 1974.

Blanco-Dávila, F., and Vasconez, H. C. The cleft earlobe: A review of methods of treatment. Ann. Plast. Surg. 33:677, 1994.

Woodforde, J. The History of Vanity. New York: St. Martin's Press, 1992. P. 55.

Gordon, H. L. (Ed.). Maimonides: The preservation of youth. Essays on health. New York: Philosophical Library, 1958. P. 5.

Holman, A. J. (Ed.). The Holy Bible. Miami: Editorial Vida, 1997. P. 61.

Buncke, H. J., and Conway, H. Surgery of decorative and traumatic tattoos. Plast. Reconstr. Surg. 20:67, 1957.

Ellis, A. The Essence of Beauty: A History of Perfume & Cosmetics. New York: Macmillan Press, 1960. P. 91.

Dirckx, J. H. Ovid's dermatologic formulary. Am. J. Dermatopathol. 2:327, 1980.

Rod, J., Rohrich, L. and Joel, E. Pessa. (2009) 'The anatomy and clinical implications of perioral submuscular fat', 124, 1, 266-71. DOI: 10.1097/PRS.0b013e3181811e2e.

Farkas, J. P., Pessa, J. E., Hubbard, B. and Rohrich, R. J. (2013) 'The science and theory behind facial ageing', *Plastic and Reconstructive surgery*.
Guyuron, B., Rowe, D. J., Weinfeld, A. B., et al. (2009) 'Factors contributing to the facial ageing of identical twins', Plast Reconstr Surg., 123, 1321-133.

Reece, E. M., Pessa, J. E. and Rohrich, R. J. (2008) 'The mandibular septum: anatomical observations of the jowls in ageing implications for facial rejuvenation', *Plast Reconstr Surg.*, 121, 1414-20.

Hellman, M. (1927) 'Changes in the human face brought about by development', *Int J Orthod.*, 13, 475.

Perrett, K. I., May, K. A. and Yoshikawa, S. (1994) 'Facial shape, and judgments of female attractiveness', *Nature*, 368, 239.

J Exerc Nutrition Biochem. 2017 Sep 30; 21(3): 55–61. The role of glycation in the pathogenesis of aging and its prevention through herbal products and physical exercise Chan-Sik Kim, Sok Park, and Junghyun Kim

Harman D. The aging process. Proc Natl Acad Sci U S A. 1981; 78:7124–8. Maillard L. Action des acides amines sur les sucres; formation des melanoidines par voie methodique. C R Acad Sci. 1912; 154:66–8.

Philippov, Michelle (2016). Fats: A Global History. London: Reaktion Books.p. 45.

Glenn, J.; Stitt, A. (2009). "The role of advanced glycation end products in retinal ageing and disease". Biochimica et Biophysica Acta (BBA) - General Subjects. 1790 (10): 1109–1116.

Semba, R. D.; Ferrucci, L.; Sun, K.; Beck, J.; Dalal, M.; Varadhan, R.; Walston, J.; Guralnik, J. M.; Fried, L. P. (2009). "Advanced glycation end products andtheir circulating receptors predict cardiovascular disease mortality in older community-dwelling women". Aging Clinical and Experimental Research. [7] Brownlee M. Advanced protein glycosylation in diabetes and aging. *Annu Rev Med.* 1995; 46:223–34.

Peng X, Ma J, Chen F, Wang M. Naturally occurring inhibitors against the formation of advanced glycation end-products. *Food Funct.* 2011; 2:289–301 Dermatoendocrinol. 2012 Jul 1; 4(3): 259–270 Advanced glycation end products Key players in skin aging? Paraskevi Gkogkolou and Markus Böhm

Characteristics of the Aging Skin Adv Wound Care (New Rochelle) 2013 Feb. 2(1): 5–10 Miranda A. Farage, Kenneth W. Miller, Peter Elsner, Howard I. Maibach Glycation and Skin Aging by Dr Sanchari Sinha Dutta, Ph.D. News Medical LifeSciences https://www.news-medical.net/health/Glycation-and-Skin-Aging.aspx

Sadowska-Bartosz I, Bartosz G. Effect of glycation inhibitors on aging and age-related diseases. *Mech Ageing Dev.* 2016; 160:1–18.

Dermatoendocrinol. 2012 Jul 1; 4(3): 259–270 Advanced glycation end products Key players in skin aging? Paraskevi Gkogkolou and Markus Böhm

Chapter 13: Vit D

Institute of Medicine Dietary Reference Intakes for Calcium and Vitamin D, (2010) S-11 and 8-7, National Academies Press.

Duesberg, P., Koehnlein, C. and Rasnick, D. (2003) 'The chemical bases of the various AIDS epidemics: recreational drugs, anti-viral chemotherapy, and malnutrition', *J Biosci*, 28, 4, 383-412.

Looker, A. C., Johnson, C. L., Lacher, D. A., Pfeiffer, C. M., Schleicher, R. L. and Sempos, C. T. (2011) 'Vitamin D status: United States, 2001-2006', *NCHS Data Brief*, 59.

Huldshinsky, K. (1928) 'The ultraviolet light treatment of rickets'. Heilung von rachitis durch kunstlich hohen-sonne. Deut Med Wochenscher 1919; 45:712-3; http://dx.doi.org/10.1055/s-0028-1137830 [CrossRef] [Google Scholar] Alpine Press New Jersey, USA.

Keevil, J. (1954) 'The illness of Charles, Duke of Albany (Charles I), from 1600 to 1612: an historical case of rickets', *Hist Med Allied Sci.*, 9, 4 407-19.

Burland, C. (1918) 'An historic case of rickets. Being an account of the remains of Princess Elizabeth, daughter of King Charles I, who died at Carrisbrooke Castle, 1650', *Practitioner*, 100, 391-5.

Huldschinsky, K. (1928) *The Ultraviolet Light Treatment of Rickets*, New Jersey: Alpine Press.

Jeffrey L. H. O'Riordana and Olav L. M. Bijvoet. (2014) 'Rickets before the discovery of vitamin D', *Bonekey Rep.*, 3, 478. Published online: 8 Jan 2014. DOI: 1038/bonekey.2013.212.

Theodosius Baptista Epistola, 42, 1553. See Hess AF Rickets. London: Kimpton, 1930, p 25.

Peter Brain, Galen. (1986) 'Galen on bloodletting: a study of the origins, development and validity of his opinions, with a translation of the three works', Cambridge University Press. ISBN 0-521-32085-2.

'The asphyxiating and exsanguinating death of President George Washington', *The Permanente Journal*, 8, 2, 79. Retrieved on 11 November 2012.

Moore, S. (1728) *Dissertatio medica inauguralis de rachitide*, Edinburgh: Balfour et Smellie.

Chapter 13a: Vit D Deficiency

Eijkman, C. (1897) 'Ein beri-beri anliche der hühner', *Virchows Arch*, 148, 523-7.

Schutte, D. (1824) Archiv fur medizinche Erfahrung.

Holst, A. (1907) 'Experimental studies relating to ship-beriberi and scurvy', *Frölich T J Hyg (Lond)*, 7, 5 634-7

Angeline, M. E., Gee, A. O., Shindle, M., Warren, R. F. and Rodeo, S. A. (2013) 'The effects of vitamin D deficiency in athletes', *Am J Sports Med*, 41, 2, 461-4.

Sniadeki, J. (1939) See Mozolowski, W. and Jedrzej Sniadeki (1768-1838) on the cure of rickets. *Nature*, 1822, 143, 121-1.

Mellanby, E. (1919) 'An experimental investigation on rickets', *Lancet*, 1, 407-12.

McCollum, E. V., Pitz, W., Simmonds, N., Becker, J. E., Shipley, P. G. and Bunting, R. W. (2002) *J Biol Chem.*, 277, 19, E8.

Hulshinsky, K. (1919) 'Heilung von rachitis durch künstlich hohen-sonne', *Deut. Med. Wochenscher*, 45, 712-3. Z. Orthopad. Chir. 1920; 39:426 as described in Bills CE. In: Sebrell WH Jr, Harris RS (eds). The Vitamins. Vol. II. Academic Press: New York, 1954, pp 162.

Wulff, Eugene C. *The New Holstein Story*, p 43.

Mowery, David C. (2004) *Ivory Tower and Industrial Innovation*, Stanford University Press.

Chapter 14: The Sun

Avoidance of sun exposure is a risk factor for all-cause mortality: results from the Melanoma in Southern Sweden cohort. Lindqvist, P. G., Epstein, E., Landin-Olsson, M., Ingvar, C., Nielsen, K., Stenbeck, M. and Olsson, H. J. (2014) *Intern Med.*, 276, 1, 77-86.

David, G., Hoel, Marianne Berwick, b., Frank, R., de Gruijl, c. and Michael, F. Holick, d. (2016) 'The risks and benefits of sun exposure',

Dermatoendocrinol, 8, 1, e1248325. Published online: 19 Oct 2016. DOI: 10.1080/19381980.2016.1248325.

The Surgeon General's Call to Action to Prevent Skin Cancer, US Department of Health and Human Resources, Office of the Surgeon General, Washington, D.C. 2014: http://www.surgeongeneral.gov.

Chapter 15: Skin and Structure

Bonifant H, Holloway S. A review of the effects of ageing on skin integrity and wound healing. Br J Community Nurs. 2019 Mar 01;24(Sup3):S28-S33.

Herskovitz I, Macquhae F, Fox JD, Kirsner RS. Skin movement, wound repair and development of engineered skin. Exp Dermatol. 2016 Feb;25(2):99-100.

Ravara B, Hofer C, Kern H, Guidolin D, Porzionato A, De Caro R, Albertin G. Dermal papillae flattening of thigh skin in Conus Cauda Syndrome. Eur J Transl Myol. 2018 Nov 02;28(4):7914.

Rzepka K, Schaarschmidt G, Nagler M, Wohlrab J. [Epidermal stem cells]. J Dtsch Dermatol Ges. 2005 Dec;3(12):962-73.

Karim N, Phinney BS, Salemi M, Wu PW, Naeem M, Rice RH. Human stratum corneum proteomics reveals cross-linking of a broad spectrum of proteins in cornified envelopes. Exp Dermatol. 2019 May;28(5):618-622

Brown TM, Krishnamurthy K. StatPearls [Internet]. StatPearls Publishing; Treasure Island (FL): May 10, 2021. Histology, Dermis.

O'Connell RL, Rusby JE. Anatomy relevant to conservative mastectomy. Gland Surg. 2015 Dec;4(6):476-83

Chapter 15a: Skin and Microbiome

Andersson T, Ertürk Bergdahl G, Saleh K, Magnúsdóttir H, Stødkilde K, Andersen CBF, Lundqvist K, Jensen A, Brüggemann H, Lood R. Common skin bacteria protect their host from oxidative stress through secreted antioxidant RoxP. Sci Rep. 2019 Mar 05;9(1):3596.

Scharschmidt, T. C. & Fischbach, M. A. What lives on our skin: ecology, genomics and therapeutic opportunities of the skin microbiome. Drug Discov. Today Dis. Mech. 10, e83–e89 (2013).

Belkaid, Y. & Segre, J. A. Dialogue between skin microbiota and immunity. Science 346, 954–959 (2014).

Grice, E. A. The intersection of microbiome and host at the skin interface: genomic- and metagenomic-based insights. Genome Res. 25, 1514–1520 (2015).

Kong, H. H. et al. Temporal shifts in the skin microbiome associated with disease flares and treatment in children with atopic dermatitis. Genome Res. 22, 850–859 (2012). This is the first study in which the skin of individuals with atopic dermatitis was longitudinally sampled and sequenced.

Paulino, L. C., Tseng, C. H., Strober, B. E. & Blaser, M. J. Molecular analysis of fungal microbiota in samples from healthy human skin and psoriatic lesions. J. Clin. Microbiol. 44, 2933–2941 (2006).

Cell. 2014 Mar 27; 157(1): 121–141. Role of the Microbiota in Immunity and inflammation Yasmine Belkaid and Timothy Hand

Cell. 2016 Jan 28; 164(3):337-40. Are We Really Vastly Outnumbered? Revisiting the Ratio of Bacterial to Host Cells in Humans. Sender R, Fuchs S, Milo R

Revised Estimates for the Number of Human and Bacteria Cells in the Body. Sender R, Fuchs S, Milo R PLoS Biol. 2016 Aug; 14(8):e1002533.

Host-bacterial mutualism in the human intestine. Bäckhed F, Ley RE, Sonnenburg JL, Peterson DA, Gordon JI Science. 2005 Mar 25; 307(5717):1915-20.

Unidentified curved bacilli in the stomach of patients with gastritis and peptic ulceration. Marshall BJ, Warren JR Lancet. 1984 Jun 16; 1(8390):1311-5.

The Integrative Human Microbiome Project. Integrative HMP (iHMP) Research Network Consortium. Nature. 2019 May; 569(7758):641-648.

Gibson GR, Scott KP, Rastall RA, Tuohy KM, Hotchkiss A, Dubert-Ferrandon A, Gareau M, Murphy EF, Saulnier D, Loh G, Macfarlane S, Delzenne N, Ringel Y, Kozianowski G, Dickmann R, Lenoir-Wijnkook I, Walker C, Buddington R. Dietary prebiotics: current status and new definition. Food Sci Technol Bull Funct Foods. 2011;7:1–19.

What are the consequences of the disappearing human microbiota? Blaser MJ, Falkow S.

Helminths and harmony. Weinstock JV, Summers R, Elliott DE Gut. 2004 Jan; 53(1):7-9

Alteration of the intestinal microbiota as a cause of and a potential therapeutic option in irritable bowel syndrome. König J, Brummer RJ Benef Microbes. 2014 Sep; 5(3):247-61.

Chapter 16: Treating Skin Cancer- SCC

Goldman, G. D. (1998) 'Squamous cell cancer: a practical approach', *Semin Cutan Med Surg.*, 17, 2, 80-95.

Alam, M. and Ratner, D. (2001) 'Cutaneous squamous-cell carcinoma', *N Engl J Med.*, 344, 13, 975-83.

Rowe, D. E., Carroll, R. J. and Day, C. L. Jr. (1992) 'Prognostic factors for local recurrence, metastasis, and survival rates in squamous cell carcinoma of the skin, ear, and lip. Implications for treatment modality selection', *J Am Acad Dermatol*, 26, 6, 976-90.

Chollet, A., Hohl, D. and Perrier, P. (2012) 'Risk of cutaneous squamous cell carcinomas: the role of clinical and pathological reports', 8, 335, 743-6. PMID 22545495.

Kay, D., Brantsch, MD., Christoph Meisner, PhD., Birgitt Schönfisch, PhD., Birgit Trilling, Dipl Inform Med., Jörg Wehner-Caroli, MD., Martin Röcken, ProfMD. and Helmut Breuninger, ProfMD. 'Analysis of risk factors determining prognosis of cutaneous squamous-cell carcinoma: a prospective study', *The Lancet Oncology*, 9.

Maula, Sanna-Mari., Luukkaa, Marjaana., Grénman, Reidar., Jackson, David., Jalkanen, Sirpa. and Ristamäki, Raija. (2003) *Intratumoral Lymphatics Are Essential for the Metastatic Spread and Prognosis in Squamous CellCarcinomas of the Head and Neck Region.*

Chapter 16a: Treating Skin Cancer- Melanoma

Treacy, Patrick J., Popescu, N. A. and Kurland, L. T. (1990) 'Cutaneous malignant melanoma in Rochester, Minnesota: trends in incidence and survivorship, 1950 through 1985', *Mayo Clin Proc.*, 65, 10, 1293-302.

'Diagnosis and treatment of early melanoma', NIH Consensus conference, JAMA, 268 10, 1314-9.

Balch, C. M, Urist, M. M., Karakousis, C. P., Smith, T. J., Temple, W. J., Drzewiecki, K., et al. (1993) 'Efficacy of 2-cm surgical margins for intermediate-thickness melanomas (1 to 4 mm): results of a multi-institutional randomised surgical trial', Ann Surg, 218, 3, 262-7.

Veronesi, U., Cascinelli, N., Adamus, J., Balch, C., Bandiera, D., Barchuk, A., et al. (1988) 'Thin stage I primary cutaneous malignant melanoma. Comparison of excision with margins of 1 or 3 cm', N Engl J Med., 318, 18, 1159-62.

Veronesi, U., Adamus, J., Aubert, C., Bajetta, E., Beretta, G., Bonadonna, G., et al. (1982) 'A randomised trial of adjuvant chemotherapy and immunotherapy in cutaneous melanoma', N Engl J Med., 307, 15, 913-6.

Rager, E. L., Bridgeford, E. P. and Ollila, D. W. (2005) 'Cutaneous melanoma: update on prevention, screening, diagnosis and treatment', Am Fam Physician, 72, 2, 269-76.

Whiteman, D. C., Whiteman, C. A. and Green, A. C. (2001) 'Childhood sun exposure as a risk factor for melanoma: a systematic review of epidemiologic studies', Cancer Causes Control, 12, 1, 69-82.

Anderson, W. F., Pfeiffer, R. M., Tucker, M. A. and Rosenberg, P. S. (2009) 'Divergent cancer pathways for early-onset and late-onset cutaneous malignant melanoma', *Cancer*, 115, 18, 4176-85. DOI: 10.1002/cncr.24481. PubMed PMID: 19536874; PubMed Central PMCID: PMC2741537.

Cohn-Cedarmark, G., Rutqvist, L. E., Anderson, R. et al. (2000) 'Long-term results of a randomised study by the Swedish Melanoma Study Group on 2-cm versus 5-cm resection margins for patients with cutaneous melanoma with a tumour thickness of 0.8-2.0 mm', *Cancer*, 89, 1495-501.

Marsden, J. R., Newton-Bishop, J. A., Burrows, L., Cook, M., Corrie, P. G., Cox, N. H., Gore, M. E., Lorigan, P., MacKie, R., Nathan, P., Peach, H., Powell, B. and Walker, C. (2010) 'Revised UK guidelines for the management of cutaneous melanoma', *BJD*, 163, 2, 238-56.

Wang, S. Q., Setlow, R., Berwick, M., Polsky, D., Marghoob, A. A., Kopf, A. W. and Bart, R. S. (2001) 'Ultraviolet A and melanoma: a review', *J Am Acad Dermatol*, 44, 837-46.

Newton Bishop, J., Bataille, V., Gavin, A., Lens, M., Marsden, J., Mathews, T., Ormerod, A. and Wheelhouse, C. (2007) 'The prevention, diagnosis, referral, and management of melanoma of the skin: concise guidelines', *Royal College of Physicians and British Association of Dermatologists*: Concise guidance to good practice series, 7.
Rager, E. L., Bridgeford, E. P. and Ollila, D. W. (2005) 'Cutaneous melanoma: update on prevention, screening, diagnosis, and treatment', *Am Fam Physician*, 72, 2, 269-76.

Abrahamsen, H. N., Hamilton-Dutoit, S. J., Larsen, J. and Steiniche, T. (2004) 'Sentinel lymph nodes in malignant melanoma: extended histopathological evaluation improves diagnostic precision', *Cancer*, 100, 1683-91.

Balch, C. M., Buzaid, A. C., Soong, S. J., et al. (2001) 'Final version of the American Joint Committee on cancer staging system for cutaneous melanoma', *J Clin Oncol*, 19, 3635-48.

Edwards, B. K., Howe, H. L., Ries, L. A., Thun, M. J., Rosenberg, H. M., Yancik, R., Wingo, P. A., Jemal, A. and Feigal, E. G. (2002) 'Annual report to the nation on the status of cancer, 1973-1999, featuring implications of age and ageing on U.S. cancer burden', *Cancer*, 94, 10, 2766-92.

Gandini, S., Sera, F., Cattaruzza, M. S., Pasquini, P., Picconi, O., Boyle, P. and Melchi, C. F. (2005) 'Meta-analysis of risk factors for cutaneous melanoma: I. Common and atypical naevi', *Eur J Cancer*, 41, 28-44.

Wang, S. Q., Setlow, R., Berwick, M., Polsky, D., Marghoob, A. A., Kopf, A. W. and Bart, R. S. (2001) 'Ultraviolet A and melanoma: a review', *J Am Acad Dermatol*, 44, 837-46.